Keio University Symposia
for Life Science and Medicine 3

Springer

*Tokyo*
*Berlin*
*Heidelberg*
*New York*
*Barcelona*
*Hong Kong*
*London*
*Milan*
*Paris*
*Singapore*

Y. Ono, A. Janca
M. Asai, N. Sartorius (Eds.)

# Somatoform Disorders
## A Worldwide Perspective

With 38 Figures

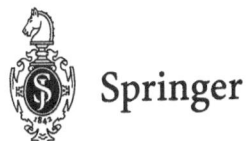 Springer

Yutaka Ono, M.D.
Assistant Professor, Department of Neuropsychiatry, Keio University School of Medicine
35 Shinanomachi, Shinjuku-ku, Tokyo 160-8582, Japan

Aleksandar Janca, M.D.
Associate Professor, Department of Psychiatry and Behavioural Science
Medical Research Foundation Building, Royal Perth Hospital
50 Murray Street, Perth WA 6000, Australia

Masahiro Asai, M.D.
Professor and Chairman, Department of Neuropsychiatry
Keio University School of Medicine
35 Shinanomachi, Shinjuku-ku, Tokyo 160-8582, Japan

Norman Sartorius, M.D.
Professor, Department of Psychiatry, University of Geneva
1201 Geneva, Switzerland

ISBN-13: 978-4-431-68502-9     e-ISBN-13: 978-4-431-68500-5
DOI: 10.1007/978-4-431-68500-5

Library of Congress Cataloging-in-Publication Data

Somatoform disorders : a worldwide perspective / Y. Ono ... [et al.].
    p. cm. — (Keio University symposia for life science and
  medicine ; 3)
    Includes bibliographical references and index.
    ISBN-13: 978-4-431-68502-9
    1. Somatoform disorders Cross-cultural studies Congresses.
  2. Somatoform disorders—Social aspests Congresses.  I. Ono, Y.
  (Yutaka), 1950–  .  II. Series.
    [DNLM: 1. Somatoform Disorders Congresses.   WM 170 S693 1999]
  RC552.S66S68   1999
  616.08—dc21
  DNLM/DLC
  for Library of Congress

Printed on acid-free paper

SPIN: 10676811

# Foreword

This volume contains the proceedings of the third symposium of the Keio University International Symposia for Life Sciences and Medicine under the sponsorship of the Keio University Medical Science Fund. As stated in the address by the President of Keio University at the opening of the symposium, the fund was established by the generous donation of Dr. Mitsunada Sakaguchi. The Keio University International Symposia for Life Sciences and Medicine constitute one of the core activities of the fund. The objective is to contribute to the international community by developing human resources, promoting scientific knowledge, and encouraging mutual exchange. Every year, the Committee of the International Symposia for Life Sciences and Medicine selects the most interesting topics for the symposium from applications received in response to a call for papers to the Keio medical community. The publication of these proceedings is intended to publicize and distribute information arising from the lively discussions of the most exciting and current issues during the symposium. We are grateful to Dr. Mitsunada Sakaguchi, who made the symposium possible, the members of the program committee, and the office staff whose support guaranteed the success of the symposium. Finally, we thank Springer-Verlag, Tokyo, for their assistance in publishing this work.

Akimichi Kaneko, M.D., Ph.D.
Chairman
Committee of the International Symposia for Life Sciences and Medicine

# Preface

This book brings together papers presented at the international conference entitled "Rethinking Somatoform Disorders," which was organized in collaboration with the World Health Organization (WHO), Division of Mental Health and Prevention of Substance Abuse, and the World Psychiatric Association (WPA), Section on Measurement Instruments in Psychiatric Care, in February 1998 in Tokyo. The conference took place in the New North Building (Kita-shinkan) at the Mita Campus of Keio University and was the third international meeting in the series of the Keio University International Symposia for Life Sciences and Medicine sponsored by the Keio University Medical Science Fund. The purpose of the meeting was to provide an international platform for the exchange of knowledge, experience, and research results in the field of somatoform disorders.

About 70 experts from a dozen countries working in the field of somatoform disorders, psychiatric nosology, epidemiology, and biological and cross-cultural psychiatry were invited to present their views on the current concepts of somatization, exchange their scientific results, and discuss future directions and strategies in clinical work and research on somatoform disorders. The participants in the conference also included representatives from a number of Asian countries as well as participants in WHO and WPA projects and activities.

The first part of the book contains papers discussing the concepts of somatization including the mind–body dichotomy, diagnosis, classification and description of specific syndromes of somatoform disorders as well as their characteristics in children and in the elderly. The second part of the book brings together papers presenting methods and results of a number of research projects carried out in different parts of the world, including the WHO International Study of Somatoform Disorders. Part three of the book provides an overview of different approaches to the management and treatment of somatoform disorders, taking into account the economic burden they create in different cultures and settings. Summarizing the current views on medically unexplained somatic symptoms from a sociocultural perspective, the last part of the book presents an outlook on future directions in clinical and research work in the field of somatoform disorders.

The editors wish to thank all participants for their interesting presentations and stimulating discussions at the conference as well as for their contributions to the book. Our thanks and gratitude also go to all the members of the Organizing Committee;

to Fumiko Maeda and Mitsue Mitanai, who served as the Conference Assistants; and especially to Hiroshi Ohin, Junko Shimane, and Hajime Ebihara, the members of the Symposium Secretariat. Finally, we would like to express our immense appreciation for the help and support we received from the staff of Springer-Verlag, Tokyo. Without their assistance and hard work in collecting and editing the manuscripts, our task of assembling this book would have been impossible.

Yutaka Ono
Aleksandar Janca
Masahiro Asai
Norman Sartorius
EDITORS

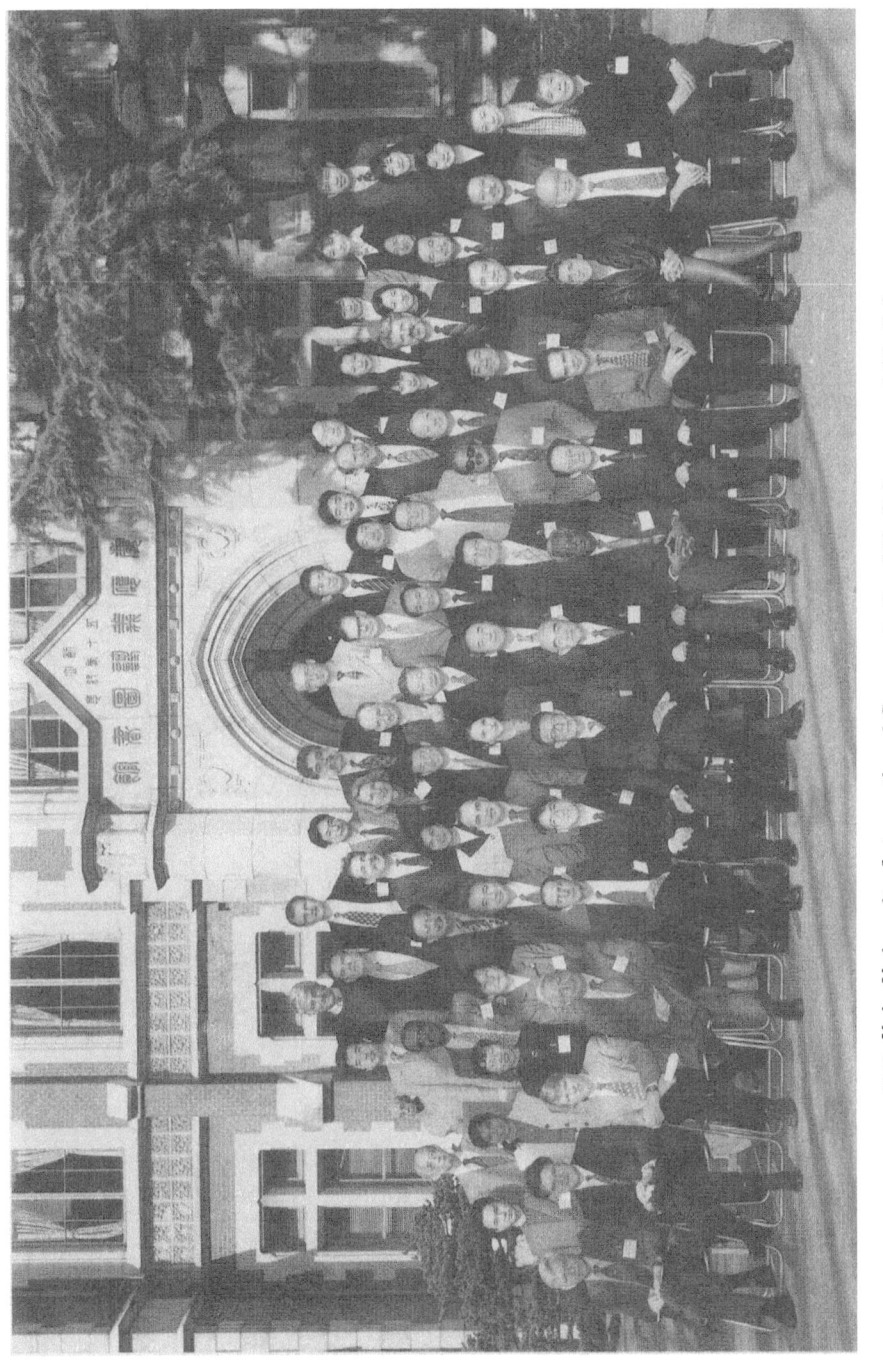

Keio University International Symposia for Life Sciences and Medicine
Rethinking Somatoform Disorders
*February 23-25, 1998*

# Contents

## Part 2  Studies on Somatoform Disorders in Different Cultures

# Part 3  Management and Economic Aspects of Somatoform Disorders

# Part 4  Summary and Outlook

# List of Contributors

# Opening Remarks*

Professor Yasuhiko Torii
President, Keio University
Chairman, Keio University Medical Science Fund

Dr. Sartorius, President of the World Psychiatric Association, Distinguished Guests, Ladies and Gentlemen:

On behalf of Keio University, I have the very great pleasure of welcoming all guests and participants to the Third Keio University International Symposium for Life Sciences and Medicine. I am particularly grateful to those clinicians and scientists who traveled such a long distance to participate in this symposium, and I deeply thank the World Psychiatric Association and the World Health Organization for their assistance.

The topic of our symposium this year is "Rethinking Somatoform Disorders." I am not a medical scientist but an economist; however, I think I can understand that we have now recognized that we should pay more attention to somatoform disorders for not only clinical but also economic reasons. There are many issues to be discussed from the economic as well as the medical viewpoint. Therefore, this seems an auspicious time to hold a symposium to discuss current dilemmas in the field of somatoform disorders.

I have a very personal reason to be interested in somatoform disorders. My personal memory goes back to more than 50 years ago, to the time of World War II. My mother was a medical doctor and she was running her own hospital after my father was drafted into the military service. She suffered from frequent somatoform disorders, such as rapid heartbeat, salivation, and other symptoms. There were neither psychiatric therapists around her nor tranquilizers, certainly not Prozac at that time, only some primitive sedative. I remember some compound of bromine was her cure.

When I was young, I myself experienced a few years of the same symptoms. A tranquilizer really rescued me. After I had suffered my disorder for 30 years, one of my daughters complained of a similar type of general malaise. Thus, I came to be very curious, with the experience of three generations of my family. Is my family's somato-

---

*This opening address was given by Professor Yasuhiko Torii, President of Keio University, at the opening session of the Keio University International Symposium for Life Sciences and Medicine, "Rethinking Somatoform Disorders: International Conference Organized in Collaboration with WPA and WHO," on the morning of Monday, February 23, 1998, in the conference hall of the New North Building on the Mita campus of Keio University.

form disorder a matter of learning? Did I learn my disorder from my mother? Or is my family's disorder a matter of genetic heredity? In any case, I am now very happy because my mother, my daughter, and I myself have overcome the disorder.

Thanks to all invited speakers for kindly accepting our invitation to this symposium. I'm sure that this unique meeting will be both exciting and successful.

Now let me briefly tell you what Keio University is and why we host such an international symposium for life sciences and medicine. Keio Gijuku, which is an educational corporation including Keio University, was founded in 1858 by Yukichi Fukuzawa. He was a pioneer of modern civilization in Japan. I assume some of you are already familiar with his personal appearance because his portrait is printed on the Japanese 10,000 yen note. In these 140 years after its establishment, we are proud that Keio, as the oldest university among 604 universities in this country, has played a major role in developing leading human resources in the academic, business, and political fields as well as in life science. The present prime minister, Ryutaro Hashimoto, is one of our alumni, for example. Among the eight faculties and nine graduate schools of Keio University, the School of Medicine is one of the most highly regarded in Japan and also, hopefully, throughout the world.

Fukuzawa, our founder, was a member of the very first mission of the Tokugawa Shogunate government to the United States in 1860 and to the European countries in 1862. Before that time, Japan's government had closed her doors to the outside world in self-isolationism for almost 300 years, until American Admiral Perry knocked on our door. During his visit to the United States and Europe as a member of the Japanese official mission, Fukuzawa realized that education was crucially important for the future of Japan. Thus, Keio has its origins in international exchanges. I hope all participants can understand that international exchanges such as this symposium have been among the most important academic and social missions of Keio University since its foundation.

In the fall of 1994, four years ago, Dr. Mitsunada Sakaguchi, an alumnus of the class of 1940 of our medical school, donated five billion yen to the university. It was his wish that the fund should be used to encourage research in life sciences and medicine at Keio University and to promote worldwide advancement in the sciences. I totally agreed with his proposal, and thus launched the Keio University Medical Science Fund in April of 1995. The International Symposium of Life Sciences and Medicine has thus been organized as one of the several projects supported by the fund. The objective of our symposium is to contribute to the international community by developing human resources, promoting scientific knowledge, and encouraging mutual exchanges of scholars. We also inaugurated the Keio Medical Science Prize. In 1996 we awarded the Keio Medical Science Prize to Dr. Prusiner of the University of California, San Francisco, and to Dr. Nakanishi of Kyoto University. And in 1997, last year, we awarded our prize to Dr. Weinberg of MIT and to Dr. Taniguchi of Tokyo University.

Now we are witnessing the dawn of the 21st century and the third millennium. We realize that our society faces many problems from this century that will be carried over into the next. In the field of life sciences and medicine alone, we are still unable to cure many kinds of cancer, AIDS, and neurological and psychiatric disorders. In addition, many new and unknown problems await us in the new century. I believe that exploring new horizons in life sciences is a vital task that we face at the dawn of the 21st century. It is equally important to ensure that the knowledge obtained through these pursuits should be used in a way which brings genuine happiness to humankind.

It is therefore more than a pleasure, indeed it is an honor, for me to meet such distinguished medical researchers and clinicians from world-renowned institutions and to share in the exchanges of valuable views. I'm also grateful for the efforts of the organizing committee, chaired by Dr. Yutaka Ono, who devoted themselves to making this symposium a high-quality and enjoyable event. I do hope this symposium will be a fruitful and productive one for all of you.

Let me close by wishing you further success in your research and clinical work. Thank you very much.

# Keynote Address

NORMAN SARTORIUS

Dear Colleagues and Friends,

It is my pleasant duty to thank the Keio University, Prof. Torii, its President and the Keio University Medical Science Fund for making this meeting possible; and Prof. Asai, Dr. Ono, and their colleagues for organizing it. Allow me also to greet the presidents of psychiatric societies from several Asian countries who are attending this meeting. I am very pleased that they could join us and hope that the results of this meeting will be helpful for the work of their psychiatric associations.

By organizing this meeting Dr. Ono continues to be an ambassador of Japan in the field of science—a role that he has played so well as an investigator in the International Study of Personality Disorders and on many other occasions. In this way, he is joining the illustrious group of Japanese colleagues who have helped to build bridges between science and culture in Japan and those in other countries. Among them are Professors M. Asai, M. Kato, Y. Nakane, R. Takahashi, and others who have all helped people in other countries to better understand the many contributions that Japanese psychiatry, science, and culture have made and will make to the world in future. I hope that these bridges will continue to grow and that they will permit Japan and the rest of the world to learn and benefit from each other. I wish to thank all of them for building these important connections and for their excellent participation in them.

I am very pleased to have with us also Prof. Shinfuku, who has returned to his country after many years of work with the World Health Organization. The achievements of Dr. Shinfuku during his time with the WHO are many, and the support that he gave to the development of mental health programmes in the Western Pacific region and worldwide is highly respected and of lasting importance.

I see this meeting as a first in a series for two reasons: first, because the topic is complex and issues relevant to it are too many to be resolved in a single meeting; and second, because a group of psychiatrists, regardless of its excellence, is not sufficiently representative of those that deal with somatoform disorders, e.g., general practitioners, internists, psychologists, and anthropologists. This first meeting should explore whether psychiatrists have a common understanding of the issues involved and

Department of Psychiatry, University of Geneva, 16-18, Bd. de St. Georges, 1205 Geneva, Switzerland whether there is a clear consensus among them about the role of psychiatry in the management of somatoform disorders. It should also define what is known and what is not yet explored so as to build an agenda of future activities in the field of psychiatry. Once this is done, discussion and collaboration with representatives of other disciplines should become easier and more fruitful.

I look forward to my participation in this meeting because of the excellence of its participants and because of its subject. The discussion about somatoform disorders opens many important questions—some epistemological (e.g., that of brain/mind relationship), some nosological (e.g., whether somatoform disorders are an idiom of distress or an independent morbid entity), some professional (e.g., that of who is responsible for the treatment of these disorders—psychologists and internists, psychiatrists, or some other professionals), and some practical (e.g., what are the best ways of recognizing somatoform disorders in the presence of physical illness). The debate on somatoform disorders is also relevant to the question of the future of psychiatry: will psychiatry become a discipline that deals exclusively with schizophrenia and states of chronic deficit, or will it maintain and expand its engagement and competence to deal not only with these problems but also with issues in the wider fields of mental health science, e.g., somatoform disorders, "subthreshold" problems seen in liaison psychiatry, and psychosocial aspects of health?

This meeting, however, also has another important task before it: it should help us to answer the question whether somatoform disorders are a problem of public health importance. If the answer to this question is yes, further research will not be a sufficient course of action: we shall also have to marshall facts that will convince decision-makers that they should give the resolution of the problems posed by somatoform disorders the priority that issues of public health importance deserve.

In order to be considered as a problem of public health importance a disorder must be frequent; stable or growing in importance; severe in its consequences; and amenable to effective health service interventions acceptable to those concerned and the population.

Do we have the evidence that we need to assess whether somatoform disorders satisfy the criteria of public health importance? Concerning frequency, for example, studies that have been done in general health services show that somatoform disorders are a frequent reason for consulting a doctor. Unfortunately, these studies have not examined the situation in all countries nor in all settings: we do know whether there are differences between urban and rural populations in this respect and we do not know whether these problems are equally frequent in different sociodemographic and cultural groups. From several studies and anecdotal reports we know that these problems are not diminishing in importance nor in visibility: however, precise data on this topic, e.g., from studies in the same population over longer periods of time, are still lacking.

The evidence to reach a decision concerning the second criterion of public health importance—that of severity of the negative consequences for the welfare of the individual and the society—is also insufficient. Statistics concerning nonpermanent disability are notoriously unreliable and specific studies on this issue are rare. Studies that would help in assessing to what extent these disorders contribute to the disability resulting from the presence of other (comorbid) disorders present at the time are lacking.

The evidence about the efficacy of treatment for somatoform disorders is also insufficient. What we know comes from studies in a few countries only. What is happening in other countries? How effective is, for example, alternative medicine in the treatment of somatoform disorders? Is it perhaps better to rely on traditional medical practitioners for the treatment of such disorders? In Africa, people who have appendicitis most often seek help from surgical departments while those with neurotic conditions first visit traditional healers. Is there some wisdom in this or is it just customary to behave in this way? Have the populations learned where the best treatment for them is? There is some evidence that some forms of psychotherapy are helpful in the management of somatoform disorders: does the effectiveness of these treatments depend on who provides it? Are psychologists just as effective or more effective than psychiatrists using such psychotherapies?

The days before us should allow us to pool the knowledge that is available and to reach consensus about the public health importance of somatoform disorders. They should also help us to find some answers to the questions mentioned before, and provide us with practical guidance about the management of these disorders and the directions of future research.

These are tall orders: I am, however, convinced that the excellence of this group will make it possible to reach the objectives outlined above, and I thank you again for accepting to participate in this meeting and in the search for new knowledge and better ways of helping those affected by mental disorder in general, and somatoform disorders in particular.

# Part 1
# Understanding the Concept of
# Somatoform Disorders

# The Concept of Somatoform Disorders: A Comment on the Mind-Body Problem in Psychiatry

Assen Jablensky

*Summary.* Notwithstanding claims to the contrary, both DSM-IV and ICD-10 are based on theoretical concepts about mind and body and the nature of their connectedness that originate in 19th century psychology and philosophy. The description and delineation of somatoform disorders and related conditions such as dissociation, conversion and dysmorphophobia is predicated on implicit psychophysical dualism which persists today in the DSM-IV and ICD-10 definition of somatisation/somatoform disorders. This essentially "negative" definition (i.e. a definition relying primarily on the lack of a medical explanation of the patient's symptoms) fails to take into account the fact that somatoform symptoms represent a small segment within the large area of psychopathology reflecting abnormal phenomena of body awareness. A scientific "phenomenology of the body", especially if coupled with research into underlying neurocognitive and neurophysiological mechanisms, may eventually render concepts such as somatisation and somatoform disorders obsolete.

*Key words.* Somatoform disorders, Psychophysical dualism, Mind/body dichotomy

## Introduction

As psychiatrists we often find ourselves in the position of de facto practitioners of psychophysical dualism, of a dichotomy between mind and body which stems from the theoretical underpinnings of our profession that date back to the 19th century or even earlier. We are not always aware that the tools of our profession—the methods we employ to elicit clinical data and the concepts we use to make sense of the data— have significant epistemological implications. The title of this conference, "Rethinking Somatoform Disorders", will hopefully prompt us to take a critical look at the concepts and terms which we still use to address the problem of mind and body in day-to-day professional discourse and clinical practice. The key words defining the scope of this conference—somatisation and somatoform disorders—are just two

Department of Psychiatry, University of Western Australia, MRF Building, 50 Murray Street, Perth 6000, Australia

nodal points within a wide semantic network that encompasses concepts such as conversion, hypochondriasis, body dysmorphic disorders, illness behaviour, factitious disorders, malingering and psychosomatic disorders. The network will probably also include terms like "chronic fatigue syndrome", "neurasthenia", "total allergy syndrome", "mitral valve prolapse" and "fibromyalgia".

What do all these terms and concepts have in common? What are the shared features of the complaints, disorders and behaviours to which they refer? Three characteristics stand out at first glance. *First*, the clinical problems subsumed by the network of related concepts are frequent, occur in all cultures, and are associated with high direct and indirect costs to individuals and the society (this has been well documented by the WHO collaborative study by Janca et al. [1]). The *second* salient feature of these disorders is a paradox: although the majority of the patients with such clinical problems are seen and treated by general practitioners, by non-psychiatric medical specialists, or by practitioners of "alternative medicine", the definition of the nature of the problems, their diagnosis and classification are at present regarded as the prerogative of psychiatry, rather than of general medicine or neurology (as it was during most of the 19th century). Their ultimate relegation to the domain of psychiatry may have had something to do with their *third* salient characteristic, namely that the lowest common denominator for these clinical problems is that they tend to behave (to paraphrase Freud) "as though anatomy did not exist" [2].

## Conceptual Precursors and Congeners

The problems of somatisation and somatoform disorders are not of a recent origin. The concepts in which our present-day diagnoses and classifications are rooted are those of hysteria and conversion, whose history through the centuries has been traced by Mace [3]. In the Middle Ages, the Latin *conversio* was used to denote the propensity for the "suffocation of the womb" to evolve into other diseases [3]. The idea of conversion thus provided an explanatory concept that linked together all of the variable manifestations. According to Hunter and Macalpine [4], the first usage of the term "hysterical conversion" in the medical literature can be attributed to the 18th century English physician John Ferriar. Ferriar's comments on conversion are worth reading:

"Fevers often terminate into hysterical disorders, especially in women. Men, too, are sometimes hysterically inclined, upon recovery from typhus ... In hysterical conversion ... the body possesses a power of representing the most hazardous disorders without incurring danger; or counterfeiting the greatest derangement in the circulating system without materially altering its movements; of producing madness, conscious of its extravagancies, and of increasing the acuteness of sensations by opressing the common sensorium ... Nature, as if in ridicule of the attempts to unmask her, has in this class of diseases reconciled contradictions and realised improbabilities, with a mysterious versatility which inspires the true philosopher with diffidence, and reduces the systematist to despair" (Ferriar, 1795; quoted in Mace [3]).

The history of the concept continues with the writings of Sydenham and Cullen. At the end of the 18th century, Sydenham developed prototype operational criteria for hysteria: (i) characteristic signs and symptoms; (ii) a "chameleon-like" capacity to imitate other diseases; and (iii) association with disturbances of passion. Later in the 19th century, the neurologists Briquet in 1859 [5], and then Charcot in 1888 [6], proposed that this group of conditions were neurological disorders. However, it was Freud who put the psychodynamic stamp on the modern concept of conversion by proposing that, "in hysteria, the incompatible idea is rendered innocuous by its sum of excitation being transformed into something somatic" [7]. Thus, somatisation became the current idiom for conversion (the term itself, somatisation, was coined by Stekel (1868–1940), who described a process whereby a "deep seated neurosis" could cause a bodily disorder [8]. Later on, Fenichel, continuing in the psychoanalytic tradition, wrote about the "translations of specific fantasies into body language" and referred to "organ neuroses" [9].

Another, altogether different, term of relevance within the same context is *illness behaviour*. This is a recent concept, first proposed by Mechanic [10], who wrote from the perspective of a medical sociologist about "the ways in which given symptoms may be differentially perceived, evaluated and acted (or not acted) upon by different kinds of persons". More recently, Pilowsky [11] added the adjective "abnormal" and introduced the term abnormal illness behaviour with its two components: first, the doctor does not believe that the patient's objective pathology entitles him/her to be placed in the type of sick role he/she expects; and, secondly, the patient remains uninfluenced by the doctor's explanation of the problem:

"The persistence of an inappropriate mode of experiencing, evaluating and reacting to one's own state of health despite the fact that an appointed agent of society has provided an accurate and reasonably lucid view of the person's health status and treatment required (if any), following full clinical assessment, with time provided for clarification and negotiation, and taking into account social, cultural and language factors" [12].

## The Epistemological Ambiguity of the DSM-IV and ICD-10 Notions of Somatisation/Somatoform Disorders

This is, in a nutshell, the convoluted history of the concepts and terms that precede the DSM-III, DSM-IV and ICD-10 concepts of somatisation and somatoform disorder. The literature that has influenced the diagnostic criteria and the manuals accompanying the two classifications seems to converge essentially on the following defining attributes of somatisation [8]: (i) a tendency to experience and communicate distressing somatic symptoms; (ii) the symptoms presented are not accounted for by pathological findings; (ii) the patient attributes his/her complaints to physical illness; (iii) the patient seeks medical help for the symptoms; (iv) psychosocial stress, as well as personality vulnerability to stress, may be an associated feature (this is usually an observation or inference on the part of the doctor or an informant, since the "somatising" person typically does not recognise and may deny any link between the symptoms and psychological causes).

As a definition of a disorder, this probably ranks among the tallest and most complex conceptual edifices ever erected in medicine. There are three components. The first part of the definition speaks about the patient. The patient has distressing bodily experiences and communicates these experiences. There is a process of attribution and consequent help-seeking behaviour. The patient does not recognise the true nature of the problem and may deny its origin. The second part of the definition is about the doctor. The doctor is unable to account for the symptoms of the patient in terms of his/her medical knowledge and, therefore, makes an inference about the something that may be going on in the mind of the patient. The third part of the definition adds an explanatory model in terms of psychological stress and vulnerability due to personality traits. This model is adopted by the doctor (following the failure of the "medical model" to explain the symptoms) but is likely to be rejected by the patient. Thus, the definition of somatisation, far from being an operational definition of a *disorder* (as DSM-IV and ICD-10 definitions claim to be), actually describes a peculiar social transaction between patient and doctor which involves subjective, experiential events (on the part of the patient); cognitive events (on the part of both doctor and patient); theoretical concepts (on the part of the doctor); and communication. The transactional nature of the DSM-IV and ICD-10 definition and diagnosis of somatisation is strongly influenced by the concept of illness behaviour and lays a heavy emphasis on the mismatch between the patient's beliefs and the doctor's beliefs, which may result in a diagnostic and therapeutic impasse: "The degree of understanding, either physical or psychological, that can be achieved about the cause of the symptoms is often disappointing and frustrating for both patient and doctor" [13].

A remarkable feature, common to both the DSM-IV and ICD-10 definitions of somatisation/somatoform disorders is their epistemological ambiguity. Somatisation/somatoform disorder is defined in terms of what it is not (i.e. not a "medical" disorder), but both classifications fail to identify the *disorder* in somatisation/somatoform disorder. The nature of the patient's subjective symptoms, beliefs, attributions and distress remains unexplained and problematic.

## Somatisation and the Experience of the Body in Psychopathology

A sample of what ICD-10 and DSM-IV enumerate as symptoms of somatisation or somatoform disorder is given in Table 1. This list represents a small segment of the rich variety of clinically significant, subjective experiences and behaviours that refer to the body. Even a perfunctory scan of the various existing manuals and instruments for the assessment of psychopathology will reveal that, probably, no less that two-thirds of all psychopathological symptoms and signs in psychiatry involve some sort of a reference to the body. Examples are listed in Table 2. They range from common symptoms such as worrying, tension and anxiety, to relatively rare, bizarre phenomena that we usually associate with psychosis, e.g. hallucinations from one's own body. Some of these symptoms undoubtedly occupy the grey zone between psychopathology and the territories usually claimed by neurologists, e.g. perceptual disorders such as phantom limbs, neglect and agnosias, and raise the question whether a true phenomenal continuity may indeed exist between the two domains. Another issue of continuity arises when we compare the somatoform symptoms "proper" with the dissociative symptoms. Can dividing lines be validly drawn between any of the subsets of subjective and objective manifestations in this area?

TABLE 1. A selection of "narrowly defined" somatoform symptoms (WHO [13])

Chest or heart pain, discomfort, burning
Headache
Problems with movement, paralysis
Numbness, loss of sensation, tingling
Excessive and distressing fatigue
Bad taste in mouth, coated tongue
Vomiting, regurgitation
Difficulty with swallowing
Stomach or bowel pains, wind, indigestion
Churning or discomfort in stomach
Frequent loose bowels
Nausea
Pain in arms or limbs, joints, hands or feet
Genital pain, discomfort, discharge
Other pain
Blotchy or discoloured skin

TABLE 2. Other symptoms and syndromes, not usually classified as "somatoform", with significant reference to the body

*Worrying and tension*
General muscular tension
Localised tension pains
Subjective restlessness
Fatiguability and exhaustion
Sensitivity to noise

*Anxiety*
Free-floating anxiety
Panic attacks

*Obsessional symptoms*
Preoccupation with contamination, contact or
   penetration

*Eating disorders*
Dread of becoming fat
Undue preoccupation with bodily shape
Action to lose weight through self-restriction or
   purgation
Binge eating

*Dissociative disorders*
Sensory loss or anaesthesia
Paraparesis / paralysis
Astasia-abasia
Akinesia, dyskinesia
Apraxia
Aphonia
Convulsions
Possession experience

*Perceptual disorders*
Depersonalisation
Heautoscopy
Unfamiliarity of self
Dysmorphophobia
Hallucinations from body
Sexual hallucinations
Coenestopathies
Phantom limbs
Neglect and agnosias

*Delusions*
Delusion of bodily change (metamorphosis)
Delusional parasitosis
Body dysmorphic beliefs
Nihilistic delusion (Cotard)
Hypochondriacal delusions
Delusion of pregnancy (pseudocyesis)

*Passivity experiences*
Replacement of bodily control (actions, voice,
   affect, handwriting)

Following (with only slight modifications) Jaspers' schema of the phenomena related to "awareness of the body" [14], the symptoms listed in Tables 1 and 2 might be tentatively grouped into several, partially overlapping clusters:

1. Disturbances associated with a neurological lesion (e.g. phantom limbs, anosognosia)
2. Hallucinations of the specific bodily senses (thermic, haptic, kinaesthetic)
3. Experience of bodily distortion (body enlarged, swollen, one side bigger)
4. Coenestopathies or disturbances of the "vital" sensations (e.g. body feels hollow, empty, shrunk or levitating)
5. Passivity experiences in the form of vital sensations (as above but experienced as externally contrived bodily change)
6. The body as a metaphor or a tool of communication (many of the dissociative and somatoform symptoms "proper" fall into this cluster)
7. Illness behaviour (social transactions predicated on explicit or implicit roles and "rules of the game")

It may be tempting to see in these clusters an ordered continuum, with the "organic" (and hence "medically legitimate") disorders occupying one end and the "functional" (psychogenic, hypochondriacal, pseudoneurological, pseudosomatic, hence not medically legitimate) disorders at the other end. However, in the absence of secure anchor points in the underlying cognitive and pathophysiological processes, it may be prudent to abstain, for the time being, from either too rigid taxonomic subdivisions of this vast field or too easy assumptions about a continuum. Seen in the perspective of the variety of bodily experience in psychopathology, the term "somatoform" appears to be particularly unfortunate since it conveys a spurious taxonomic validity to an ill-defined segment of this experience.

The field mapped by the tentative clusters might instead be designated as the *phenomenology of the body*, which clearly requires further study with the methodologies and techniques at our disposal today [15]. Its psychological salience was first highlighted by the French 19th century philosopher Maine de Biran who wrote:

"There is an immediate knowledge of one's own body, based solely on the response to a willed effort . . . Independently of the external knowledge of the form and the figure of the parts of our body, as an object relative to the sense of touch and sight, there is an internal apperception of the presence and consistency of this body of ours . . . which cannot act and be known except *from within*, without being able to be represented *from without*" (Maine de Biran, 1818; quoted in Henry [16]).

A century later, Maine de Biran was echoed by Jaspers:

"I am aware of my body as my existence . . . The body is the only part of the world that is both felt from within and—so far as its surface goes—at the same time perceived. The body provides me with an object and I am also that body" [14].

Surprisingly, the phenomenological perspective on the body, obvious to thinkers such as Maine de Biran and Jaspers (and to perceptive writers such as Sontag [17]) is, by and large, excluded from present-day medical and psychiatric discourse. The essential distinction between the *phenomenal body* (the body as subjectively perceived and experienced, which is always *my* body) and the *biological body* (the body as an object which we observe, measure, dissect, etc.) is as relevant to understanding the medical patient suffering from metastatic cancer as it is to understanding the "somatising" patient presenting with "medically unexplained" symptoms.

## Somatisation and Somatoform Disorders from a Phenomenological Perspective

How can the phenomenological perspective inform and enrich our conceptualisation of the somatoform disorders?

It is important to realise that the phenomenal body is the arena of our daily conscious experience, of the "inward self-expression of neurophysiological activity" [18]. The Cartesian mind-body dichotomy, on which many of our medical concepts (and practices) are predicated, is totally invalidated by the immediacy of that experience. It is equally important to highlight the role of the phenomenal body as the primary medium of social communication which makes use of a vast repertoire of innate and learned sign systems. Hypothetically, we can conceive of the dissociative, somatoform and other related disorders as communication codes couched in the idiom of the prevailing, socially sanctioned representations of the "objective" or biological body. Thus, the body presenting with a "somatoform" disorder is a "medicalised" phenomenal body whose communication idiom needs to be decoded and interpreted as a preliminary step to a diagnostic analysis [19].

This has some obvious implications for the conceptual framework of the current and future classifications of psychiatric disorders. Notwithstanding statements to the contrary, neither DSM-IV nor ICD-10 are atheoretical [20]. Classifications, whether of plants, microorganisms, or human behaviour, are always guided by concepts and ideas about the "essence" of the things to be classified and about the laws or patterns that determine their interrelationships. However, a useful classification in psychiatry cannot be predicated on vexing philosophical questions: it must be pragmatic and rooted in empirical data. Phenomenology is the empirical foundation of psychopathology and, at the bottom line, the classification of the somatoform disorders must reflect the phenomenology of the experienced body. It is likely that in the coming decades the phenomenology of body awareness and consciousness will be complemented by an increasingly specific mapping of the phenomena of consciousness on neural networks. This proposition might seem ambitious, but it is already on the agenda of neuroscience research. The advances of neuroscience into the territory of consciousness may eventually render concepts and terms such as somatisation and somatoform obsolete, and replace them with specific knowledge about the neurophysiological and neurocognitive mechanisms underlying such behaviour and subjective experience.

## References

1. Janca A, Isaac M, Costa e Silva JA (1995) World Health Organization international study of somatoform disorders—background and rationale. Eur J Psychiatry 9:100–110
2. Freud S (1893) Some points for a comparative study of organic and motor paralyses. In: Strachey J (ed) The complete psychological works, vol. I (standard edn). Hogarth, London

3. Mace CJ (1992) Hysterical conversion. I: A history. II: A critique. Br J Psychiatry 161:369–389
4. Hunter R, Macalpine I (1963) Three hundred years of psychiatry. Oxford University Press, London
5. Briquet P (1859) Traité de l'Hysterie. Baillière, Paris
6. Charcot JM (1888) Clinical lectures on certain diseases of the nervous system. Trans Hurd EP, Davis GS. Detroit, Michigan
7. Freud S (1894) The neuro-psychoses of defence. In: Strachey J (ed) The complete psychological works, vol. III (standard edn). Hogarth, London
8. Lipowski ZJ (1988) Somatization: the concept and its clinical application. Am J Psychiatry 145:1358–1368
9. Fenichel O (1945) The psychoanalytic theory of neurosis. Routledge, London
10. Mechanic D (1962) The concept of illness behavior. J Chron Dis 15:189–194
11. Pilowski I (1969) Abnormal illness behaviour. Br J Med Psychol 42:347–351
12. Pilowski I (1978) A general classification of abnormal illness behaviour. Br J Med Psychol 51:131–137
13. WHO (1992) The ICD-10 Classification of Mental and Behavioural Disorders. Clinical descriptions and diagnostic guidelines. World Health Organization, Geneva
14. Jaspers K (1963) General psychopathology. Transl. Hoenig J, Hamilton MW. Manchester University Press, Manchester
15. Starobinski J (1990) A short history of bodily sensation. Psychol Med 20:23–33
16. Henry M (1975) Philosophy and phenomenology of the body. Martinus Nijhoff, The Hague
17. Sontag S (1979) Illness as metaphor. Random House, New York
18. Rado S (1946) Psychodynamics as a basic science. Am J Orthopsychiatry 16:405–409
19. Kirmayer LJ (1988) Mind and body as metaphors: hidden values in biomedicine. In: Lock M, Gordon DR (eds) Biomedicine examined. Kluwer, Dordrecht, pp 57–93
20. APA (1994) Diagnostic and statistical manual of mental disorders, 4th edn. American Psychiatric Association, Washington

# The Classification of Somatoform Disorders in ICD-10

John E. Cooper

*Summary.* The recognition of somatoform disorders as a major group in ICD-10 probably reflects the development of liaison psychiatry, and also of psychiatry in primary care. The provision of descriptions of these disorders that can be used reliably between observers should be regarded as the essential first step in studies of their distribution both in hospital groups and in the community. The differences between ICD-10 and DSM-IV for this group of disorders are largely differences in arrangement rather than differences in concepts. This agreement is partly due to the use in both classifications of the wide concept "disorder", which implies a retreat from the idea of a diagnosis which underlies the presenting complaints. In future studies it will be important to examine social and cross-cultural issues by involving medical anthropologists from the start. This is because some of these disorders can be viewed, at least in part, as disturbances of sick roles and illness behaviour. This raises the question of whether future experimental classifications should contain separate and specified sections for role disorders, psychiatric disorders and syndromes, and brain diseases.

*Key words.* ICD-10, Somatoform, Somatization, Sick role, Illness behaviour

## The Concept of Somatoform Disorders in ICD-10

As a result of the extensive process of international consultation that led to the production of ICD-10, F45 Somatoform Disorders was agreed as a section of the major "block" F4 (F40–48) Neurotic, Stress-related and Somatoform Disorders (see Figure 1). ICD-9 and its predecessor ICD-8 contained only Hypochondriasis as a means of describing patients who would now be covered by one or other of these somatoform disorders.

All the disorders in F45 share the features of "repeated presentation of physical symptoms, together with persistent requests for medical investigations, in spite of repeated negative findings and reassurance by doctors that the symptoms have

Department of Psychiatry, University of Nottingham, 25 Ireton Grove, Attenborough, Nottingham NG9 6BJ, UK

**F45.0  SOMATIZATION DISORDER**

**F45.1  UNDIFFERENTIATED SOMATIZATION DISORDER**

**F45.2  HYPOCHONDRIACAL DISORDER**

**F45.3  SOMATOFORM AUTONOMIC DYSFUNCTION**

**F45.30  HEART AND CARDIOVASCULAR SYSTEM**

**F45.31  UPPER GASTRO-INTESTINAL TRACT**

**F45.32  LOWER GASTRO-INTESTINAL TRACT**

**F45.33  RESPIRATORY SYSTEM**

**F45.34  GENITO-URINARY SYSTEM**

**F45.35  OTHER ORGANS AND SYSTEMS**

**F45.4  PERSISTENT SOMATOFORM PAIN DISORDER**

**F45.8  OTHER SOMATOFORM DISORDERS**

      **(e.g. dysphagia [globus hystericus], psychogenic pruritus**

      **psychogenic torticollis, etc).**

**F45.9  SOMATOFORM DISORDER, unspecified.**

FIG. 1. Somatoform disorders in ICD-10

no physical basis." Somatization disorder and hypochondriacal disorder are differentiated within this general concept by the emphasis given to the type and the possible causes of the complaints; in somatization disorder, the emphasis is upon the number and variety of the complaints themselves, whereas in hypochondriasis there is also a conviction that a specific serious disease (usually named by the patient), such as cancer or heart disease, is responsible for the complaints—and these are not usually so numerous and often not so spectacular as in somatization disorder.

F45.3—Somatoform Autonomic Dysfunction—is reserved for those disorders in which there is clear presentation of some symptoms of autonomic over-activity, such as flushing, sweating, or cardiac palpitations. Some conditions with a long history and special names such as "Da Costa's syndrome." "Effort syndrome" and "cardiac neurosis" are included here.

Persistent pain disorder is self-explanatory, and under the "other" category of F45.8 go a variety of other historically well-known but fairly rare conditions, as shown in Figure 1.

Neurasthenia, whose presentation can have a number of feature in common with somatoform disorders, is given a separate place in ICD-10, as F48.0 in Other Neurotic

Disorders; this is because of its historical importance, and its frequency of use as a diagnosis in some countries, such as China.

## Differences Between ICD-10 and DSM-IV

In general, the individual disorders present in each classification under the overall heading of Somatoform can be found somewhere in the other classification, and with no great differences in the way that they are described. An important exception is neurasthenia, which is absent from DSM-IV; cases of this are best recorded in DSM-IV under Undifferentiated Somatoform Disorder.

Body Dysmorphic Disorder of DSM-IV is included in Hypochondriasis in ICD-10, and there is no exact equivalent of the ICD-10 category F45.3 Somatoform Autonomic Dysfunction in DSM-IV.

For somatization disorder, in ICD-10 both the overall list of complaints and the number required to qualify for the disorder are smaller than for DSM-IV. One reason for this is the purposeful omission of overtly genital and sexual complaints from the list in ICD-10, since in some cultures these types of complaints cannot be easily and openly expressed, even if they are present.

There is an additional difference in arrangement rather than content, in that conversion disorders (motor, sensory, convulsive, and mixed types) are included as somatoform disorders in DSM-IV. This is not so in ICD-10, where these conversion disorders remain together with other types of dissociative disorders (amnesia, fugues, etc.), since the presumed mechanism of "dissociation" is common to all this group.

This difference in arrangement is not very important in itself, and it has a quite simple cause; the policy of the ICD has always been to be rather conservative, and so when choices have to be made between alternatives without any convincing evidence to favour one or the other, the ICD tends to stick to concepts and terms that are already familiar and widely accepted, rather than to favour the new and the less familiar. The WHO advisers considered that the long-standing (although not well-understood) clinical concept of "dissociation" as a basis for all types of what used to be called "hysterical conversion" (i.e., loss of memory, sensation, or movement) should not be overpowered by the comparative newcomer "somatoform," even though this latter concept is useful in other respects. Similarly, the retention of the various subdivisions of F45.3—Somatoform Autonomic Dysfunction—allows several conditions to be specified that have been accepted by psychiatrists in many countries for a long time.

In summary, the similarities between ICD-10 and DSM-IV are much greater than the differences between them, and it is important to emphasize this rather than to dwell upon the details of the differences. Both the classifications share the same data base, which is the international psychiatric literature freely available to all. The organizers of both the classifications, helped by the National Institute of Mental Health of the United States, put a great deal of effort into making them as similar as possible, and those differences that remain are due to the different sets of users at which each classification is aimed. The ICD-10 must be as acceptable as possible to a wide international audience, and the DSM-IV must give special precedence to the wishes and interests of the members of the American Psychiatric Association. Where there are still differences, they are due to interesting differences of clinical tradition and opinion, but they are not based upon robust evidence.

The ICD-10 as a whole should continue in use in its present form for general clinical and administrative purposes for many years to come. Before large changes are made there is a need for much more information about the disorders as at present described and defined. But for research purposes, the situation is quite different. Experimental classifications of groups of related disorders need to be developed and tested, so that any future changes can rest upon a firm foundation. The rest of this chapter is devoted to suggestions of this type.

## Problems for Somatoform Disorders Shared by All Sections of ICD-10

Although ICD-10 is presented as if it were one classification, it is better regarded as a mixture of several different classifications. This is due largely to the very wide concept of "disorder" upon which it is based. The definition of this is similar in both ICD-10 and DSM-IV (although not quite the same) and means little more than something which clinical psychiatrists feel they can do something about, that is, "clinically recognizable" for ICD-10 and "clinically significant" for DSM-IV. This very broad definition is justified by the present patchy and incomplete state of psychiatric knowledge about aetiology and underlying processes, but it carries with it some interesting problems. One of these can be called "the retreat from diagnosis," illustrated by Figure 2.

"Diagnosis" is used in Figure 2 and in the present discussion in the strict sense of referring to a detectable lesion or measurable process that is known to underlie the presenting complaints, as in many medical and surgical conditions and diseases. "Symptom" is also used in a special sense, to indicate a complaint or a finding that the doctor knows to be associated with a possible underlying lesion or abnormal process that could lead to a diagnosis as just specified.

"Complaint" is used to mean only what the patient says about physical or mental functioning. The complaints are very important to the patient, but they are not necessarily symptoms in the above sense; equally, they may not have anything to do with whether a diagnosis can be made or not.

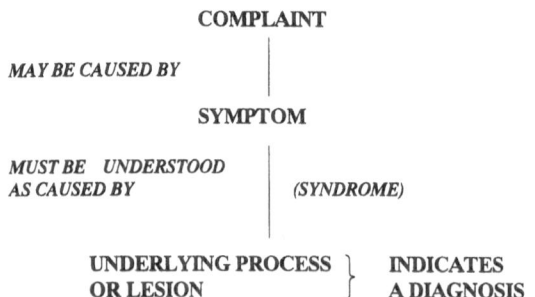

Fig. 2. The "retreat from diagnosis"

In these terms, most of the common psychiatric disorders in ICD-10 and DSM-IV are not diagnoses; they remain at the superficial level of "complaint disorders", except for those which are by definition attached to a cause such as brain damage or substance abuse. Strictly speaking, it is therefore wrong to speak of "diagnostic" criteria for large sections of ICD 10 and DSMIV. It would be much better in the future to indicate clearly that most of the descriptions, guidelines and detailed criteria in the current versions of the classifications are for the "identification of disorders", and to use the title of "diagnostic criteria" only for those categories that are diagnoses as defined here.

As an aside, if this view of complaints, symptoms, and diagnoses is kept in mind, the fact that one person is found to have more than one disorder is not at all surprising if they are disorders expressed at the level of complaints—as so many of them are. What has become known as the "co-morbidity problem" is only a serious problem to those who make the false assumption that all the disorders in the classification have the same status as medical diagnoses.

## The Contents of "Diagnostic Criteria"

An additional problem is that at the moment, under this mistaken label of "diagnostic criteria" there can often be found, in addition to the expected complaints, symptoms, and abnormal behaviours, statements about the age and the sex of the patient, the duration of the complaints, symptoms and behaviours, and the personal and social consequences of the disorder. Inclusion and exclusion statements about other disorders or possible aetiological influences also occur. It would be easier to appreciate what is involved in trying to describe disorders and diagnoses if these different types of information were separated out in clearly different sub-lists, alongside the items that describe only the disorders.

This would facilitate the next step of trying to understand more about the levels of abnormality implied by those criteria which identify the clinical syndrome itself; these may well include attitudes and interpersonal (or social) behaviour, as well as clearly abnormal psychopathological symptoms.

The point of this for the present discussion is that if all we have are complaints (but no symptoms as defined here) with which to identify somatoform disorders in general and somatization disorder in particular, we cannot necessarily assume that the most important process that is disordered is something wrong inside the presenting patient that might be an equivalent to a medical diagnosis. This is particularly clear for somatization disorder, since studies have been known for a number of years that demonstrate an association with disturbances of social and interpersonal behaviour and family functions [1–3]. These authors and others have pointed out that patients presenting with somatization and other somatoform disorders appear to be using the sick role as a way of obtaining attention, but there do not appear to have been any attempts to take this reasonable assumption any further than a general statement.

One simple way of doing this is to examine the constituent illness behaviours of the sick role in detail so as to learn more about how the sick role is being distorted by patients with somatoform disorders.

# The Sick Role and Its Constituent Illness Behaviours

Figure 3 illustrates this, using the sick role of Western European and North American societies that has been well described in the medical and sociological literature for some years [4, 5]. This list is rather larger than some that have appeared in the publications just mentioned, so as to emphasize that the performance of any social role involves a complicated and reciprocal social interaction with other persons who are at the same time carrying out their own roles. Section 3 of Figure 3 should perhaps be labelled as the role of the doctor as healer.

When a patient who meets the criteria for somatization disorder consults a doctor, many of these behaviours are blocked or distorted. It is particularly striking that most of the behaviours of the doctor (by which the healer's role is manifest) are blocked by the patient; for instance, (a) it is very difficult (although not impossible) for the doctor to believe what the patient persists in complaining about; (b) investigations and ques-

### 1. OF THE PATIENT

- COMPLAINS OF FEELING ILL, SEEKS MEDICAL CARE

- COMPLIES WITH TREATMENT & ADVICE GIVEN BY DR

- EXPRESSES HOPE OF RECOVERY

### 2. OF THE FAMILY & OTHERS (eg EMPLOYER)

- OFFER SYMPATHY AND SUPPORT

- ASSIST IN GETTING MEDICAL CARE & ENCOURAGE

    PATIENT TO FOLLOW TREATMENT AND ADVICE

- EXCUSE PATIENT OF RESPONSIBILITIES

- EXPRESS HOPE OF RECOVERY

### 3. OF THE DOCTOR

- BELIEVES WHAT THE PATIENT SAYS ABOUT COMPLAINTS

- ASKS QUESTIONS AND MAY DO INVESTIGATIONS

- TELLS PATIENT WHAT IS WRONG (DIAGNOSIS)

- GIVES TREATMENT/ADVICE AND EXPLANATION

- IMPLIES THAT TREATMENT/ADVICE WILL GIVE

IMPROVEMENT

- AGREES WITH EXCUSED RESPONSIBILITIES

FIG. 3. Illness behaviours of the sick role

tions have already given negative results, so the doctor does not want to repeat them; (c) a medical style of diagnosis, i.e., the identification of an underlying abnormal process or lesion, cannot be given to the patient; and (d) treatment or advice that should lead to recovery cannot be suggested.

In other words, large parts of the complex interactive system that constitutes the normal performance of the sick role and related social interactions cannot take place. Most of the role disturbances in this illustration of the network of behaviours are actually in the role of the doctor, rather that the patient, and it is probably correct to say that the doctor will be complaining just as much as the patient. Doctors have an urge to treat patients just as much as patients have an urge to be treated by doctors.

The next step in this social interpretation of somatization disorder is to enquire what other social roles or interactions of the patient might be disturbed, but not immediately presented by the patient and family, that could be understood as being the cause of the patient needing to obtain sympathy and support from the doctor by misusing the sick role.

There are, of course, many schedules and questionnaires in the literature which enquire into role performance, social interaction, and social support, but none of those used most frequently involve a comprehensive and systematic mapping out of the roles and the constituent sub-role behaviours of both the key individual and the most immediate family members. To do so would need an interview very different to the type of family consultation that is usually carried out by social workers, at least in the UK, so some careful interdisciplinary consultations about the design of a suitable interviewing schedule are needed.

In summary, there seems to be a good case for regarding the distortion of the sick role of the patient and the healer role of the doctor as the central features of somatization disorder, rather than merely interesting side issues that accompany a disorder of some other sort. By mapping out the other roles and their behaviours that constitute the social network in which the patient lives, and by doing this more systematically than is the custom at the moment, it may be possible to identify the non-medical source of the presenting disturbance.

If this is accepted, the next issue is whether the same applies to other disorders in ICD-10.

## Are There Other Role Disorders in ICD-10?

It seems clear that there are many. There is no time to go through all the possibilities, but a few deserve special mention because they share some characteristics with somatization disorder. The categories are:

1. F68.1 Intentional production or feigning of symptoms or disabilities (Factitious Disorder)
2. all the Dissociative (conversion) disorders, F44
3. The closely related category of Malingering Z76.5, not in Chapter V itself

In another context that is not within the remit of this paper, many of the personality disorders can clearly be interpreted as disorders of social roles, and the same applies to many of the categories in the sections of ICD-10 and DSM-IV that deal with disorders of childhood and adolescence.

# Experimental Sub-Divisions and Re-Arrangements of ICD-10

With the above suggestions and possibilities as a guide, it would be worthwhile to begin to devise some groupings of disorders by means of their social characteristics, looking at them quite overtly as disorders of social roles of inter-related persons. This would be a different approach to the present implicit assumption that goes through all of ICD-10 and DSM-IV, which is that their contents refer to disorders of individual persons.

## Conclusions

If further investigation of these possibilities confirms some of the suggestion made here, the main practical gain is likely to be an increased emphasis on social remedies for a social disorder, rather than medical procedures or medication. Possible theoretical gains are new ways of arranging the categories of our present psychiatric classifications, so as to clarify relationships between groups of related disorders.

## References

1. Cloninger CR, Guze SB (1970) Psychiatric illness and female criminality; the role of sociopathy and hysteria in antisocial women. Am J Psychiatry 127:303–310
2. Guze SB, Woodruff RA, Clayton PJ (1971) Hysteria and antisocial behaviour; further evidence of an association. Am J Psychiatry 127:957–960
3. Pilowsky I (1988) Abnormal illness behaviour. In: Henderson S, Burrows G (eds) Handbook of social psychiatry. Elsevier, Amsterdam, Chapter 24
4. Parsons T (1951) The social system. Free Press, Glencoe
5. Mechanic D (1962) The concept of illness behaviour. J Chron Dis 15:189–194

# The Differential Diagnosis of Somatoform Disorders

ALLEN FRANCES[1] and BRANDON VANCE[2]

*Summary.* Somatoform disorders lie on the boundary between medicine and psychiatry and have been relatively ignored by both. Though quite common, these disorders have received little systematic research. Misdiagnosing these disorders results in morbidity, expense, and the possibility of missing more treatable medical or psychiatric diagnoses. The differential diagnosis of somatoform disorders is a difficult but important task that we will discuss in some detail.

*Key words.* Mental illness, Somatoform disorder, Differential diagnosis, DSM-IV

## Introduction

In many cultures across the world, a patient who experiences stress and/or has a psychiatric disorder will often present with somatic complaints. The section of the Diagnostic and Statistical Manual of Mental Disorders, Fourth Edition (DSM-IV) classification titled Somatoform Disorders includes Somatization Disorder, Conversion Disorder, Pain Disorder, Hypochondriasis, and Body Dysmorphic Disorder [1]. These conditions share the following features: the patient is preoccupied by physical complaints that significantly impair functioning in some important aspect of life; the symptoms are not intentionally produced or feigned; and the problem is not better accounted for by other specific medical or psychiatric disorders [2].

By their very nature, these somatoform disorders lie on the boundary between medicine and psychiatry. This unique position often leads to difficulties in their differential diagnosis and treatment in both the medical and the psychiatric settings. In medical settings, patients with somatoform disorders are often the recipients of unneeded tests and diagnostic procedures. False positive results from these procedures may lead to erroneous treatments, complications, unnecessary morbidity, and

---

[1] Department of Psychiatry and Behavioral Sciences, Room 4584, Box 3950, Duke South Hospital, Duke University Medical Center, Durham, NC 27710, USA
[2] Department of Psychiatry and Behavioral Sciences, Room 3547, Box 3018, Duke South Hospital, Duke University Medical Center, Durham, NC 27710, USA

wasted cost. For example, a woman with abdominal pain as part of a somatization disorder may have an exploratory laparotomy in which her uninflamed appendix is removed prophylactically and to make differential diagnosis easier in the future.

On the other hand, doctors sometimes become frustrated with the ever-complaining patient who seems to be constantly crying wolf. Consequently, they may end up refusing to embark upon an adequate medical and psychiatric workup and miss what may be a real problem. New problems that arise in someone labeled with a somatoform disorder may be written off as being "in the patient's head." The patient in the previous example may later develop adhesions from the surgery, causing bowel obstruction and consequently, more pain. Due to the patient's history of somatic complaints with heavy psychiatric influence, the patient's important new pain may be ignored. Obviously, these are difficult diagnostic problems that rely significantly on the clinician's judgment and understanding of the patient's physical and psychological functioning.

Because somatoform disorders fall on a boundary between disciplines, there has been remarkably little research on their diagnosis and treatment. Both medicine and psychiatry have tended to neglect these disorders, each leaving them for the other field to handle. As a result, there is little evidence guiding the treatment of most of these somatoform disorders. Morbidity and cost incurred by overextensive or underextensive workups, problems inherent in labeling patients with somatoform disorders, as well as lack of good treatments, make appropriate differential diagnosis all the more important.

# Differential Diagnosis of the Somatoform Disorders

Before making the diagnosis of a somatoform disorder, it is important to take into account the following possible explanations of the symptom presentation: (1) general medical conditions; (2) primary psychiatric conditions; (3) substance abuse and withdrawal; (4) cultural factors; and (5) feigned medical conditions.

## General Medical Conditions

The clinician must first rule out the possibility that the symptoms are caused by a general medical condition that has not yet clearly declared itself or that presents with an atypical course. One should be specifically alert to the possibilities of systemic lupus erythematosus, multiple sclerosis, acute intermittent porphyria, and hyperparathyroidism. All of these are medical conditions that present with a diverse symptom pattern which may mimic a somatoform disorder. Contact with the patient's primary medical provider is necessary, especially when this primary doctor has had long-term experience the patient. Careful review of the patient's medical records also helps prevent superfluous testing. Clinical judgment based on these factors along with the patient's presentation will help determine the nature and the extent of the workup.

## Primary Psychiatric Disorders

Primary psychiatric disorders must also be ruled out, especially since most of these are much better defined and more treatable than somatoform disorders. Many psychiatric disorders present with prominent physical symptoms. DSM-IV criteria for panic attacks are perhaps the clearest example. Persons experiencing panic attacks undergo a barrage of physical symptoms including palpitations, diaphoresis, hot flushes or chills, trembling, dyspnea, chest pain, choking feelings, nausea, lightheadedness, and paresthesias. Likewise, criteria for a major depressive episode include prominent physical signs and symptoms. These characteristics include significant weight loss or gain, decrease or increase in appetite, insomnia or hypersomnia, psychomotor retardation or agitation, and loss of energy.

## Substance Abuse and Withdrawal

Substance use and withdrawal cause a wide range of physical and psychological signs and symptoms. These signs and symptoms can include fatigue, weight loss or gain, perceptual changes, weakness, muscle rigidity, seizures, coma, incoordination, diminished response to pain, blurred vision, chest pain, nausea, vomiting, diarrhea, and constipation. The symptoms of substance intoxication and withdrawal are additionally misleading because they may be misinterpreted by the patient as being part of a physical illness unrelated to substance use.

## Cultural Factors

Cultural factors influence the expression of somatic symptoms and must be considered in the diagnosis of somatoform disorders. In some cultures, somatic presentation is the only means of receiving attention for problems that are psychiatric or psychological in origin. A narrow focus on somatic symptoms may lead to missed psychiatric diagnoses. On the other hand, culturally sanctioned and ritualized somatic or dissociative experiences must be distinguished from psychiatric disorders. The clinician must also consider the possibility that the patient has a medical disease related to the patient's regions of residence or visitation. Endemic infections, malnutrition, or other recurrent illnesses may present atypically with symptoms in multiple organ systems.

## Feigned Medical Conditions

Finally, one must differentiate between somatoform disorders and disorders of feigning such as malingering and factitious disorder. The main difference here is intentionality, i.e., persons with somatoform disorders do not consciously and intentionally produce their symptoms. This distinction is often difficult to make because conscious and unconscious feigning lie on a continuum, and clinicians are not particularly good at spotting either end.

# Somatization Disorder

Persons with somatization disorder present with numerous and varied physical complaints that begin before age 30 and persist over time. The symptoms cause social or occupational impairment and are not feigned or intentionally produced. To meet criteria for somatization disorder, a patient must have four pain symptoms, each relating to a different bodily part or system. The patient also must express symptoms other than pain related to sexual or reproductive function (one symptom), the gastrointestinal system (two symptoms), and neurological function (one symptom). If these complaints occur as part of a medical condition, they must be out of proportion to what would be expected for the condition. The patient often describes the complaints in exaggerated and sometimes inconsistent ways.

The differential diagnosis of somatization disorder is difficult but important. Patients with systemic lupus erythematosus, for example, often have intermittent symptoms in multiple organ systems including gastrointestinal pain, arthritis, visual changes, as well as central nervous symptoms such as seizures, depression, and psychosis. Confusion and frustration occasioned by these seemingly random symptoms as well as the appearance of the neuropsychiatric findings associated with lupus may lead a clinician to believe the patient is somatizing. This belief may result in a prematurely discontinued and incomplete workup.

Patients with chronic mood disorders and generalized anxiety disorder often present with multiple somatic complaints. These disorders must therefore be ruled out when considering the diagnosis of somatization disorder. The presence of somatic symptoms regardless of state of mood and anxiety may suggest a somatization disorder rather than a mood or anxiety disorder. Panic disorder is frequently missed with a consequent overdiagnosis of somatization disorder due to the occurrence of physical complaints in multiple organ systems during panic attacks. Strict use of the diagnostic criteria for somatization disorder, however, usually prevents misdiagnosing what is really a panic disorder. The workup of possible somatization disorder depends on the clinician's judgment and knowledge of the patient over time in addition to a careful and appropriate search for medical etiologies.

## Conversion Disorder

Conversion disorder refers to a set of unintentional symptoms causing impairment in the voluntary motor or sensory systems which are preceded by, exacerbated by, or associated with psychological factors or stressors. These symptoms must cause marked distress or impairment and must not be an expression of an underlying medical or neurological condition.

As defined in the DSM-IV, conversion disorder comprises symptoms occurring only in the voluntary motor and sensory systems. Thus, it excludes presentations of autonomic nervous system dysfunction (such as persistent vomiting), other neurological symptoms (such as fainting), and non-neurological symptoms (such as pseudocyesis). Conversion episodes usually do not lead to physical damage or to disability.

Psychological factors must play a role in the pathogenesis of conversion disorder. However, this role is difficult to evaluate. Psychological factors are so totally ubiquitous in human existence that psychological causality is impossible to prove. For example, patients with conversion disorder often appear overly calm (*la belle indifférence*) or overly dramatic about their symptoms, but people with medical illnesses also may act this way. People with true medical illnesses often have psychological problems that are caused by or incidental to the illness rather than causative of it. In attempting to sort out this causality, it may be useful to establish a temporal relationship between the onset of the symptoms and the experience of a current stressor. This relationship together with a knowledge and understanding of the patient's psychological issues and conflicts may aid the clinician in assessing the role of psychological factors in the patient's presentation.

The clinician must also take into account the patient's cultural and religious practices. For example, seizure-like activity or change in conscious state are common in rituals of some cultures and would not be considered a disorder if it occurs in those contexts.

The diagnosis of a conversion disorder should be made only after a cautious process of exclusion with careful evaluation and a nonphysiological pattern of symptoms. Historically, clinicians have often mistaken conversion disorders for underlying neurological disease. Multiple sclerosis, myasthenia gravis, and substance-induced dystonias have been often mistaken for conversion disorders. On the other hand, a patient may have both an underlying neurological disease and a conversion disorder. For example, a patient with epilepsy may have pseudoseizures in addition to epileptic seizures. The surprisingly high frequency of underlying physical disease that eventually accounts for the symptoms of a previously diagnosed conversion disorder highlights the importance of a thorough medical and neurological workup.

## Pain Disorder

A pain disorder may be diagnosed when pain is the presenting symptom and when it causes an impairment in the patient's life. The clinician must judge psychological factors to be important in the onset, exacerbation, or persistence of the pain. If the patient has an existing medical condition, the pain must be out of proportion to what would be expected for the condition. The pain must not be feigned or intentionally produced.

The experience of pain is by definition subjective and varies with individual personality and cultural expectations. A general medical condition may generate pain with or without psychological causation, exacerbation, exaggeration, or maintenance. To differentiate these issues, the clinician may investigate chronicity and pervasiveness of the pain as well as its repercussions on the rest of the patient's life.

It may be particularly difficult to distinguish a pain disorder from malingering given that the clinician must rely to a large extent on the patient's report of symptoms and their intensity. Often there are issues at stake of disability insurance, employment, compensation, and tort liability which must figure into the clinician's judgment.

## Hypochondriasis

Hypochondriasis is a persistent preoccupation with the belief that one has a serious medical disease due to the misinterpretation of bodily symptoms. This belief persists in spite of medical reassurance to the contrary. The preoccupation lasts for at least 6 months and causes significant distress or impairment.

After ruling out medical conditions, and especially some of the diseases with atypical presentations mentioned earlier, a diagnosis of hypochondriasis must be differentiated from other psychiatric disorders. A patient with hypochondriasis is often able to admit the possibility that his or her preoccupation is exaggerated or unfounded. If the patient does not have this insight, the clinician must consider whether the beliefs are of delusional proportion. Beliefs that are of delusional proportion would imply a diagnosis of delusional disorder, somatic type, as opposed to a diagnosis of hypochondriasis with poor insight.

Hypochondriasis is differentiated from a phobia because the fear is of currently having a disease rather than a fear of becoming diseased. Somatization disorder can share many features with hypochondriasis. However, patients with hypochondriasis are preoccupied with the conviction that they have a serious illness whereas persons with somatization disorder are preoccupied with the actual symptoms they are experiencing.

Like anyone else, people with hypochondriasis may have or develop underlying medical or mental illnesses, making careful examination essential and an appropriate extent of diagnostic testing challenging. Frequent "doctor-shopping" by patients with hypochondriasis makes it more difficult for a given clinician to differentiate the medical from the psychiatric aspects of the patient's presentation.

## Body Dysmorphic Disorder

Persons suffering from body dysmorphic disorder are preoccupied with the thought that they have an anomalous or ugly appearance. The preoccupation must cause significant distress or impairment in the patient's life and must not be accounted for by another mental or physical disorder.

The clinician must ensure that the patient's concern about his or her appearance is not in the normal range. Almost everybody has at least some concern about and dissatisfaction with physical appearance. Individuals with body dysmorphic disorder, however, are tormented by their appearance and this preoccupation becomes a focus of their lives. It is sometimes difficult to distinguish between body dysmorphic disorder and somatic delusion since views concerning one's personal physical appearance are so highly subjective. For a belief of a bodily anomaly to be considered delusional, it should be extremely unusual or result in destructive or bizarre behavior. Patients with other mental disorders such as anorexia nervosa, gender identity disorder, and obsessive compulsive disorder also often have concerns about appearance, but a separate diagnosis of body dysmorphic disorder is not ordinarily given.

## Discussion

Patients with somatoform disorders use a disproportionately large share of diagnostic and treatment resources. Overtesting and overtreating can lead to complications, morbidity, and wasted expense. Once a patient is thought to have a somatoform disorder, other more treatable medical and psychiatric diagnoses may be overlooked or dismissed. Though we include a section for somatoform disorders in the DSM-IV, the disorders are not well understood. Consequently, we must be cautious about making this diagnosis and about what are its implications.

Though most of these conditions are chronic and do not have specific accepted treatments, there are some general principles for dealing with patients with somatoform disorders. One should accept the importance of the patient's experience and accept that the symptoms will not just go away. By definition, somatoform disorders exclude feigning. Once feigning and malingering are ruled out, the sensations and perceptions experienced by the patient need to be treated as real to him or her. Dismissing or diminishing the importance of the patient's experiences, preoccupations, or concerns will prevent building a therapeutic relationship. Instead, the clinician should teach coping skills to lessen the disorder's impact on the patient's life.

Patients can also be taught new approaches to coping with physical fears such as distraction, relaxation, and meditation. Finding useful activities and increasing interpersonal contacts can reduce preoccupations. Cognitive restructuring to help reduce catastrophization and to change mental constructs that perpetuate somatoform illnesses has been used successfully. Additionally, rationing care to these patients, as may happen in a managed care environment, may actually be helpful.

Though they are relatively common and much money is spent in their diagnosis and treatment, somatoform disorders are among the most unresearched areas in Psychiatry and Medicine. Descriptive studies in real-life settings are needed to accurately track the incidence and cost of these conditions and to help develop improved methods of diagnosis. Controlled interventional studies need to be performed to investigate effective treatments. In this way, the medical and psychiatric fields may work on their mutual border for better diagnosis and treatment of these common, expensive, distressing, and complex disorders.

## References

1. American Psychiatric Association (1994) Diagnostic and statistical manual of mental disorders, 4th edn. American Psychiatric Association, Washington
2. Frances A, First MB, Pincus HA (1995) DSM-IV Guidebook. American Psychiatric Press, Washington, pp 275–292

# European Concepts

RICHARD MAYOU

*Summary.* Historical European concepts of the nature and causes of physical symptoms without clear explanation have caused considerable confusion. This chapter argues that, in recent years, there has been increasing awareness of the need for a broader approach based on understanding all unexplained symptoms in a general population and all medical settings. Aetiology should be viewed as an interaction of physical, psychological, and social factors. Current definitions of somatoform disorders are unhelpful and need to be revised in a manner not based on mind/body separation. There have been major advances in showing the efficacy and cost-effectiveness of treatments.

## Introduction

Most of the historical concepts and terminology that underlie present discussion, at least in Western countries, derive from European concepts of great antiquity [1]. Whilst some of what has been written remains useful, historical views are a great barrier to our current understanding [2]. It is unhelpful to dwell too much on the history, especially in a book intended to provide an international perspective. Countries and cultures whose approach to psychiatry does not share the Western assumption of separation of mind and body have no need to master outdated views which will only divert them from developing a better understanding of very major theoretical and clinical issues.

There are great practical problems in presenting a European view in that Europe is a large and diverse group of cultures. In addition, academic material is fragmented and unsatisfactory and there is, at present, no comprehensive view of disparate problems which relate to a major part of everyday clinical medicine. It is also artificial to separate European research and clinical developments from those in North America and other countries following similar models. This chapter is therefore a discussion of a number of key issues as seen by a rather small number of European psychiatrists and psychologists. It argues that European research has made a distinctive contribu-

Department of Psychiatry, University of Oxford, Warneford Hospital, Oxford OX3 7JX, UK

tion in all these areas, not least because it is less hindered than North America by the imposition of rigid classification and also because publicly organised systems of health care make research and clinical innovation with patients' groups much more straightforward.

I consider five themes:

- The concept of medically unexplained symptoms
- Epidemiology
- Classification
- Aetiology
- Treatment

I argue that we now have an opportunity to bring together current knowledge in an overview which might be accepted by most of those clinically and academically active in the field. It would be unrealistic to expect that we shall eliminate all the confusions between different disciplines or be able to agree a single terminology. However, we can highlight these problems so that the difficulties and disagreements are made explicit.

## Unexplained Medical Symptoms

Most widely used terms, such as somatization or functional symptoms or somatoform symptoms, have aetiological connotations. In particular, there is an implication that somatic symptoms are an alternative means of expressing distress to psychological symptoms. Originally apparent in the original nineteenth century formulation of conversion disorder, it persists within the increasingly widely used word somatization. This term has been very variously defined as a category and process. It is often used as a very general term as, for instance, in the widely-quoted definition by Lipowski [3], "a tendency to experience and communicate somatic distress and symptoms unaccounted for by pathological findings, to attribute them to physical illness and to seek medical help for them". This covers a substantial area of medicine, some very diverse behaviours and, implicitly, an idea of expression of psychological distress as transformed physical symptoms. Kleinman applied these concepts to cross-cultural understanding emphasising somatization as an idiom of distress [4]. In contrast, Bridges and Goldberg [5] and others have defined somatization as physical symptoms associated with standard psychiatric diagnoses of anxiety and depression. It may now be difficult to achieve an agreed definition and it would be best to drop the term altogether; at its very least, it is essential that the limitations are widely recognised.

There is much to be said for using the increasingly widely used term medically unexplained symptoms for all non-specific symptoms which are widespread in the general population and in all medical settings and for which there is no precise medical answer. An alternative is the synonym for somatoform disorders in the primary care version of ICD-10: unexplained physical symptoms. The term is not without cultural bias and is not completely satisfactory in that all somatic symptoms do, in fact, have explanations. Even so, it is probably the best and most straightforward English term that we have. It is consistent with recognition in many cultures that there are non-specific physical symptoms which are common and, if persistent, may be disabling and difficult to treat. For example, in Japan the word *futeishuso* refers to non-specific physical symptoms, and is widely understood as referring to complaints whose precise cause is difficult to identify. Other countries and cultures have similar concepts and terms.

"Unexplained medical symptoms" is a term that has the advantage of having no aetiological implications and relates directly to the clinical problem experienced by patients and presented to those who treat them. It is one that makes no aetiological assumptions and may be seen as a "bottom up" approach, in contrast to the "top down" approach of starting with psychiatric theory or highly selective and specialised experience and attempting to generalise from this.

# Epidemiology

Research on the epidemiology of medically unexplained symptoms has expanded greatly in all parts of the world. Perhaps the most influential European contributions have been in relation to defined clinical syndromes and primary care research [6].

## Clinical Syndromes

In Western medicine there are many clinically recognised syndromes which have no single accepted medical explanation. Some of the syndromes are purely descriptive (headache, pelvic pain), but many long-standing terms have aetiological connotations (post-traumatic syndrome, irritable bowel). They include syndromes discussed elsewhere in this book, such as chronic fatigue and fibromyalgia. European epidemiological surveys in the community have been principally concerned with particular syndromes, for example, chronic fatigue [7] and irritable bowel [8]. Taken together with other studies of primary and secondary care, they have added to understanding of symptoms which are common in the general community and medical practice. Although there is some doubt about the validity of these syndromes [9], they should be an important focus of our clinical and research attention in that they represent the clinical problems which present to doctors.

There is undoubtedly variation between European countries and many other syndromes have been described in non-Western countries. We need to know more about operational defined syndromes and their cross-cultural and more local validity. I believe that there have been advantages in operational definitions which have been developed for severe syndromes, for example, chronic fatigue [7]. These are definitions which make no assumption about aetiology but enable discussion of a clinical problem that requires assessment and treatment. We clearly need to know more about the epidemiology of these syndromes; in particular, it is only recently that there has been systematic cross-cultural research, and this tends to suggest that unexplained symptoms are common in all cultures but that there may be some differences in patterns of symptoms or in syndromes. It may also be that there are cultural differences in reporting symptoms in surveys and in everyday consulting.

There is also a very considerable tendency for lay groups to coin new terms for poorly understood syndromes and many of these make assumptions about possible causes. Examples are the various synonyms for chronic fatigue syndrome, Gulf War syndrome and repetitive strain injury. Such terms have been profoundly unhelpful in that they make assumptions, publicise them and often arouse anxiety which may be needless. They also prevent a considered evidence-based approach to understanding and to the development of treatment.

## Primary Care

Another very major theme in British and other European research has been the epidemiology of unexplained symptoms in primary care [5, 10–13]. There has been increasing evidence on the significance of somatic symptoms. Research on a restricted definition of somatization by Bridges and Goldberg is well known [5]. More recent studies have included a survey by Peveler and colleagues who looked at patterns of psychiatric disorder [14]. Their findings have replicated those of Kirmayer and Robbins in Canada [15]. These studies suggest that unexplained symptoms of a severity that might be regarded as fitting the diagnosis of somatoform disorders, can be considered as showing three main groupings: chronic personality-related syndromes with multiple symptoms, complaints related to effects of anxiety disorder, hypochondriacal or health anxiety symptoms. These categories overlap to some extent but do not fit well with our current nosology.

One very often neglected finding of a number of studies, including the very large and important WHO Primary Care Study [13], is that persistent somatic symptoms can occur without there being any conventional psychiatric disorder. These are people who may be worried and limited but there are no grounds for making a psychiatric diagnosis. We need to stress that straightforward psychiatric disorder is not an adequate explanation for the problems discussed in this book.

# Aetiology

The Western mind/body split, viewing physical and psychological explanations as alternatives, and the search for single aetiologies has been very harmful but remains extremely common. However, there has been increasing awareness of the need to see aetiology as multicausal, the interaction of physical and psychological factors.

We have proposed a model (Fig. 1) [16, 17] which resembles, but is more comprehensive than, some other models showing the interaction of psychological and social factors as influencing the ways in which bodily sensations or worries are interpreted to result in physical symptoms, distress, behavioural change, and disability [6]. The model is an oversimplification of the complex interaction of many factors but provides a useful basis for discussion and understanding. It enables us to combine the distinctly different models which in the past have been seen as having possible aetiological significance—behavioural, psychodynamic, cognitive, psychiatric [18]. Other authors in this book describe models which refer to sections of the model shown in this chapter; I believe it is possible to reconcile the various approaches described.

European research has elucidated many components of the model. These have included the importance of unexplained symptoms in association with undoubted major physical disorder, pathophysiological mechanisms [19], the significance of lay

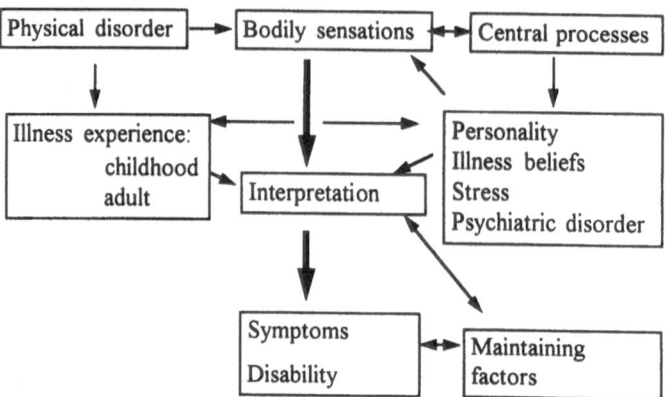

Fig. 1. Model of psychological and social factors that influence somatic symptoms

beliefs about symptoms and illness, and biological research on possible central mechanisms. In this chapter I want to bring out three topics:

• Childhood developmental factors
• The cognitive theory of health anxiety
• Iatrogenic maintaining factors

Increasing retrospective evidence suggests that childhood factors such as illness experience, parental attitudes, and sexual abuse may be determinants of later unexplained physical symptoms. It would seem that they increase vulnerability and concern. This data is largely retrospective [20]. However, we have recently been able to make use of data from a population-based birth cohort established in 1946. This had 19 waves of data gathering, including information at the ages of 36 and 43 years. One set of analyses has identified children with persistent abdominal pain throughout childhood [21]. This was associated with parental poor health and emotional disorder, often persisted in adult life and was associated with an increased risk of adult psychiatric disorder. Perhaps more interesting are analyses which examined childhood predictors of later adult medically unexplained symptoms as judged by self-report and hospital admission and diagnosis [22]. The clearest predictors appeared to be family ill health but not chronic physical illness in childhood. Psychiatric disorder itself only accounted for a proportion of adult unexplained symptoms. A specific example is chest pain. Chest pain was common, with a prevalence of 17.2% at the age of 36, but exertional chest pain was relatively rare and not due to ischaemic heart disease. There was a striking relationship with psychiatric disorder in adult life. In addition, childhood experience of poor health reported by the parents during childhood and experience of fatigue during childhood were both associated with adult chest pain.

There have been various attempts to describe the interaction of personality, mental state, and physical symptoms. Theories of symptom perception involving attention, amplification, and other possible mechanisms have largely been based on normal subjects or people with clear physical disorder. The theory of cognitive health anxiety had been developed to explain the possible mechanisms in psychiatric disorder such as hypochondriasis and panic [23]. It is supported by experimental evidence and appears to be of value as a basis for effective treatment. The cognitive theory suggests that personality and experience result in dysfunctional assumptions which can be activated by a critical incident and results in distorted interpretation of bodily sensations or health information. The consequences are cognitive, physiological, behavioural, and emotional. Psychiatric outcomes include panic in those who have catastrophic interpretations and hypochondriasis. There is already substantial evidence to suggest the validity of the cognitive theory and its value as a basis for designing effective treatment. However, its relationship to the very largely separate areas of health psychology research is not entirely clear. Further progress to try and bring together parallel conceptual models and experimental evidence would be helpful.

Maintaining factors can be of different types. One important group relate to medical care itself. Medical assessment and treatment can often exacerbate problems, increasing concern rather than reassuring the subject. This is especially so in those with high health anxiety [24, 25]. Inconsistent, ambiguous advice or information, lack of an explanation and over-investigation can all perpetuate problems. This has been apparent in patients with chronic pain [26] and in our programme of research on non-cardiac chest pain [27, 28]. For example, in a recent audit of consecutive referrals to Oxford cardiac clinics, many patients had been told that they had heart disease and had been treated as having heart disease before referral to cardiologists. Thereafter, investigation was frequently prolonged, and reassurance appeared to be ambiguous or inconsistent. We concluded that there is a need to provide rapid access to specialist investigation, to try and prevent provisional diagnosis and treatment as heart disease, and for simple improvements in oral and written advice within clinics together with review and access to extra care.

# Classification

The rival approaches to classification, medical and psychiatric, become confused and confusing. We believe that there are advantages in moving away from the idea of alternative single aetiologies to the acceptance of multiple physical and psychological causes. These are best considered in terms of clinical syndrome, psychiatric diagnosis, and other dimensions.

## Clinical Syndromes

There are, in fact, several ways of diagnosing unexplained medical symptoms. One already discussed is by clinical syndrome, such as irritable bowel, chronic fatigue, and atypical chest pain. These are apparent syndromes presented to doctors. European research has defined many of these and usefully so; the example given in the chapter by Wessely (this volume) demonstrates this. Even so, acrimonious discussion between those favouring either a physical or a psychiatric aetiology has been unhelpful. In contrast, a growing number of syndromes are defined in terms of their suggested aetiology; many of them suggested by lay pressure groups. These are generally unhelpful and invalid, and there is a need for operational syndrome definitions, such as those of chronic fatigue. These are important because they describe what people suffer from, and require treatment for, but they do not have unjustifiable implications about causation.

## Psychiatric Diagnoses

In parallel with clinical syndromes we need to consider the significance of psychiatric disorder. For many, many years the classification of disorders such as hypochondriasis and conversion disorder preoccupied European writers. In recent years, argument has been less vociferous but has been concerned with the syndromes imposed first by DSM-III and continued by DSM-IV and ICD-10. In particular, the group introduced in DSM-III—somatoform disorders. DSM-IV introducing this section states "The grouping of these disorders in a single section is based on clinical utility . . . rather than assumptions regarding shared aetiology or mechanism".

Unfortunately, a tentative attempt to provide for clinical problems that could not be easily contained within better established categories has frequently been interpreted as a rigid solution, having greater validity than the evidence warrants. Outside the countries familiar with the traditional European/North American concepts of a separation of mind and body, the whole category has caused very considerable bewilderment and dismay. The term has little meaning in the many countries where it is assumed that mind and body should always be considered as parts of the same whole. For example, national classifications in China, Japan, and elsewhere have struggled to maintain compatibility.

Apart from the lack of a satisfactory organising principle, the whole grouping and its subcategories have proved unreliable and unsatisfactory in practice. There are significant differences between ICD and DSM, and the use of both categories results in a minority of patients being classified within non-specific groupings. The combination of tightly defined specific categories and large vague non-specific subcategories is unfortunate. It has resulted in much of the literature and research being focused on subgroups which are relatively unimportant in the total picture of somatic complaints falling within the overall definition of somatoform disorders. Thus a very great deal has been written about somatization disorder, which is extremely uncommon, and rather little about the moderately distressed and disabled patients which make up much of everyday primary care and other medical practice.

The more specific categories have also attracted criticism. Somatization disorder has been widely seen as having the greatest validity but, in fact, it probably has the highest reliability and is an arbitrary extreme of a continuum or indeed a series of dimensions. It has been cogently argued that it is best seen as a personality disorder [29, 30]. More recent concepts, such as abridged somatisation disorder, may have had some practical value but are equally arbitrary.

Hypochondriasis is essentially a syndrome of abnormal degrees of health anxiety. Its particular criteria are not easy to apply, especially that relating to reassurance by doctors. Personality is important [29, 30]. Many would argue that patients who have been regarded as hypochondriacal have not in fact had explanation and reassurance that meets their needs. Analysis of the WHO Primary Care Study has suggested that there may be more value in a broader concept of health anxiety which omits the reassurance criterion [31]. We should perhaps echo a comment made a number of years ago by Kirmayer and Robbins, "somatoform disorders appear to be best thought of as

TABLE 1. A proposed classification of non-specific unexplained symptoms [16]

| |
|---|
| Physical symptoms: |
|     number of symptoms (single symptom, multiple symptoms) |
|     type (e.g., sensory, motor) |
| Mental state: |
|     depression |
|     anxiety and panic |
|     other psychiatric disorder |
| Cognitions: |
|     fear of disease |
|     conviction of disease |
| Behavioural and functional impairment: |
|     avoidance |
|     illness behaviour |
|     use of health services |
| Pathophysiological disturbance: |
|     identifiable mechanisms (e.g., hyperventilation) |
|     organic disease |

Disorders are classified as acute (less than 6 months' duration) or chronic (greater than 6 months).

symptoms or patterns of reactions rather than discrete disorders ... we might shift our attention from efforts to characterise disorders to attempts to understand the underlying pathological processes that may result in functional somatic distress".

Scepticism about the current definition and validity of hypochondriasis should not detract from the importance of a significant amount of research on the characteristics and treatment of patients who have been diagnosed as having this disorder. Rather, we need now to apply this evidence to a wider range of patients with and without health anxiety.

It is difficult to believe that abandoning the present official classification would, at the present time, be helpful. There is a lack of empirical evidence about the epidemiology, severity, and course of clinical problems, and no agreement about the principles which might underlie a classification which could be applicable across cultures. It may well be that guidance and caveats about the present classification would be valuable.

## Dimensions

We have suggested that, rather than trying to modify unsatisfactory psychiatric categories to include a variety of different types of information, it would be better to think in terms of multidimensional classification [6], as shown in Table 1.

## Treatment

There has been considerable European research on treatment which has included detailed clinical studies, randomised controlled trials, and a variety of attempts to improve delivery to large numbers of people [16]. To some extent, the current problem is one of applying what we already know as much as seeking further evidence of effectiveness [32].

## General Principles

Clinical experience suggests that providing an explanation should, wherever possible, provide an account of underlying minor pathological or physiological causes of body sensations together with a clear message to the patient that the whole syndrome is common, familiar, and treatable. It is not necessary for patient and doctor to share a substantially psychological explanation, and many patients who remain convinced that they may have a physical problem will, nonetheless, accept that they have been adequately investigated and that they can expect no specific physical treatment. In these circumstances they welcome assurances that there are a number of ways in which doctors and others can help and also ways in which they can help themselves. Establishing a joint understanding of the aims and scope of treatment is in itself helpful to the patient who is uncertain, concerned by doctors' apparent inability to make a diagnosis and who has lost confidence in medical care.

## Specific Intervention

Approaches to management include:

- Drug treatments, especially antidepressants
- Cognitive behavioural treatments
- Other behavioural treatments
- Psychotherapy
- Educational approaches
- Self-help treatments

A number of studies suggest a role for antidepressants in some types of pain syndrome [33, 34]. However, there appear to be limitations for their use in syndromes such as chronic fatigue, fibromyalgia, and other common clinical problems unless there are very clear symptoms of major depressive problems. Cognitive behavioural treatment has been shown to be effective in the treatment of hypochondriasis [35, 36] and in a number of specific clinical syndromes [26, 37, 38]. Several psychotherapies and other interventions have also been evaluated [39].

There is convincing evidence that cognitive behavioural and other psychological treatments are effective. Although at first sight there are substantial differences between some of the approaches that have been proposed, it is also evident that there are common elements in terms of providing an explanation and advice and encouraging graded return to full activities.

Most of the treatments that have been evaluated are relatively complex, and it is likely that they will never be appropriate for anything other than highly specialist treatment of selected subjects. There is every reason to think that, like other psychological treatments for psychiatric disorders, it would be possible to simplify them and to make them available in a form that could be provided by less specialised therapists. There is limited evidence on the value of self-help treatments, on the use of specialist nurses and on the training of doctors.

## Delivery

The European comprehensive health care systems have emphasise the needs for improvements in treatment in primary care and in outpatient clinics. This has led to a number of accounts of basic principles such as the acceptance of reality of symptoms, providing an explanation, providing advice, and discussing misconceptions. In addition, some patients have other significant psychiatric or social problems which require individual attention.

# Conclusion

Traditional views of unexplained medical symptoms and of psychiatric disorders such as hypochondriasis and hysteria have been found inadequate and largely unhelpful. In recent years there has also been dissatisfaction with terminology and classification, and lack of agreement about the role of psychological and psychiatric factors. However, there are also some signs of new and flexible concepts. European countries have probably been less dominated than North America by the rigid financial consequences of the introduction of the concept of somatoform disorders in DSM-III. There remains a considerable need to re-examine thinking and to develop an agreed approach to theory and clinical practice.

This chapter argues that the comprehensive approach to all unexplained medical symptoms is a valuable starting point for discussion and that we need to develop an interactive and multicausal view of aetiology, a view which is applicable to all cultures and health care systems. This new understanding of causes has immediate implications for designing and delivering treatments. Whilst it remains difficult to treat many of those with severe or chronic unexplained symptoms, there is much encouraging clinical experience and evidence about the efficacy of a range of types of psychiatric and psychological treatment. However, there are as many problems in implementing what we already know as there are in devising new, effective treatments. This book is a sign of increasing interest in somatic complaints and somatoform disorders. Whilst the very considerable conceptual and practical problems are conspicuous, it is also apparent that there is much common ground and that there is now an opportunity to develop wider agreement about the priorities for research and especially about the priorities for developing and providing treatments.

## References

1. Berrios GE (1997) The history of mental symptoms. Cambridge University Press, Cambridge
2. Janca A, Isaac M, Costa e Silva JA (1995) World Health Organization international study of somatoform disorders—background and rationale. Eur J Psychiatry 9(2):100–110
3. Lipowski ZJ (1988) Somatization: the concept and its clinical application. Am J Psychiatry 145:1358–1368
4. Kleinman A (1977) Depression, somatization and the "new cross-cultural psychiatry". Soc Sci Med 11:3–10
5. Bridges KW, Goldberg DP (1985) Somatic presentation of DSM-III psychiatric disorders in primary care. J Psychosom Res 29:563–569

6. Mayou R, Bass C, Sharp M. Overview of epidemiology, classification and aetiology. In Mayou R, Bass C, Sharpe M (eds) (1995) Treatment of functional somatic symptoms. Oxford University Press, Oxford, pp 42–65

7. Wessely S, Hotopf M, Sharpe M (1998) Chronic fatigue and chronic fatigue syndromes. Oxford University Press, Oxford

8. Creed F. Psychological treatment of irritable bowel syndrome and abdominal pain. In Mayou RA, Bass C, Sharpe M (eds) (1995) Treatment of functional somatic symptoms. Oxford University Press, Oxford, pp 255–270

9. Robbins JM, Kirmayer LJ, Hemami S (1997) Latent variable models of functional somatic distress. J Nerv Ment Dis 185(606):615

10. Faravelli C, Salvatori S, Galassi F, Aiazzi L, Drei C, Cabras P (1997) Epidemiology of somatoform disorders: a community survey in Florence. Soc Psychiatry Psychiatr Epdemiol 32:24–29

11. Goldberg D (1995) Epidemiology of mental disorders in primary care settings. Epidemiol Rev 17(1):182–190

12. Üstün TB, Sartorius N (1995) World Health Organisation. Mental illness in general health care. An international study. Wiley, Chichester

13. Kisely S, Goldberg D, Simon G (1997) A comparison between somatic symptoms with and without clear organic cause: results of an international study. Psychol Med 27: 1011–9

14. Peveler R, Kilkenny L, Kinmonth A (1997) Medically unexplained physical symptoms in primary care: a comparison of self-report screening questionnaires and clinical opinion. J Psychosom Res 42:245–252

15. Kirmayer LJ, Robbins JM (1991) Three forms of somatization in primary care: prevalence, co-occurence, and sociodemographic characteristics. J Nerv Ment Dis 179: 647–655

16. Mayou RA, Bass C, Sharpe M (1995) Treatment of functional somatic symptoms. Oxford University Press, Oxford

17. Mayou RA (1976) The nature of bodily symptoms. Br J Psychiatry 129:55–60

18. Barsky AJ, Klerman GL (1983) Overview: hypochondriasis, bodily complaints, and somatic styles. Am J Psychiatry 140:273–283

19. Sharpe M, Bass C (1992) Pathophysiological mechanisms in somatization. Int Rev Psychiatry 4:81–97

20. Benjamin S, Eminson DM (1992) Abnormal illness behaviour: childhood experiences and long-term consequences. Int Rev Psychiatry 4:55–70

21. Hotopf M, Carr S, Mayou R, Wadsworth M, Wessely S (1998) Why do children have chronic abdominal pain, and what happens to them when they grow up? Population based cohort study. Br Med J 316:1196–1200

22. Hotopf M, Mayou RA, Wessely S (1997) Childhood risk factors for adult medically unexplained symptoms: results from a prospective cohort study. Academy of Psychosomatic Medicine Proceedings 44th Annual Meeting, p 32

23. Salkovskis PM, Clark DM (1993) Panic disorder and hypochondriasis. Adv Behav Res Ther 15:23–48

24. Lucock MP, Morely S, White C, Peake MD (1997) Responses of consecutive patients to reassurance after gastroscopy: results of self administered questionnaire survey. Br Med J 315(572):575

25. Coia P, Morley S (1998) Medical reassurance and patients' responses. J Psychom Res (in press)

26. van Dulmen AM, Fennis FM, Bleijenberg G (1996) Cognitive-behavioral group therapy for irritable bowel syndrome: effects and long-term follow-up. Psychosom Med 58:508–514

27. Mayou R, Bryant B, Forfar C, Clark D (1994) Non-cardiac chest pain and benign palpitations in the cardiac clinic. Br Heart J 72:548–553

28. Mayou R, Bryant B, Sanders D, Bass C, Klimes I, Forfar C (1997) A controlled trial of cognitive behavioural therapy for non-cardiac chest pain. Psychol Med 27:1021–1032
29. Tyrer P, Fowler-Dixon R, Ferguson B, Kelemen A (1990) A plea for the diagnosis of hypochondriacal personality disorder. J Psychosom Res 34:637–642
30. Bass C, Murphy M (1995) Somatoform and personality disorders: syndromal comorbidity and overlapping developmental pathways. J Psychosom Res 39(4):403–427
31. Gureje O, Üstün TB, Simon GE (1997) The syndrome of hypochondriasis: a cross-national study in primary care. Psychol Med 27:1001–1010
32. Mayou R, Sharpe M (1997) Treating medically unexplained physical symptoms. Br Med J 315:561–562
33. McQuay HJ, Tramèr M, Nye BA, Carroll D, Wiffen PJ, Moore RA (1996) A systematic review of antidepressants in neuropathic pain. Pain 68:217–227
34. Wilson JJ, Gil KM (1996) The efficacy of psychological and pharmacological interventions for the treatment of chronic disease-related and non-disease-related pain. Clin Psychol Rev 16(6):573–597
35. Warwick HMC, Clark DM, Cobb AM, Salkovskis PM (1996) A controlled trial of cognitive-behavioural treatment of hypochondriasis. Br J Psychiatry 169:189–195
36. Avia MD, Ruiz MA, Olivares ME, Crespo M, Guisado AB, Sanchez A, Varela A (1996) The meaning of psychological symptoms: effectiveness of a group intervention with hypochondriacal patients. Behav Res Ther 34(1):23–31
37. Speckens AEM, Van Hemert AM, Spinhoven P, Hawton KE, Bolk JH, Rooijmans HGM (1995) Cognitive behavioural therapy for medically unexplained physical symptoms: a randomised controlled trial. Br Med J 311:1328–1332
38. Sharpe M, Hawton K, Simkin S, Surawy C, Hackman A, Klimes I, Peto T, Warrell D, Seagroat V (1996) Cognitive behaviour therapy for the chronic fatigue syndrome: a randomised controlled trial. Br Med J 312:22–26
39. Guthrie E, Creed A (1991) Controlled trial of psychological treatment for the irritable bowel syndrome. Gastroenterology 100:450–457

# Somatoform Disorders—
# An Arab Perspective

A. OKASHA and T. OKASHA

*Summary.* The inclusion of the diagnosis of "unexplained somatic symptoms" in the primary version of ICD-10 and DSM-IV is a cornerstone in identifying somatization. The majority of our psychiatric patients (80%–90%) are not aware that their somatic symptoms can be secondary to a psychiatric disorder. Therefore their first encounter is usually either with primary care physicians or with traditional or religious healers depending on attributing factors. Religion plays an important role in symptom formation, attribution, and management of somatization disorders. In our culture physical symptoms are more socially accepted than are psychological ones, as psychological ones can be taken to indicate personal weakness or lack of faith. The pubic would accept, tolerate, and sympathize with suffering of somatic symptoms more than psychological complaints, which people tend to perceive more as under the control of the person's will. In the countryside somatization is attributed to the wrath of God, possession of evil spirits, and magical doing. The treatment may vary from a pseudoreligious or traditional intervention, to cognitive or behavioral therapy, or psychotropic medication, the latter preferably by parenteral route. Our religious culture with its external locus of control, extended family, family care and concern of the elderly, disabled children, and the attribution of illness to God's will and the solid belief in the determined fate, can color and affect somatization. There is, however, increasing evidence that somatization as such is not necessarily a culturally bound phenomenon. What may be unique for every country is its clinical image and the challenges it puts on the existing mental health care facilities. The later should be a prime area of input and concern, to the benefit of a considerable percentage of our psychiatric population.

*Key words.* Somatoform, Cross-cultural, Religious therapy, Locus of control, Arab region

Little is known about the cultural differences in psychological adjustment and perception of illness. Illness perception is a culture-dependent factor and appears to influence psychological adjustment very differently. The cultural impact on illness

---

Institute of Psychiatry, Ain Shams University, 3 Shawarby St., Kasr Elnil, Cairo, Egypt

perception does not only affect the clinical presentation of the illness, but also the psychological coping mechanisms, the most appropriate lines of management, and the patients' expectations from their therapist.

Somatization is one form of illness presentation that implies several cultural connotations. The term has been used in medical sociology and anthropology, to describe a pattern of illness behavior, especially a style of clinical presentation, in which somatic symptoms are presented to the exclusion or eclipse of emotional distress and social problems [1]. In official psychiatric nosology, somatization refers to a family of psychiatric disorders (the somatoform disorders in DSM-IV or ICD-10) presenting with somatic complaints. The use of the term in both references is not equivalent. It involves varying degrees of inference about underlying processes that are, at present, unmeasurable. Kirmayer et al. refer to three different ways of operationalizing research on somatization [2]: (a) somatization in the sense of medically unexplained somatic symptoms (for example, in the somatization disorder module of the DIS, the Composite International Diagnostic Interview or the WHO Somatoform Disorders Schedule [3, 4]; (b) as hypochondriacal worry or somatic preoccupation [5]; and (c) as somatic clinical presentations of affective, anxiety or other psychiatric disorders [6]. An attempt to distinguish between the three different definitions of somatization may help to resolve some of the contradictory findings in gross cultural literature.

Recent evidence shows that somatization, in each of its definitions, is present in all cultural groups and societies. This wide prevalence challenges the notion that somatization is indicative of some special form of psychopathology. Differences among groups may reflect cultural styles of expressing distress (idioms of distress) that are influenced not only by cultural beliefs and practices, but also by familiarity with health care systems and pathways to care.

The notion that somatization is more common among or characteristic of patients from certain non-Western cultures, particularly Asians and Africans, has been repeatedly emphasized [7]. However, Kirmayer and Isaac argue that somatization is a universal phenomenon and that somatic symptoms are the most common clinical explanation of emotional distress worldwide [8, 9].

Epidemiological research on somatization in the United States has been dominated by the construct of "somatization disorder" and a *forme fruste* thereof termed "subsyndromal somatization disorder". The diagnosis is given based on a lifetime count of four medically unexplained symptoms for men and six for women in somatization section of the NIMH Diagnostic Interview schedule (termed the Somatic Symptom Index and denoted as "SSI 4,6") [3].

Kirmayer and colleagues criticized the concept of somatization as the product of Western mind-body dualism [8, 9]. Manson also criticized the artificial differentiation and separation of mental manifestations into "psyche" and "soma" [10]. It is only because clinicians expect patients to adopt exclusively psychological idioms for their distress, that they treat the persistent expression of distress in physical terms as a special diagnostic category [9]. Results of regression analysis showed that somatization is related to both anxiety and depression and also to the duration of symptoms. However, all those factors explained only 30% of the variance, meaning that the other factors contribute to the phenomenon. This supports the view that somatization is a common final pathway for expression of different types of psychological distress.

It is interesting to know that ancient pharaonic Egyptian medicine did not recognize a specialty called mental disorders. They attributed all mental phenomena to disorders in the heart (Eber's papyrus) or the uterus (Kahun papyrus). There was no psyche, only soma [11].

Somatization disorder was estimated as "rare" in the general population. The Epidemiological Catchment Area (ECA) studies, found a diagnosis of somatization disorder in 0.01% of the population, mostly among African American women (0.8%) and by African American men (0.4%). This difference in prevalence may be accounted for by differences in educational status. Somatization disorder was no more prevalent among Hispanic Americans than other groups. However, levels of both somatization disorder and "SSI4,6" were some 10 times higher in the Puerto Rican ECA study than in the U.S. population [12].

Epidemiological studies have used measures of somatization that are insensitive to culture-specific symptoms and mode of expressing distress. Few efforts have been made to develop expanded inventories of somatic symptoms in Nigeria, Pakistan, India, and England [14]. However, the scales resulting from those studies have not yet been widely applied. Several studies with symptom checklists have disputed the higher rate of somatization among non-Western groups [14, 15]. Available literature should be reviewed and conclusions attempted to answer this question: is there a culturally specific attribute to the disorder of somatization? And if so does culture impact the prevalence, the clinical picture, treatment response, etc.?

Escobar et al. studied 700 patients attending medicine clinics in Montreal and found that more than 75% of patients with major depression, panic disorder, or milder forms of mixed depression and anxiety presented with somatic complaints, and that 17% of patients had a lifetime history of medically unexplained symptoms [3]. Across all ethnocultural groups 26% of patients met the study criteria for one or more forms of somatization. This high prevalence in a North American city challenges the notion that Asians or other "non-Western" groups are more prone to somatize their distress than Europeans or Americans. Similar findings have been made in primary care in Britain [6], Spain [16], Nigeria [17], and elsewhere [18]. Furthermore, the ICD-10 concept of somatoform disorders was generally appropriate for use across cultures (23 countries) [19].

The WHO Cross-National Study of Mental Disorders in Primary Care studied 5438 patients from 15 centers in 14 countries. While a high prevalence of somatization was found across all centers, the rates varied markedly [20]. The overall prevalence of somatization disorder was 0.9%, but this varied from zero to 3.8% at specific centers; the overall frequency of abridged somatization (based on the SSI) was 19.7% and this varied almost fivefold from 7.6% to 36.8%. The authors emphasize the similarity of the relationship between somatic, affective, and anxiety symptoms across sites but their own data also provide evidence of significant cultural variation.

Arab culture has general features. It is a culture that tends to believe in supernatural forces: devils, djinnis, evil eye, etc. (delusional cultural beliefs). The family structure is characterized by affiliated behavior at the expense of differentiating behavior. Also, rearing is oriented towards accommodation, conformity, cooperation, affection, and interdependence as opposed to individuation, intellectualization, independence, and compartmentalization, which may be more characteristic of western cultures.

The extended family helps in managing intergenerational conflicts. Young individuals vacillate between two worlds of values: one world is felt to be dying, the other is not yet born. These intrafamilial ties may provide for inclusion rather than exclusion of the mentally sick, the disabled, and the old. This attitude may indicate good intrafamilial mental health, and leads to a lower rate of referral and a general preference of caring for the sick in their natural and warm environment at home. However, it also implies that cases which do need referral may suffer a worse prognosis than they would have if they had been referred at an earlier point in their disease process.

For Arabs "pain" is the main indication of illness. It is usually attributed to a neighboring organ, as in headache, tightness of chest, etc. Emotional and behavioral problems are not perceived as a mental illness. Sometimes they are explained in terms of delusional cultural beliefs, low level of endurance or low level of patience. A number of writers have stressed the importance of viewing pain as a multidimensional experience with more similarity to emotional states than sensory processing. The Arabic language tends to be overemphatic and hyperbolic. It expresses emotivity at the expense of rationality. Patients and relatives exaggerate their verbal reports of distress. Somatizers are usually young, more histrionic, and exposed to a multitude of stress factors [22].

Demographic factors have been suggested as determinants of the prevalence of somatization. Rural and urban dichotomies proved irrelevant to the prevalence of somatization. This may be explained by the fact that the rural/urban dichotomy itself is inaccurate in several places of the world. This is especially the case in those countries where urbanization of the countryside and ruralization of cities are taking place. Gender and population studies of prevalence has shown that female patients outnumbered males in the presentation of somatoform disorders [2, 23]. The authors argue that the higher prevalence of women among somatizers may be explained by a female pattern of help-seeking behavior. Expectations from housewives and mothers would attribute more respect to a somatic complaint that a psychological one. While the former is frequently respected, the latter is frequently discarded as irrelevant. Katon et al. have found that almost 60% of the high utilizers of primary health care suffered from less sever forms of somatization [23]. Swartz et al. defined a subsyndromal form of somatization that was associated with higher rates of seeking health care, that is intermediate between that of somatizers in the general population and patients with somatization disorder [24].

Somatization was found to be associated with both anxiety and depression in other studies as well. Goldberg, in a WHO study, recommends that somatization be better described in dimensional rather than categorical terms [25].

Soliman studied all patients presenting to the outpatient psychiatric clinic of an Upper Egyptian University Hospital over a 4-month period [26]. Out of 620 Egyptian psychiatric outpatients, somatoform disorders were present in 17.8%. Among those, 76.6% were diagnosed as Undifferentiated Somatoform. Other diagnoses included somatization disorder (9.5%), persistent pain disorder (8.7%), and hypochondriasis (5.4%). The most frequently reported symptoms were headache, pain in other parts of the body, autonomic symptoms, abdominal symptoms, and sensory complaints. SCAN comorbidity was 85%–90%, where depression came first (58.7%), followed by anxiety (36.9%), and then anxiety/depression (6.5%). The total number of somatization symptoms was highest in somatization disorder and least in pain disorder, with undifferentiated somatoform and hypochondriacal disorders occupying an intermediate position.

Okasha and Okasha studied 120 Egyptian patients (84 men and 36 women) with ages ranging between less than 20 years and over 60 years of age [27] (12 subjects under 20, 54 from 20–29, 27 from 30–39, 18 from 40–49, 3 from 50–59 and 6 > 60) . Symptom clusters involved CNS symptoms (90%), gastrointestinal symptoms (87.5%), pain and headache (80%), fatigue (90%), chest symptoms (82%), cardiovascular symptoms (72.5%), genito-urinary symptoms (52.5%), and muscular symptoms (52.5%). Diagnoses given to the 72 inpatients were as follows: depressive disorder (31.9%), schizophrenia (29.1%), anxiety and phobic disorder (13.8%), delusional disorder (12.5%), somatoform disorder (8.3%), and acute polymorphic psychotic disorder (7.1%). Among the 48 outpatients 25% had depressive disorder, 25% had somatoform disorder, 25% had anxiety and phobic disorder, 18.75% had bipolar manic disorder, and 6.25% had neurasthenia.

In Bahrain, Haddad and Charlotte applied the general health questionnaire (GHQ) and the BSI (Bradford Somatic Inventory) and showed psychiatric morbidity presenting with somatization in 19.4% of general hospital patients [28]. The prevalence of psychological morbidity in the general hospital was in agreement with other studies conducted in India and the UK, where it has been estimated that approximately 20% to 25% of the patients attending the general medical outpatient department and the primary care facilities do so for symptoms due to psychological or social factors [29, 30]. Symptoms involved tension, fatigue, abdominal symptoms, panic, pain all over, urinary symptoms, symptoms in lower limbs, and cold and heat sensations. A similar study in Saudi Arabia revealed a prevalence of 56% for somatic symptoms and 16% somatization in a sample of 270 patients. Also, Fahmy investigated 100 somatizers, and found 34% to suffer from depression, 30% from anxiety, 16% from adjustment disorders, 4% from Somatoform disorders, and 2% from somatization. Women with somatization were significantly more illiterate, culturally deprived, and depressed [31].

Hamdi et al. argue that cross-cultural variation in the frequencies and modes of expression of depressive symptoms may influence the validity of depression rating scales [32]. Evaluation of the face validity of HDRS by studying symptom frequency, factor structure and symptom clusters in 100 UAE depressed patients showed that the Hamilton Depression Rating Scale was sensitive to severity of depression in UAE culture. However, it was found to measure heterogeneous aspects of the disorder and its internal consistency suffered as a result. High levels of retardation and somatization contributed significantly to the total score in socially developing countries. In agreement with this are the findings of Ragurum et al., who studied Indian patients and found depressive symptoms unlike somatic symptoms to be construed as socially disadvantageous depending on the degree of stigma associated with particular symptoms [33].

Somatizers in primary care are usually characterized by low level of psychological distress, are less introspective, show less concern about having an emotional problem, are less likely to attribute their suffering to psychological causes. They show little use of mental health services, and are usually unable to talk about personal problems, and are less likely to seek help for anxiety or sadness.

# Nosological Implications

The very existence of a discrete category of somatoform disorders in psychiatric nosology implies a separation of affective, anxiety, dissociative, and somatic symptoms that is not reflected in the co-occurrence of these symptoms in syndromes worldwide [17]. This separation largely reflects the persistent mind-body dualism of western medicine: psychiatric disorders are perceived as mental disorders, notwithstanding their prominent somatic symptoms. The somatoform disorders are then a residual category lying between the somatic and the psychic to make the nosological system complete. This is particularly useful in consultation-liaison psychiatry. As a result, diagnostic categories that combine somatic and psychological symptoms have continued to be popular in many countries. An example of that is the glossary of culture-related syndromes included as Appendix (I) in DSM-IV [34]. Many of these syndromes have predominately somatic symptoms and so might be viewed as forms of somatization (e.g., bilis or cholera, hwa-byung, brain fog, dhat, shenkui, falling out, koro, shenjing shuairuo, and neurasthenia). These culture-related syndromes illustrate how ethnophysiological ideas about the body can give rise to culture-specific somatic symptoms and complaints like "heat in the head," "loss of semen in the urine," and specific types of conversion symptoms [8].

Several pieces of research have revealed a different prevalence for symptoms than that of disorders. When, then , should functional symptoms be worthy of clinical attention? When do they require specific treatments? When do they take a chronic and invalidating course affecting quality of life? In an attempt to answer those questions Fava believes that the DSM-IV or ICD-10 criteria for somatoform are of little help in prognostic and therapeutic terms for approaching these symptoms [35]. This awareness led an international group of experts on psychosomatic illness to introduce alternative criteria for somatoform disorders. Although these criteria are still tentative and are still in need of appropriate validation, it may be useful to mention them at this point. They include:

1. Functional somatic symptoms secondary to a psychiatric disorder (subtype for anxiety—depression and adjustment disorders)
2. Persistent somatization (like undifferentiated somatoform disorders in ICD-10 and DSM-IV)
3. Conversion symptoms (histrionic personality not essential)
4. Disease phobia (high overlap with panic and hypochondriasis)
5. Health anxiety
6. Thanatophobia
7. Illness denial: irrelevant in somatoform disorders

The entity of "functional somatic symptoms secondary to psychiatric disorder" is very practical in diagnosing the more frequently observed type of somatization disorder. It is consistent with the suggestion that somatization disorder would include a subtype often associated with anxiety and depression as well as another type associated with adjustment [23]. Taking into consideration the comorbidity between somatization, anxiety, and depression, it is clear that this entity could serve a lot, especially that it does not require a specific duration or age of onset. Also, the disorder termed "persistent somatization" could easily include the common disturbance that in the DSM-IV and ICD-10 would be subsumed under the rubric of undifferentiated somatoform. The entity of "health anxiety" is easily applicable and deficient in the other current classifications. It does not necessitate the 6 months duration so it coincides with the request made by Barsky et al. that the picture of transient hypochondriasis, frequently encountered, should be respected [36].

In spite of this contribution which solves some problems in both DSM-IV and ICD-10 criteria, it does have some drawbacks. The entity of "illness denial" is alien to the somatoform disorders. Its features are against the core presentation of somatoform disorder, which is the patients' preoccupation that they are sick despite all negative findings and reassurance. Secondly, although the criteria for "disease phobia" respect the comorbidity between panic attacks and hypochondriasis, yet this category may increase the overlap in diagnosis and may add to the confusion of hypochondriacal related disorder. This may also be the case with an entity like Thanatophobia.

## Policy Implications

Other than the interesting nosological debate that the nature of somatization disorders can invoke, somatization can be challenging in other disciplines. It leads to particular health care-seeking behavior and may demand relevant intervention strategies. The Egyptian example can be demonstrative.

Egypt has a special, rather unique demographic feature. It has a population of 60 million unevenly distributed over 24 governorates, 5 of which have no psychiatric services. There are 120,000 physicians (1/500 citizens), 500 psychiatrists (1/130,000 citizens) and 9000 psychiatric beds (15/100,000), constituting less than 10% of total hospital beds.

As in so many other developing countries challenged by the maintenance of their infrastructure and subsidy of the basic needs of their people, priorities of health care services and planning are not for mental health. Since 75%–80% of Egyptian psychiatric patients present with somatic symptoms, the majority of them tend to seek help with traditional and religious healers.

Religion plays an important role in symptom formation, attributions (God's will), and management. Psychological symptoms are usually attributed to weakness of personality, lack of faith, lack of conformity, and laziness. Also, In the Arabic the word "Wiswas" refers to both obsessions and the devil, and 60% of obsessive compulsive symptoms in Egyptian patients are religious in nature. The first referral is therefore to religious leaders. Religiously based cognitive psychotherapy (If God is willing—I seek refuge to God from the accursed Satan—God is the healer) or warding off blasphemous thoughts by Koranic verses (thought stopping: don't postpone death. you will gloriously meet God) are some of the mechanisms used in "therapy." Religious and group therapies (El Zar), suggestion, devices such as amulets, and incantations are popular remedies for unexplained illnesses [11]. The health profession cannot ignore these actors. Since they cannot be overruled in the traditional societies of our countries, agreements should be made that draw the line where professional help should be sought.

Also, physicians in primary care settings frequently have to deal with minor neurotic, psychosomatic, and transient psychotic states. Patients presenting with somatic complaints are usually referred to a long list of investigations and specialists with the psychiatrists being the last on the list, in case none of the former referrals prove useful. This should not necessarily be the case. General practitioners should be able to manage a great majority of psychiatric disorders presenting with somatic complaints. It would therefore be considered prudent that in the training of the general physicians, due emphasis is put upon somatic presentation of psychological ill-health, not only as far as diagnosis is concerned, but also to the inclusion of management.

In conclusion, we would argue that evidence is accumulating that somatization as such is not necessarily a culturally bound phenomenon. What may be unique for every country is its clinical image and the challenges it puts on the existing mental health care facilities. The latter should be a prime area of input and concern, to the benefit of a considerable percentage of our psychiatric population.

## References

1. Kleinman AM (1977) Depression, somatization and the "new cross-cultural psychiatry". Soc Sci Med 11:3–10
2. Kirmayer LJ, Robbins JM (1991) Three forms of somatization in primary care: prevalence, co-occurrence and sociodemographic characteristics. J Nerv Dis 179:647–655
3. Escobar JL, Rubio-Stipec M, Canino G, Karno, M (1989) A new and a bridged somatization construct. J Nerv Ment Dis 177:140–146
4. Janca A, Burke JD Jr, Issac M et al (1995) The World Health Organization somatoform disorders schedule. A preliminary report on design and reliability. Eur J Psychiatry 10:373–378
5. Barsky AJ (1992) Amplification, somatization, and the somatoform disorders. Psychosomatic 33:28–34
6. Goldberg DP, Bridges K (1988) Somatic presentations of psychiatric illness in a primary care setting. J Psychosom Res 32:137–144
7. Gaw AC (1993) Culture, ethnicity and mental illness. American Psychiatric Press, Washington
8. Kirmayer JJ, Young A (1998) Culture and somatization: clinical, epidemiological and ethnographic perspectives. Psychosom Med (in press)
9. Issac M, Janca A, Orley J (1996) somatization—a culture-bound or universal syndrome? J Ment Health 5:219–222
10. Manson SM (1996) Culture and DSM-IV, Implications for the diagnosis of mood and anxiety disorders. In: Mezzich JE, Kleinman A, Faberga H Jr et al (eds) Culture and psychiatric diagnosis. A DSM-IV perspective. American Psychiatric Press, Washington, pp 99–114
11. Okasha A, Karam E (1998) Mental health services and research in the Arab World. Acta Psychiatr Scand 98:406–413
12. Canino IA, Rubio-Stipec M, Canino G, Escobar JI (1992) Functional somatic symptoms: A cross comparison. Am J Orthopsychiatry 62:605–612
13. Ebigbo PO (1986) A cross-sectional study of somatic complaints of Nigerian females using the Enugu somatization scale. Culture Med Psychiatry
14. Mumford DB (1991) Somatic sensations and psychological distress among students in Britain and Pakistan. Soc Psychiatry Psychiatr Epidemiol 24:321–326
15. Mumford DB, Bavington JT, Bhatnagar KS, Hussain Y, Mirza S, Naeaghi MM (1989) The Bradford somatic inventory: a multi-ethnic inventory of somatic symptoms reported

by anxious and depressed patients in Britain and the Indo-Pakistan subcontinent. Br J Psychiatry 158:379–386, 1991

16. Lobo A, Garcia-Campayo J, Campos R, Marcos G, Perez-Echeverria MJ (1996) The GMPPZ: somatization in primary care in Spain. I. Estimates of prevalence and clinical characteristics. Br J Psychiatry 168:344–353

17. Ohaeri JU, Odejide OA (1994) Somatization symptoms among patients using primary health care facilities in a rural community in Nigeria. Am J Psychiatry 151:728–731

18. Ustun TB, Sartorius N (1995): Mental health in general health care: an International study. Wiley, Chichester

19. Janca A, Issac M, Bennett LA et al (1995) Somatoform disorders in different cultures— a mail questionnaire survey. Soc Psychiatry Psychiatr Epidemiol 30:44–48

20. Gureje O, Simon GE, Ustun TB, Goldeberg DP (1997) Somatization in cross—cultural perspective: a World Health Organization study in primary care. Am J Psychiatry 154:989–995, 1997

21. Pearce S, Miles A (1993) Chronic pain. In: Kenneth Granville—Grossman (ed) Recent advances in clinical psychiatry. Churchill Livingstone, Edinburgh

22. de Leon J, Saiz-Ruiz LA, Chinchilla A et al (1987) Why do some psychiatric patients somatize? Acta Psychiatr Scand 76:203–209

23. Katon W, Lin E, Von Korff M, Russo J, Lipscomb P (1991) Somatization: a spectrum of severity. Am J Psychiatry 48:34–40

24. Swartz M, Blazer D, George L et al (1986) Somatization disorder in a community population. Am J Psychiatry 143:1403–1408

25. Goldberg D (1996) A dimensional model for common mental disorders. Br J Psychiatry 168(suppl. 30):44–49

26. Soliman H (1997) Comorbidity of somatoform disorder. Egypt J Psychiatry 20:129–140

27. Okasha A, Okasha T (1998) somatoform disorders. An Arab perspective. Read at Tokyo conference on Somatoform disorders. Feb

28. Haddad M, Charlotte K (1996) Aspects of somatization in Bahraini patients. Egypt J Psychiatry 19:61–67

29. Wig NN, Verma SK (1973) A cross cultural study of psychiatric patients on Carnell Medical Index. Indian Psychiatry 15:363–366

30. Lipowski ZJ (1988) Somatization: the concept and its clinical application. Am J Psychiatry 145:1358–1368

31. Fahmy M (1996) Somatic presentations of psychiatric illnesses in outpatient psychiatric clinic in Jeddah. Egypt J Psychiatry 19:61–67

32. Hamdi E, Amin Y, Abou-Saleh MT (1997) Performance of Hamilton Depression Rating Scale in depressed patients in United Arab Emirates. Acta Psychiatr Scand 96:416–423

33. Ragurum R, Weiss MG, Channabasavanna SM et al (1996) Stigma, depression and somatization in south India. Am J Psychiatry 153(8):1043–1049

34. American Psychiatric Association (1994) Diagnostic and statstical manual of mental disorders (4th edn.) (DSM-IV). American Psychiatric Association, Washington

35. Fava GA (1995) New diagnostic approaches to somatization. Int Psychiatry Today, 5(2):1–4,8

36. Barsky AJ, Wyshak G, Klerman GL (1990) Transient hypochondriasis. Arch Gen Psychiatry 47:746–752

# Classification of Somatoform Disorders in Japan

Yoshibumi Nakane

*Summary.* It is less than 20 years since the term "somatoform disorder" was introduced in Japan. Owing not only to its short history but also to the difficulty in understanding the meaning of its concept, it has not been appropriately used in Japan yet. In this chapter, the author introduces the history of the categorization of neurotic disorders in Japan, and particularly refers to Japan's traditional classification system of mental disorders with physical symptoms. Furthermore, by analyzing our data concerning the related field (the results of the PPGHC study and a study on the mental health of atomic bomb survivors), the dissociation between the understanding of the term and the actual use in diagnosis is clarified, concluding that it would take some more time until "somatoform disorder" is understood and used appropriately in Japan.

*Key words.* Somatoform disorder, Neurasthenia, Japan, Traditional classification, Atomic bomb survivors

## Introduction

When discussing in a general way psychiatric symptoms which appear as physical symptoms, it has to be understood that these symptoms vary across a wide range, including symptoms from suspected hypochondriasis to hysteria, conventionally called psychosomatic disorder, physical symptoms in psychotic disorder, affective disorder, and factitious disorders.

Somatoform disorder first appeared as a disease category in DSM-III [1] including some of the symptomatologies I have mentioned. Later the category was developed into a series of disorders in DSM system. However, when somatoform disorder was introduced in Japan, it was such a new category that four or five kinds of different Japanese terms were suggested for its translation. Here, I would first like to summarize the history of the concept of neurosis in Japan.

Department of Neuropsychiatry, Nagasaki University School of Medicine, 1-7-1 Sakamoto, Nagasaki 852-8501, Japan

# Historical Progress

Looking at the table of contents of *Lehrbuch der Psychiatrie* [2] written by Noboru Ishida, the first professor of the psychiatric department of our Medical School, in 1910, which is known as a classic medical textbook in Japan, he listed "Chronische nervöse Erschöpfung" as one of the subcategories of "Das Erschöpfungsirresein." There he gave a description, saying

This is what usually called acquired neurasthenia, and when conducting mental tasks, first fatigue appears, comprehension ability is lowered, memory is disturbed, and then agony, anxiety, dizziness and headaches appear. Physical symptoms such as insomnia, back pains, fatigue in the legs and arms, heart weakness, digestion disorders and reproductive difficulties appear.

He also listed "Konstitutionelle Neurasthenie" along with "Zwangsirresein", "Konstitutionelle Versimmung," and "Pathologische Charakter" under a subcategory "Entartungsirresein," and described the condition as "constitutional neurasthenia, when even with high-level psychiatric task ability, a patient has hypochondriac mood, deprecates him/herself and visits many doctors for consultation about his/her illness" (Table 1).

However, in the ninth version [3] of his book, published in 1922 (Table 2), "Psychoneurosen" was established as one chapter and was divided into three categories, "die Tatigkeitsneurosen", "die Verkehrspsychosen," and "die Schicksalspsychosen." "Neurasthenie" is listed under the first category, and he reported that it had been described as "Neurasthenia" by Beard in 1880. Abnormal personality gradually developed into an independent chapter over the course of various versions, and its relationship to "Psychoneurosen" was often referred to.

Around 1950, the historical course of the general concept of neurosis in Europe came to be appreciated more adequately in Japan. For example, it was realized that the term "neurosis" had been advocated by Cullen in 1776, and the concept then had been quite general and included all nervous diseases, mental and neurotic disorders. Among other things, it was also understood that Janet had named all the neurotic disorders induced by a lowering of psychological energy as "Psychoneurose" in general, that Dubois (1905) had also advocated calling psychological disorders "Psychoneurosis", that neurosis had been classified into two types "Aktualneurose"

TABLE 1. Contents relating to neurotic disorders in the *Lehrbuch der Psychiatrie* 4. Auflage, 1910 [2]. Section II: Psychiatric disorders

| | |
|---|---|
| Chapter 6 | "Histerische Irresein" |
| Chapter 8 | "Das Erschöpfungsirresein" |
| | 1. "Collapsdelirium" |
| | 2. "Amentia, die acute Verwirtheit" |
| | 3. "Chronische nervöse Erschöpfung (ervorbene Neurasthenie)" |
| Chapter 12 | "Entartungsirresein" |
| | 1. "Abnorme Sexualempfindung" |
| | 2. "Konstitutionelle Neurasthenie" |
| | 3. "Zwangsirresein" |
| | 4. "Konstitutionelle Verstimmung" |
| | 5. "Pathologische Character" |

TABLE 2. Contents relating to neurotic disorders in the *Textbook of Mental Diseases* 9th Edition, 1922 [3]. Section II: psychiatric disorders

| | |
|---|---|
| Chapter 8 | "Die Psychogenen Erkrankungen, Psychoneurosen" |
| | 1. "Die Tätigkeitsneurosen (Ponopathien)" |
| | ① "die nervöse Erschöpfung, Neurasthenie" |
| | ② "die Erwartungspsychose' (Nervous disorders resulting from expectation) |
| | 2. "Die Verkehrspsychosen (Homilopathien)" |
| | ① "das induzierte Irresein" |
| | ② "Der Verfolgungswahn der Schwerhörigen" |
| | 3. "Die Schicksalspsychosen (Symbantopathien)" |
| | ① "Die Unfallsneurosen" |
| | (1) "Die Schreckneurose" (Nervous disorders resulting from fright, Dread neurosis) |
| | (2) "Die traumatische Neurose" (traumatic neurosis) |
| | ② "Die psychogenen Geistesstörungen der Gefangenen" |
| | ③ "Querulantenwahn" |
| Chapter 14 | "Die originären Krankheitszustände (Entartungsirresein)" |
| | Original or Constitutional Conditions |
| | 1. "Die Nervosität (Nervosity)" |
| | 2. "Das Zwangsneurose" (Imperative psychoses) |
| | 3. "Das impulsive Irresein" (Impulsive insanity) |
| | 4. "Die geschlechtlichen Verirrungen" (Sexual psychopathia) |
| Chapter 15 | "Die psychopathischen Personlichkeiten" (Psychopathic personalities) |
| | 1. "Der geborene Verbrecher" (The born criminal) |
| | 2. "Die Haltlosen" (The unstable) |
| | 3. "Die krankhaften Lügner und Schwindler" (The morbid liars and frauds) |
| | 4. "Die Pseudoquerlanten" (The pseudoquerlants) |

and "Psychoneurose," and that these had been classified into several subtypes by Freud. It also became widely known in Japanese psychiatry that in 1868 GMB Beard advocated the term "neurasthenia" for a disorder with irritable weakness as the main symptom.

With various concepts for neurosis being advocated in Japan, the subclassifications also varied. For example, as shown in Table 3, Matsumoto introduced various classifications of neurosis in his book [4] in 1964, taking account of international trends: classification according to onset condition including traumatic neurosis, classification according to a technological viewpoint, classification according to major symptoms, classification from the viewpoint of reaction, classification concerning personality trait mainly, and classification by age.

He also considered classification mainly by condition state as being clinically convenient, and classified psychiatric neurosis as a major neurosis into eight states as shown in Table 4. He noted that not many cases could be clearly categorized in only one subtype condition, but that cases often showed a combination of several subtypes. He also considered organ neurosis and psychosomatic disease as borderline disorders. Complaints of somatic symptoms in neurasthenic states and in hypochondria were particularly significant in this classification system, so it was often difficult to make a distinction between the two states. As for neurasthenia, its position as a disease concept had been uncertain, and then the category developed a very wide sense; however, in recent years it has not been used by psychiatrists.

TABLE 3. Various categorizations of neuroses [4]

I. Classification by onset condition
    Traumatic neurosis / accident neurosis
    War neurosis
    Environmental neurosis / prison neurosis
II. Classification by technological viewpoint
    Rentenneurose / Pensionsneurose
    Wunschneurose / Begehrungsneurose / Erwartungsneurose
    Zweckneurose
III. Classification by major symptoms
    1. Classification according to psychiatric symptoms
      Anxiety neurosis/ obsessive-compulsive neurosis/ depressive neurosis/ hypochondriasis/
        neurasthenia/ psychyasthenia
    2. Classification according to somatic symptoms
      Organneurose/ vegetative Neurose/ Angioneurose/ Herzneurose/ Magenneurose/
        Gesclechtneurose/ vasomotorishe Neurose
IV. Classification from the viewpoint of reaction
    neurotishe Reaktion / hysterische Reaktion / psychogene Reaktion
    Erlebnisreaktion / Konfliktreaktion
    Milieureaktion / Personlichkeitsreaktion
    primitive Reaktion
V. Classification by personality trait
    Nervosität / Charakterneurose / neurotische Personlichkeit
    nervöse Psychopathie / asthenische Psychopathie / geltungsbedürftige Psychopathie
VI. Classification by age
    Childhood neurosis/ neurosis in climacterium
    Presenile neurosis/ senile neurosis

TABLE 4. Classification by clinical condition state

| | |
|---|---|
| Neurasthenic states | Depressive states |
| Anxiety states | Sensitive states |
| Hysterical states | Hypochondria |
| Obsessional-compulsive states | Depersonalization states |

TABLE 5. Classification of "Shinkeishitsusyo (nervosity)" by Morita theory

Ordinary *shinkeishitsu* (so-called neurasthenia)
Paroxysmal neurosis (anxiety neurosis)
Obsession (phobia)

When referring to the classification of neurosis in Japan, an independent system based on the theory of Masatake Morita [5] should be discussed (Table 5). Morita advocated a disease unit called "Shinkeishitsu or Shinkeishitsusho (Nervosity)" as a general category of neurosis. He argued that it was not a kind of personality characteristic, nor did it correspond to neurasthenia or to hypochondriasis in the European sense. He thought that there was a certain common psychiatric tendency at the base of the onset of "Shinkeishitsusyo," which he called the "hypochondriac temperament." He described its features to be introversion, strong self-reflection, precise awareness of physical and mental discomfort or abnormalities or abnormal feeling, particularly being attached to these, self-awareness, and worry about them. He said that an onset of "Shinkeishitsusyo" was induced by these tendencies. Furthermore, he said that the condition would develop into "psychic interaction," which was the name he gave to the process in which a concentration on a certain sense would sharpen the sense, and then this sharpened sense would attract attention more and more strongly towards itself, the sense and the attention would interact mutually, and this interaction would strengthen the sense more. Therefore, he classified Shinkeishitsusyo into three types as shown in Table 5, ordinary *shinkeishitsu*, paroxysmal neurosis, and obsession, and stated that these types could develop into one another or merge. Ordinary *shinkeishitsu* is nervosity in a narrow sense and the core type. Its symptoms vary from heavy feeling of the head, dizziness, tinnitus, insomnia, destructiveness, stomach atony, habitual constipation, palpitation, fatigue, and impotence.

## ICD and DSM Systems

On the other hand, the neurosis study group [6], which was funded by the scientific research fund of the Ministry of Education and started in 1957, published a classification draft which added "others" to Matsumoto's eight-type classification. This classification was used for over 25 years after that, and is recognized as the conventional neurosis classification in Japan. This classification is based on clinical states, and in essence accords with the ICD-8 [7] established in 1965.

Soon after the ICD-8 was published in 1965, the American Psychiatric Association established DSM-II, revising DSM-I, and in it the classification of neurosis was adopted from ICD-8. When ICD-8 was revised to ICD-9 [8], as shown in Table 6, the section on neurosis was left as it was in ICD-8.

In Japan, there has been a tendency for the ICD classification which is similar to that of the study group of the Ministry of Education to be accepted without question.

TABLE 6. Subcategories of neurosis in ICD-8 and ICD-9 [7, 8]

| | |
|---|---|
| 300 Neurosis | 300 Neurotic disorder |
| 300.0 anxiety neurosis | 300.0 anxiety state |
| 300.1 hysterical neurosis | 300.1 hysteria |
| 300.2 phobic neurosis | 300.2 phobic state |
| 300.3 obsessive-compulsive neurosis | 300.3 obsessive compulsive disorder |
| 300.4 depressive neurosis | 300.4 neurotic depression |
| 300.5 neurasthenia | 300.5 neurasthenia |
| 300.6 depersonalization syndrome | 300.6 depersonalization syndrome |
| 300.7 hypochondriacal neurosis | 300.7 hypochondriasis |
| 300.8 other | 300.8 other specified neurotic states |
| 300.9 unspecified neurosis | 300.9 unspecified neurosis |

However, since the publication of DSM-III, in which the category of neurosis was broken up, there has been some confusion concerning the classification of neurosis into three types, anxiety disorder, somatoform disorder, and dissociative disorder. That is, the category of neurosis could be classified into these subtypes, which could be regarded as independent categories. Particularly, the concept of somatoform disorder had not appeared in the textbooks in Japan prior to DSM-III.

Receiving impetus from the publication of DSM-III, the Japanese Committee of International Diagnostic Criteria in Psychiatry, the present Japanese Society of Psychiatric Diagnosis, was established in Japan. There, DSM-III was thoroughly discussed and field work was conducted to examine the possibility of the adoption of DSM-III in Japan. Based on the results of the field work, the society also prepared a draft of diagnostic criteria adequate for use in Japan and examined the possibility of developing a classification system which Japanese psychiatrists could use. In the course of the work, a subcommittee on neurotic disorder published the results of some of their studies.

One of their studies is on the breakdown of neurosis as a category in DSM-III, the later DSM-III R, ICD-10 [9], and DSM-IV [10]. They gave questionnaires to 70 leading members of the society in 1985, and many of them answered that the classification in ICD-9 was easier to adapt. Again in September, 1989, they conducted an investigation nationwide, collected 389 neurosis cases from 29 institutions, and gave them three kinds of disease titles according to a diagnostic system conventionally used in Japan, DSM-III-R and the draft version of ICD-10. The most frequent diagnosis given according to the conventional diagnostic system was anxiety state in 107 cases, accounting for 25.4%, followed by obsessive compulsive disorder in 63 cases (14.9%), hysteria in 46 cases (10.9%), phobic state in 46 cases (10.9%), neurotic depression in 45 cases (10.7%), hypochondriasis in 39 cases (9.2%), and psychotic reaction in 13 cases (3.1%). There were no cases diagnosed as neurasthenia. Based on the results, the subcommittee [11] made a draft classification of neurotic disorders as shown in Table 7, and also proposed a draft of the relevant diagnostic criteria.

Although this is the most current classification of neurotic disorders in Japan, unfortunately the disease title "somatoform disorder" cannot be seen. In the textbooks

---

TABLE 7. Tentative classification of neurotic disorders prepared by the JCIDCP (1989) [11]

I. Situational reaction (308, 309)
   1. Acute situational reaction (308)    2. Adjustment reaction (309)
II. Neurosis (300)
   1. Anxiety neurosis (300.0)   ① anxiety attack   ② generarized anxiety   ③ mixed type
   2. Phobia (phobic neurosis) (300.2)
      ① agoraphobia   ② social phobia   ③ nosophobia   ④ unitary phobia
   3. Obsessive-compulsive neurosis (300.3)
   4. Hysteria (hysterical neurosis) (300.1)
      ① conversion type   ② dissociative type   ③ regression type   ④ mixed type
   5. Hypochondria (hypochondriacal neurosis) (300.7)
      ① disease-adhesive type      ② multiple complaint type
      ③ autonomic dysfunction type   ④ pain-type
   6. Depressive neurosis (300.4)
   7. Depersonalization (neurosis) (300.6)
   8. Other (300.8)

used in Japan recently, it is often listed in the introduction of ICD and DSM systems, but it has not been fully introduced in Japan.

## Data from Nagasaki Center

We have the results of a study on neurosis among the atomic-bomb survivors which was conducted by our predecessors at our Medical School at the time of ICD-7. I do not think that these can be used as data to see the frequency of various subcategories of neurosis, but since we also have the results of a study conducted with the same atomic bomb survivors 40 years later, I would like to summarize the results of this early study for a comparison with the later study.

Right after the atomic bombing in August 1945, few psychiatric studies were conducted. There is only one study conducted within the following 2 years. This was a report on a psychiatric investigation of 50 patients selected among 192 inpatients of the Nagasaki National Hospital 3 months after the bombing. In 1956, 11 years later, Nishikawa [12] and his colleagues of Nagasaki University conducted a study with 7287 atomic bomb survivors who visited for an atomic-bomb survivors' health consultation, and reported that 533 of them (7.3%) had neurosis. As shown in Table 8, more than 90% of them were diagnosed as suffering from the subtype "neurasthenia." The frequency of symptoms seen in the 533 people is shown in the table, but the construction of symptoms for an individual case is not clear, so we cannot confirm the validity of the diagnosis. The percentage of neurasthenia is surprisingly higher than we would expect. Such a high frequency of neurasthenia does not seem unique to this study in the period.

Now I would like to discuss the diagnostic classification of somatoform disorder in Nagasaki, presenting the latest data from our department. We have participated in the WHO International Study on Psychological Problems in General Health Care (PPGHC) as one of 15 centers from 14 countries. The purpose of the project was to examine the classification and frequency of psychological psychiatric problems in patients visiting general health care settings, and to develop proper measures and treatments for those patients. We conducted the study with patients who were between 15 and 60 years old and who had visited the internal departments of a national

TABLE 8. Psychiatric survey of the atomic-bomb survivors (Nagasaki, 1956)

|  | Group I $n = 4269$ | Group II $n = 3038$ | Total $n = 7287$ |
|---|---|---|---|
| Cases with neurosis: | 415 (9.7%) | 118 (3.9%) | 533 (7.3%) |
| Sub-classification |  |  |  |
| Neurasthenia | 93.0% | 93.2% | 93.1% |
| Anxiety neurosis | 3.9 | 0.8 | 3.2 |
| Reactive depression | 1.2 | 0.8 | 1.1 |
| Hysteria | 1.0 | 0.8 | 0.9 |
| Obsessive neurosis | 0.5 | 0.8 | 0.6 |
| Organ neurosis | 0.5 | 3.4 | 1.1 |

hospital or a municipal hospital in Nagasaki for the first time during the 6 months from March to September, 1991. We selected 336 subjects among 1555 patients who had been screened by the General Health Questionnaire 12-item version, and evaluated them using the World Health Organization/ Composite International Diagnostic Interview [13]/ Primary Health Care Version (WHO-CIDI/PHC), as revised for this project, and the Groningen Social Disabilities Scale, then conducted 3- month and 12- month follow-ups. About 20% of the subjects were regarded as having a clinical psychiatric condition on the basis of a clinical interview with a psychiatrist. Table 9 shows the diagnosis given according to CIDI, and compared to the average of all the participating centers, the percentage of patients with clinical diagnosis was lower in the Nagasaki center [14]. About one-quarter of the patients had some kind of psychological disorders in the average of all the centers, while the proportion was only one-seventh in the Nagasaki center. Particularly, the frequency of somatoform disorder including somatization disorder and hypochondriasis was significantly low in the Nagasaki center.

Next, I would like to introduce the results of a study [15, 16] on the frequency of neurotic disorder among the atomic-bomb survivors in Nagasaki. The method of the study was similar to that used in the previously discussed PPGHC study. We conducted the study for 3 years from 1994, and the total number of subjects was 7670. About 300 of them were considered as subjects for CIDI interviews and clinical interviews by psychiatrists, but finally a CIDI interview was completed with 225 people and a clinical interview with 212 people. The relationship between the CIDI interviews and the clinical interviews can be seen in Table 10.

TABLE 9. Prevalence of neurotic disorders in the PPGHC study

|  | All centers | Nagasaki center |
|---|---|---|
| F45 Somatoform disorder |  |  |
| F45.0 Somatization disorder | 2.7% | 0.1% |
| F45.2 Hypochondriasis | 0.8 | 0.4 |
| F48.0 Neurasthenia | 5.4 | 3.4 |
| Any CIDI DX | 24.0 | 14.8 |

TABLE 10. Prevalence of "F4: neurotic, stress-related and somatoform disorders" among the atomic-bomb survivors

|  | CIDI interview ($n = 225$) | | | Clinical psychiatric interview ($n = 212$) | | |
|---|---|---|---|---|---|---|
|  | Male | Female | Total | Male | Female | Total |
| 41.1 General anxiety disorder | 4.76 | 10.83 | 8.00 | 2.0 | 1.79 | 1.89 |
| 41.2 Mixed anxiety-depressive disorder | 2.86 | 2.5 | 2.67 | 0.0 | 0.89 | 0.47 |
| 45.0/3/8/9 Somatoform disorder | 3.81 | 8.33 | 6.22 | 1.0 | 2.68 | 2.36 |
| 45.2 Hypochondriacal disorder | 3.81 | 0.83 | 2.22 | 3.0 | 0.89 | 1.89 |
| Other mixed | 1.90 | 1.67 | 1.78 | 0.0 | 0.89 | 0.47 |
| Total | 7.14 | 24.17 | 20.89 | 6.0 | 7.14 | 6.60 |

It is rather surprising that there were significant differences between the frequencies found in CIDI and those in clinical interviews. It was shown in the PPGHC that according to CIDI interviews the prevalence of neurotic disorder including the somatoform disorder was lower in the Nagasaki center compared to other centers, but it was shown in this study that the prevalence rates were much lower according to the clinical interviews. Among the subclassification of somatoform disorders and related disorders, the prevalences of neurasthenia are rather similar among two kinds of evaluation; however, the rest of the subgroup is quite different, such as about only one-third of CIDI patients are recognized clinically as such by psychiatrists. The CIDI interview is a fully structured interview and is designed to be used even by nonspecialists and to reach automatically ICD-10 diagnoses, while conventional clinical interviews vary even using the same diagnostic classification system, such as ICD-10, which suggests that the classification system has not been fully understood or is not yet fully used by psychiatrists.

## Conclusion

The category of "somatoform disorder" is considered very useful in research and clinical sites [17]. However, for psychiatrists in Japan, this title is not familiar, and cases which could be diagnosed in the category are still diagnosed according to traditional Japanese diagnostic titles or ICD-9 classification. I believe we need some more time to have a disease concept, such as somatoform disorder according to the ICD-10F, understood and used efficiently among psychiatrists in Japan.

## References

1. American Psychiatric Association (1980) Diagnostic and statistical manual of mental disorders (3rd edn), American Psychiatric Association, Washington
2. Ishida N (1910) Lehrbuch der Psychiatrie, 4 Auflage (in Japanese). Nanko-do, Tokyo
3. Ishida N (1922) Textbook of mental diseases, 9th edn (in Japanese). Nanko-do, Tokyo
4. Matsumoto Y (1964) Neurosis and its borderline (in Japanese). Kanehara, Tokyo
5. Kora T (1964) Morita therapy. In: Research anthology dedicated to Takchisa Kora, Professor Emeritus. Tokyo Jikeikai Medical School, Tokyo, pp 1–33
6. Kakeda K, Sato M (1957) Categories of neurosis (in Jananese). In: Uchimura Y, Kasamatsu A, Shimazaki T (eds) Advances in psychiatric research. Ishiyaku, Tokyo, pp 229–237
7. World Health Organization (1974) Glossary of mental disorders, and guide to their classification, for use in conjunction with the International Classification of Diseases, 8th revision. World Health Organization, Geneva
8. World Health Organization (1978) Mental Disorders: glossary and guide to their classification in accordance with the ninth revision of the International Classification of Diseases. World Health Organization, Geneva
9. World Health Organization (1993) The ICD-10 Classification of mental and behavioural disorders: diagnostic criteria for research. WHO, Geneva
10. American Psychiatric Association (1994) Diagnostic and statistical manual of mental disorders, 4th edn. American Psychiatric Association, Washington
11. Yamashita I, Iwasaki T, Oguchi T et al (1989) Tentative classification criteria of neurotic disorders prepared by the JCIDCP (in Japanese). Clin Psychiatry 31:345–352

12. Nishikawa T, Tsuiki S (1961) Psychiatric investigations of atomic bomb survivors (in Japanese). Nagasaki Igakkai Zasshi (Nagasaki Med J) 36:717-722
13. World Health Organization (1993) Composite international diagnostic interview (CIDI) (core version 1.1). American Psychiatric Association, Washington
14. Nakane Y, Michitsuji S (1995) Results from the Nagasaki Centre. In: Ustun TB, Sartorius N (eds), Mental illness in general health care: an international study. Wiley, New York, pp 193-209
15. Nakane Y, Honda S, Mine M et al (1996) The mental health of atomic bomb survivors. In: Nagataki S, Yamashita S (eds), Nagasaki symposium radiation and human health. Elsevier, Tokyo, pp 239-249
16. Nakane Y, Takada K, Imamura Y et al (1998) Mental health among atomic bomb survivors in Nagasaki. In: WHO/HICARE symposium on radiological accidents and environmental epidemiology: a decade after the chernobyl accident—proceedings. World Health Organization, Geneva, pp 93-106
17. Nakane Y (1997) The concept of somatoform disorders and psychosomatic diseases in ICD-10 and DSM-IV (in Japanese with English abstract). Jpn J Psychosom Med 37:21-27

# Somatization in the Elderly

Scott Henderson

*Summary.* Clinicians working with older persons are familiar with the pattern of somatic symptoms of psychological origin. But it is unknown if older persons are indeed more prone to somatization after allowing for the higher level of physical morbidity in that age group. It is also unknown if there is an interaction effect between age and culture, whereby the elderly might differ in either direction from younger adults between cultures. In epidemiological surveys using community samples, in contrast to studies based on patients in primary care or clinics, it is very rare for adequate data to be obtained, with sufficient numbers across the whole age range to make stable estimates. But even if there were good epidemiological data, showing that older persons tend to have more, or to have less somatization than younger adults, what use would such information be? What is important for public health purposes is to improve the capability of primary care staff, and of other clinicians, to recognize and manage the somatic presentation of psychological distress or depression in all age groups.

*Key words.* Somatization, Epidemiology, Elderly, Community surveys, International comparisons

## Introduction

Let us start with the assumption that the phenomenon being discussed occurs in the general population in measurable amounts. Somatization as a psychological and behavioural phenomenon can be considered as a continuous variable, where most individuals have no symptoms and a decreasingly small number have one or more. The frequency distribution of symptoms in a population is therefore markedly skewed. But for clinicians, the presentation of somatization is categorical: it is either present or absent in any individual. For somatization disorder to be present, the symptoms and history must fulfill the diagnostic criteria for this syndrome in ICD-10 [1].

National Health and Medical Research Council, Psychiatric Epidemiology Research Centre, The Australian National University, Canberra, A.C.T. 0200, Australia

Persons fulfilling the diagnostic criteria for being a "case" will always lie far on the right of the frequency distribution of symptoms. Over time, some individuals at all levels of severity may move up or down the horizontal axis of severity. Others will stay more or less fixed at some point from zero to a maximum. Most of the population will remain at having no or only one or two symptoms from time to time, while a small minority will consistently have severe symptoms, either all the time or only in episodes. Note that so far, we have considered only symptoms and behaviour: we have not considered the amount of disablement that may accompany either the symptoms or the diagnosis.

To obtain good information about somatization in later life, one starting point is to consider what questions could be answered by epidemiological data; and why such questions are worth asking. As always, epidemiological data can be at three levels: samples of the general population, of persons reaching primary care, or of persons who have reached psychiatric services. Note that for present purposes, little can be said about the data unless these include both the elderly and younger adults, sampled in the same way. Let us bravely assume that such data do exist. It is then necessary to deal with the problem of ascertainment, or of recognizing persons who truly do have it, or who truly do not. By "it," I am referring to symptoms of somatization. There is indisputably more physical morbidity in older than younger persons. This may lead to false positives in diagnosis, whereby somatic symptoms may have a medical origin, but be attributed to a psychological cause. Conversely, it might lead to failure to diagnose somatization states, or false negatives, through the clinician's mistakenly attributing the psychologically determined somatic symptoms to a medical origin, or to aging itself. In a similar manner, patients themselves may attribute somatization symptoms to advancing years, not recognizing their psychological or medical origins.

This is clearly a situation in which, for research purposes, a standardized clinical assessment may be useful. In the Composite International Diagnostic Interview (CIDI) [2, 3] there is a module specifically for identifying somatization states. Indeed, there are a number of variants of that module. In all other parts of the interview, the algorithm for rating symptoms requires that symptoms be discounted if a medical or physical basis is likely. A further issue in instrument development to be aware of, is that there is some overlap between symptoms of somatization and aging itself. In the Symptom Checklist prepared by Janca, Isaac and Tacchini for the WHO International Study of Somatoform Disorders, there are 60 items in all. The following 8 of these symptoms are likely to be age-related in their frequency of endorsement: blindness, blurred vision, deafness, tinnitus, shortness of breath, weakness, tiredness, and sleep problems. The instrument may not perform in the same way in younger as in older persons, just as it may not perform the same for men and women. In psychometric terms, such items are biased and exhibit differential item functioning. And this is prior to the introduction of cultural variables, or the interaction of age or gender with culture. So any data obtained with the Symptom Checklist or similar instruments would need to be cautiously interpreted before comparisons are made across age groups.

Let us now assume that some of these issues can be overcome, or at least allowed for in the analysis of epidemiological data. In this presentation, there is time to consider only one research question: does the prevalence of somatization states increase or decrease with age? That is, what are the age-specific estimates for the 1-month prevalence of somatization disorder; or of somatization symptoms not reaching the arbitrary diagnostic criteria? This basic question is a start to determining if the aging process, or the biomedical and psychosocial context of late life, promote or decrease prevalence. In his recent monograph, "Abnormal Illness Behaviour," Pilowsky [4] has provided a scholarly examination of the presentation and causes of this group of disorders. It might be expected that rates might be higher in the elderly because of comorbidity with physical disorders. What about comorbidity with neuropsychiatric disorders such as dementia, stroke, or depression? On the risk factor side, the list that might promote somatization can be extended with ease: an accentuation of premorbid personality traits; the behaviour of relatives and carers in rewarding abnormal illness behaviour; and iatrogenic factors such as medication, polypharmacy, overemphasis on special investigations, and the motivation of remuneration. To my knowledge, the data for the question, "does the prevalence increase or decrease with age?" are not yet available; and even if they were, their interpretation is likely to be challenging.

But an opposing argument is also reasonable. Counter-intuitively, the prevalence in the elderly might be found to be lower than in younger adults. This seems to be the case for depression and anxiety [5–7]. It may be that the elderly have less neurotic disorders than younger adults, and this may not be a cohort effect. Speculatively, this may be due to attenuation of some of the risk factors recently found which we have to decrease in late life [7] as shown in Figure 1. Alternatively, the elderly may have acquired an increased resistance through repeated exposure to the trammels of life.

## The Available Evidence

Some of the major epidemiological studies have given estimates of prevalence for somatization disorders by age group, but the scientific significance of these is very slight. In a pioneering study in Baltimore, Pasamanick et al. [8] reported an overall prevalence of 3.7% for psychophysiological, autonomic, and visceral disorders, with a M:F ratio of 1:3. The rate was twice as high in whites as blacks, and was more common in mid-life, not old age. In Stirling County, Leighton et al. [9] found a rate of 69% of the population showing "psychophysiological symptom patterns." The rate rose with age. For socioeconomic status, Hollingshead and Redlich [10] found that in contrast to the neuroses, psychosomatic reactions were inversely related to class. In a study of hypochondriasis in a series of 60 patients assembled at the Massachusetts General Hospital, Barsky et al. [11] found no relationship with age, but acknowledged the small sample size. It was, of course, a sample of cases referred to a major teaching hospital, and therefore open to considerable selection effects, including Berkson's bias [12].

In the Epidemiologic Catchment Area (ECA) studies, the overall prevalence of somatization was found to be 0.2%. The National Comorbidity Study chose an upper age-limit of 59 years, making it unable to contribute information on this national sample. In the recent British Survey of over 10,000 persons [13–15], no increase with age was found in fatigue, irritability, somatic symptoms, depression, or anxiety. There was a slight trend towards more worry about physical health in the elderly, but only in men.

In the Australian National Survey of Mental Health and Wellbeing, a section on neurasthenia was included and the sample is of the total population with

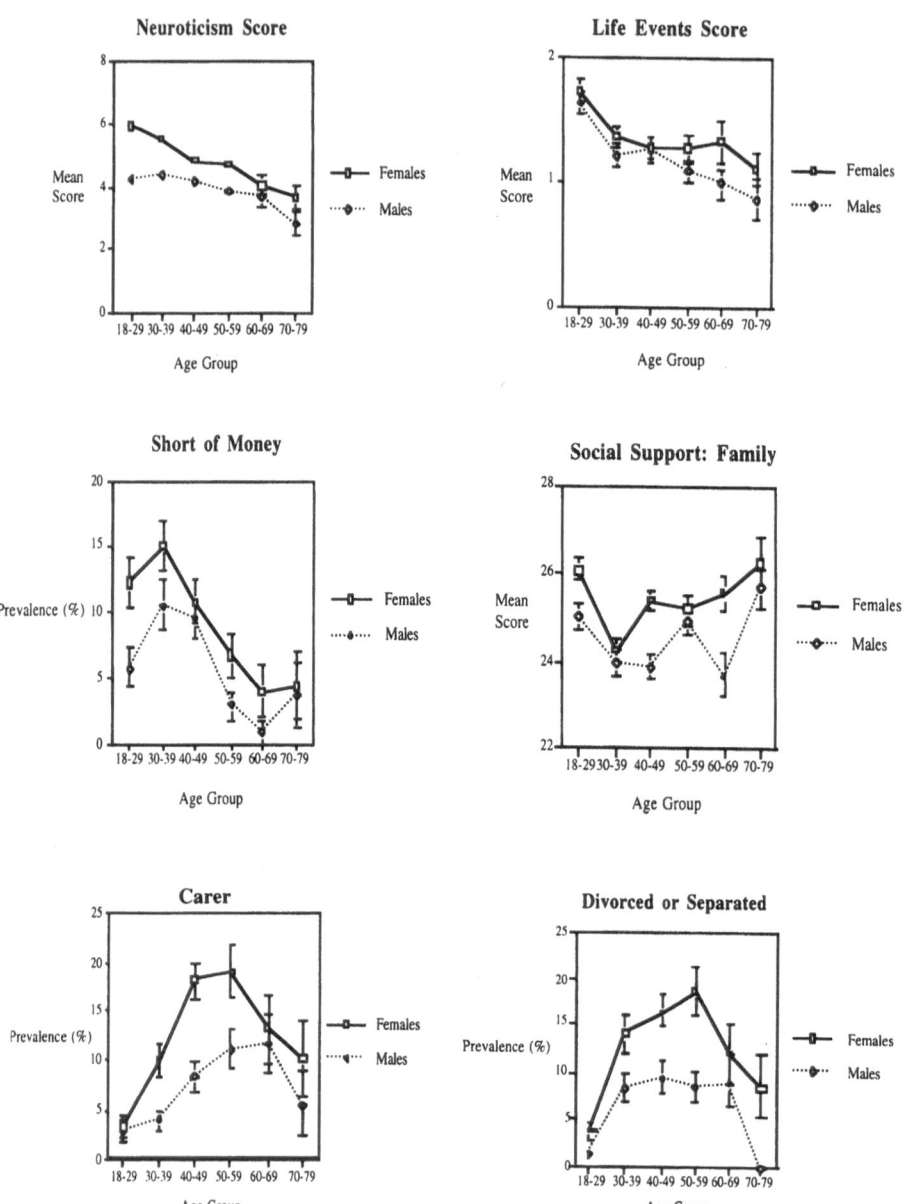

FIG. 1. Frequency distribution of risk factors by age group

FIG. 2. Tiredness. *Squares*, men (*n* = 891); *diamonds*, women (*n* = 1121). Data and Figure by A.F. Jorm

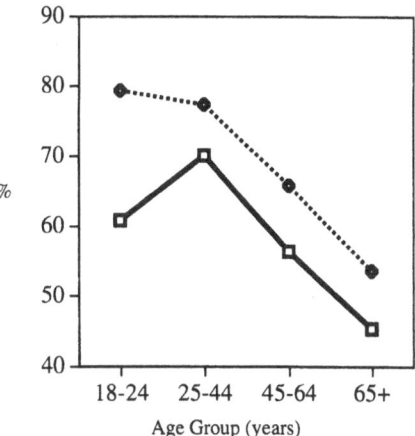

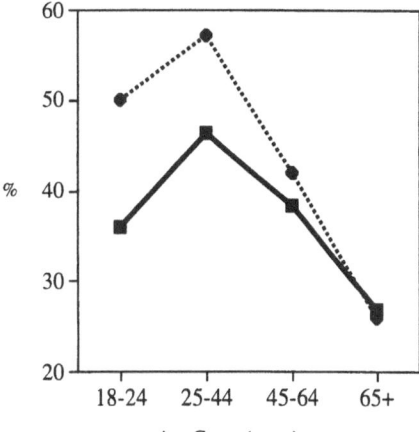

FIG. 3. Irritability. *Squares*, men (*n* = 889); *diamonds*, women (*n* = 1115). Data and Figure by A.F. Jorm

representation of all ages from 18 years. The findings will be published later this year. Meanwhile, our center has data on a national sample of adults who were interviewed for a study of mental health literacy [16–18]. Jorm and colleagues have provided me with data for the age groups 18–24, 25–44, 45–64, and 65+ years. The elderly consistently reported lower rates for the following: colds, sore throat, flu, headache, palpitations, breathlessness, depression, tiredness, and irritability. The latter two symptoms change with age, as shown in Figures 2 and 3.

## International Comparisons

In their much-cited review of epidemiological studies in psychosomatic medicine, Kessel and Munro [19] said that international comparative studies are not profitable for aetiological purposes: "While at first sight they seem very attractive, such a host of uncontrollable variables is introduced that any observed differences cannot be properly interpreted; much expenditure of money and effort is involved which could yield important information if it were put to studying differences *within* rather than *between* populations." But that was some 35 years ago. In the WHO International Study of Somatoform Disorders, we should consider what methodological issues need to be considered in interpreting the findings.

## Clinical Significance of the Epidemiological Data

If the prevalence of somatization disorder or neurasthenia is higher or lower in the elderly than other age groups, what use is this information? On its own, not much. But if the difference also applied to depression, anxiety, alcohol misuse, and other forms of psychiatric morbidity, a very interesting question emerges. Is there a true drop, or are there other interpretations? If there is a decrease, to what might it be attributed? These are matters that my colleagues and I have recently examined [7], but for which an explanation remains elusive.

For treatment, and for the development of better services for all age groups, a much more important issue is how adequately somatization states—whether at ICD-10 case level or not—are recognised in primary care [20]; and how such patients are offered treatment that has been demonstrated to be effective [4]. For both of these, recognition and treatment, the situation is usually unfavourable, sometimes inexcusably so and often very costly as a consequence. My impression is that the somatization disorders lead to very great expenditure by patients and by governments, because of repeated and unnecessary medical consultations, endoscopies, blood tests, X-rays, and imaging procedures.

## Economic Rationalism and Its Anti-Hippocratic Heresy

Under the contemporary zeitgeist of economic rationalism, epidemiology is being called upon to present evidence that there are, or are not, benefits to be gained by some specified intervention; and, as Kessler [21] has put it, that there is evidence that the benefits of treatment—and that includes benefits to the national economy—clearly exceed the sum of its direct costs and any expected risks. I urge you as scientists, as clinicians, and as health service administrators, to pause at this point, because of the implications for the practice of decent medicine.

Kessler says, "There is no necessary relationship between level of need and appropriateness of intervention." The decision to treat or not to treat is to be determined by a ratio. The prospect is awesome. For somatization disorders, if no treatment that is both effective and financially beneficial is available, what is an acceptable professional response? At best, we can hope that clinicians will be able to continue behaving as they have for many centuries. But what will they say to the patients? For those who are not to be treated, there must be some professional obligation to interpret the verdict of economic rationalism so as not to induce hopelessness and further demoralization. Then suppose that treatment is available but will cost more than leaving the condition untreated? Are we to understand that neither Governments nor commercial organizations would fund such treatment? That would mean that the patient pays or goes untreated. Countries with such a system face difficult times: there, unmet need may reach new levels, at least until treatments emerge that are both scientifically and financially effective. As Whiteford [22] concisely writes, ". . . the challenge for governments is to influence the allocation of scarce resources on a rational basis to optimise the health status of the population for both humane and economic reasons." For somatization disorders in any age group, we should hope that an acceptable balance between the humane and the economic will prevail.

## References

1. World Health Organization (1992) The ICD-10 Classification of Mental and Behavioural Disorders. Clinical descriptions and diagnostic guidelines. World Health Organization, Geneva
2. Robins LN, Wing J, Wittchen HU, Helzer JE, Babor TF, Burke J, Farmer A, Jablensky A, Pickens R, Regier DA, Sartorius N, Towle LH (1988) The Composite International Diagnostic Interview. Arch Gen Psychiatry 45:1069–1077
3. Peters L, Andrews G (1995) Procedural validity of the computerized version of the Composite International Diagnostic Interview (CIDI-auto) in the anxiety disorders. Psychol Med 25:1269–1280
4. Pilowsky I (1997) Abnormal Illness Behaviour. John Wiley & Sons, Chichester
5. Wittchen H-U, Knäuper B, Kessler RC (1994) Lifetime risk of depression. Br J Psychiatry 165:16–22
6. Henderson AS (1994) Does ageing protect against depression? Soc Psychiatry Psychiatr Epidemiol 29:107–109
7. Henderson AS, Jorm AF, Korten AE, Jacomb P, Christensen H, Rodgers B (1998) Symptoms of depression and anxiety during adult life: evidence for a decline in prevalence with age. Psychol Med 28:1321–1328
8. Pasamanick B, Robert DW, Lemkau PV, Krueger DE (1957) A survey of mental disease in an urban population. I. Prevalence by age, sex, and severity of impairment. Am J Publ Health 47:923–929
9. Leighton DC, Harding JS, Macklin DB, Hughes CC, Leighton AH (1963) Psychiatric findings of the Stirling County Study. Am J Psychiatry 119:1021–1026
10. Hollingshead A, Redlich FC (1958) Social Class and Mental Illness. Wiley, New York
11. Barsky AJ, Frank CB, Cleary PD, Whyshak G, Klerman GL (1991) The relation between hypochondriasis and age. Am J Psychiatry 148:923–928
12. Berkson J (1946) Limitations of the application of fourfold table analysis to hospital data. Biometrics Bull 2:47–53
13. Meltzer H, Gill B, Petticrew M (1994) OPCS Surveys of Psychiatry Morbidity in Great Britain. The prevalence of psychiatric morbidity among adults aged 16–64, living in private households, in Great Britain. OPCS Office of Population Censuses and Surveys, pp 1–16
14. Jenkins R, Bebbington P, Brugha T, Farrell M, Gill B, Lewis G, Meltzer H, Petticrew M (1997a) The National Psychiatric Morbidity Surveys of Great Britain—strategy and methods. Psychol Med 27:765–774
15. Jenkins R, Lewis G, Bebbington P, Brugha T, Farrell M, Gill B, Meltzer H (1997b) The National Psychiatric Morbidity Surveys of Great Britain—initial findings from the Household Survey. Psychol Med 27:775–789
16. Jorm AF, Korten AE, Jacomb PA, Christensen H, Rodgers B, Pollitt P (1997) "Mental health literacy": a survey of the public's ability to recognise mental disorders and their beliefs about the effectiveness of treatment. Med J Aust 166:182–186

17. Jorm AF, Korten AE, Jacomb PA, Christensen H, Rodgers B. Pollitt P (1997) Public beliefs about causes and risk factors for depression and schizophrenia. Soc Psychiatry Psychiatr Epidemiol 32:143–148
18. Jorm AF, Korten AE, Rodgers B, Pollitt P, Jacomb PA, Christensen H, Jiao Z (1997) Belief systems of the general public concerning the appropriate treatments for mental disorders. Soc Psychiatry Psychiatr Epidemiol 32:468–473
19. Kessel N, Munro A (1964) Epidemiological studies in psychosomatic medicine. J Psychosom Res 8:67–81
20. Bridges KW, Goldberg DP (1985) Somatic presentation of DSM-III psychiatric disorders in primary care. J Psychosom Res 29:563–569
21. Kessler R: Some considerations in making tesource allocation decisions for the treatment of psychiatric disorders. In: Andrews G, Henderson S (eds) Unmet need in Psychiatry. Cambridge University Press, Cambridge, UK, in press
22. Whiteford H: Unmet need: a challenge for governments. In: Andrews G, Henderson S (eds) Unmet need in Psychiatry. Cambridge University Press, Cambridge, UK, in press

# Somatic Symptoms in Children from Three Ethnic Groups

Glorisa Canino[1], Rafael Ramírez[1], María de los A. Balzac[2], Aislinn Frye[2], and Brenda Matos[2]

*Summary.* The main purpose of this study is to compare the prevalence rates of somatic symptoms associated with anxiety disorders in three ethnic groups, Hispanic, African Americans, and European Americans. Probability samples of children (aged 9 to 17 years) were obtained from four geographic areas in the United States and Puerto Rico as part of Methods for the Epidemiology of Child and Adolescent Mental Disorders (MECA) study funded by the National Institute of Mental Health.[1] Version 2.3 of the NIMH Diagnostic Interview Schedule for Children (DISC-2.3) was used at all sites to yield current diagnoses, according to DSM-III-R criteria. Nineteen somatic symptoms associated with anxiety disorders were ascertained. Results showed that after controlling for parental education, age, and gender, the average number of somatic symptoms did not differ by ethnic group, except for cardiovascular symptoms which were more prevalent in Hispanic and African American children. In all ethnic groups the most frequent symptoms were headaches and gastrointestinal problems, with the latter been more prevalent in the younger age cohort. In all age groups, females had higher rates of somatic symptoms. Results are interpreted in lieu of the main limitation of the study, that is, somatic symptoms were not ascertained independent of the diagnoses of anxiety disorders.

## Introduction

Medically unexplained physical symptoms have long been recognized as common and problematic in pediatric practice, but only since late 1980s have somatic complaints become a topic of research and discussion in the child and adolescent psychiatric literature [1]. This paucity of research may be due in part to the fact

---

[1] Behavioral Sciences Research Institute, and [2] Department of Psychiatry, University of Puerto Rico, Medical Sciences Campus, P.O. Box 365067, San Juan, Puerto Rico 00936-5067

that the psychiatric diagnostic criteria of somatization disorder was not developed for children [2]. As a consequence the diagnostic criteria are not developmental and its application in children, particularly younger ones, may be inappropriate. For example, the clinical manifestations of the symptoms vary with age, so that abdominal pain and headaches are more common in early childhood, whereas pseudoneurological, menstrual, and genitourinary and polysymptomatic symptoms are more common in adolescence [3]. In addition, although no significant differences in the distribution of somatization among the genders is found in early childhood, somatic symptoms are more prevalent in girls after the onset of pubertal development and menarche [4, 5]. It is not surprising, then, that coupled with the restrictiveness of the diagnostic criteria and the lack of developmental appropriateness of the same, the disorder is extremely rare in children. Less than 1% of children have been reported as meeting criteria for the disorder [6, 7], and most epidemiological pediatric studies prefer to report on somatic symptom levels than on the disorder per se [8].

Somatic symptoms in children have been associated with a family history of somatization, lower parental education, with chronic physical symptoms or disability in a parent, loss or death of a close family relative and other traumatic experiences and with functional impairment, and psychiatric disorders, particularly anxiety, and depression [9–12]. Yet the potential influence of culture and ethnicity on the development of somatic symptoms has not been adequately studied in the pediatric population.

A significant number of studies have been reported in the adult literature, which suggest that the prevalence of somatic symptoms in both clinical and community samples may be associated with belonging to a particular ethnic group [13–16]. Epidemiological population studies have shown that Puerto Ricans report higher rates of somatic symptoms as compared to European Americans and Mexican Americans from Los Angeles, CA, even after statistically controlling for sociodemographic factors [14, 15]. Other studies of clinical samples from 17 different countries have shown a higher prevalence of somatic symptoms among patients from Latin countries (e.g., Spain, Puerto Rico, Italy, Chile, Brazil, etc.) than in patients from other cultural heritage [17]. This higher prevalence of somatic symptoms among Latin or Hispanic populations has been explained as possibly due to the integration of somatic and psychological phenomena in the expression of symptoms in the Latino cultures as opposed to the Cartesian way of dichotomizing mind-body experiences in other cultures [14]. In addition, somatic complaints to express psychological distress may be more culturally acceptable than psychological symptoms in Latino populations, particularly for the male population.

Similar cross-cultural studies of somatic symptoms have not been reported with pediatric populations. The present study aims at filling this gap in the literature by comparing the rates of somatic symptoms associated with anxiety disorder in three ethnic groups; African American, Hispanics, and European American children. To our knowledge this is the first study that compares rates of pediatric somatic symptoms in different ethnic groups derived from four different community samples, three in the United States and one in Puerto Rico. We report the results of the analyses based on the data from the Methods for the Epidemiology of Child and Adolescent Mental Disorders (MECA*) study [18].

# Methods

## Sample

Probability samples of children were obtained in 1992 in four geographic areas in the United States and Puerto Rico: Connecticut ($n = 324$), with 78% of the sample from European American heritage, 11% African American heritage, 4% Hispanic heritage, and 7% other heritage; Georgia ($n = 299$), 64% European American, 30% African American, 1% Hispanic, and 5% other; New York ($n = 360$), 63% European American, 18% African American, 10% Hispanic, and 10% other; and Puerto Rico ($n = 312$), 100% Hispanic. Children aged 9 to 17 years, as well as their primary caretaker (96% were the mother) were interviewed in their household by two lay interviewers (each blind to the other's findings), using a computer-assisted version of the National Institute of Mental Health (NIMH) Diagnostic Interview Schedule for Children (NIMH-DISC 2.3) [19]. The analyses presented in this paper include only those parent-child dyads where DISC data allowed the determination of somatic symptoms in children by either or both informants and for which the primary caretaker identified herself and her child as European American, African American, or Hispanic (see Ref. [18] for more details on design and methods).

## Instruments

Version 2.3 of the NIMH-DISC was used by all sites as the lay-administered structured diagnostic interview. This version of the DISC generates psychiatric diagnoses as defined by the Diagnostic and Statistical Manual, Version 3-R [20]. The English version

* The MECA Program is an epidemiological methodology study performed by four independent research teams in collaboration with staff of the Division of Clinical Research, which was reorganized in 1992 with components now in the Division of Epidemiology and Services Research and the Division of Clinical and Treatment Research, of the NIMH, Rockville, MD. The NIMH Principal Collaborators are Darrel A. Regier, MD, MPH, Ben Z. Locke, MSPH, Peter S. Jensen, MD, William E. Narrow, MD, MPH, Donald S. Rae, MA, John E. Richters, PhD, Karen H. Bourdon, MA, and Margaret T. Roper, MS. The NIMH Project Officer was William J. Huber. The Principal Investigators and Coinvestigators from the four sites are as follows: Emory University, Atlanta, U01 MH46725: Mina K. Dulcan, MD; Benjamin B. Lahey, PhD, Donna J. Brogan, PhD, Sherryl H. Goodman, PhD, and Elaine W. Flagg, PhD; Research Foundation for Mental Hygiene at New York State Psychiatric Institute, New York, U01 MH46718: Hector R. Bird, MD, David Shaffer, MD, Myrna Weissman, PhD; Patricia Cohen, PhD, Denise Kandel, PhD, Christina Hoven, PhD, Mark Davies, MPH; Madelyn S. Gould, PhD, and Agnes Whitaker, MD; Yale University, New Haven, CT, U01 MH46717: Mary Schwab-Stone, MD, Philip J. Leaf, PhD, Sarah Horwitz, PhD, and Judith Lichtman, MPH; University of Puerto Rico, San Juan, U01 MH46732: Glorisa Canino, PhD, Maritza Rubio-Stipec, MA, Milagros Bravo, PhD, Margarita Alegria, PhD, Julio Ribera, PhD, Sara Huertas, MD, Michel Woodbury, MD, and Jose Bauermeister, PhD.

of the DISC has been shown to generate reliable and valid diagnoses for most diagnostic categories [21, 22]. Similar findings have been reported for the Spanish version of the instrument [23, 24].

## Measurement of Somatic Symptoms

Although most major disorders of childhood are contained in the DISC, the instrument has no measure of somatization disorder. Nevertheless, a list of 19 somatic symptoms are evaluated as part of each anxiety disorder measured by the DISC: simple phobia, social phobia, agoraphobia, panic disorder, separation anxiety, generalized anxiety, overanxious disorder, and avoidant disorder. Somatic symptoms are asked only if the respondent scores positive to at least one anxiety symptom related to any of the above mentioned anxiety disorders. The 19 somatic symptoms from the anxiety module of the DISC were categorized in five types of somatic symptoms: gastrointestinal, neurological, respiratory, nonspecific, and cardiovascular.

Comparison among groups of mean number of somatic symptoms was made controlling for age, gender, and parental education. Multiple regression analysis was performed to assess the significance of the differences found.

# Results

Figure 1 presents the mean number of somatic symptoms associated with any anxiety disorder in the three ethnic groups. Somatic symptoms are divided in to gastrointestinal, cardiovascular, neurological, respiratory, and nonspecific. As can be seen for most somatic symptoms, there are no significant differences among the three ethnic groups. Cardiovascular symptoms were the only ones significantly more prevalent in children of Hispanic origin as compared to European American. African American children showed a tendency to report more somatic symptoms but this did not reach statistical significance ($P < 0.06$). The same analyses were done for gender and age (data not shown). Significant differences among the ethnic groups were only observed for cardiovascular symptoms in males in younger children, being more prevalent among Hispanic and male children and in children between the ages of 9 to 11. The mean number of somatic symptoms by gender and by age was also estimated for the entire MECA sample disregarding ethnicity (data not shown). Females showed a significantly ($P < 0.01$) higher prevalence of somatic symptoms as compared to males for total amount of symptoms, for gastrointestinal, neurological, and cardiovascular symptoms (data not shown). Contrary to expectation, the predominance of symptoms in females as compared to males was maintained in the younger age cohort also (data not shown). When analyses were performed by age alone, only the gastrointestinal symptoms were significantly more common in the younger age cohort (9 to 11 years). The most common somatic symptoms reported in the entire MECA sample were headaches (50.8%), gastrointestinal disturbances (35.8%), palpitations (26.5%), and pain or general malaise (22.2%).

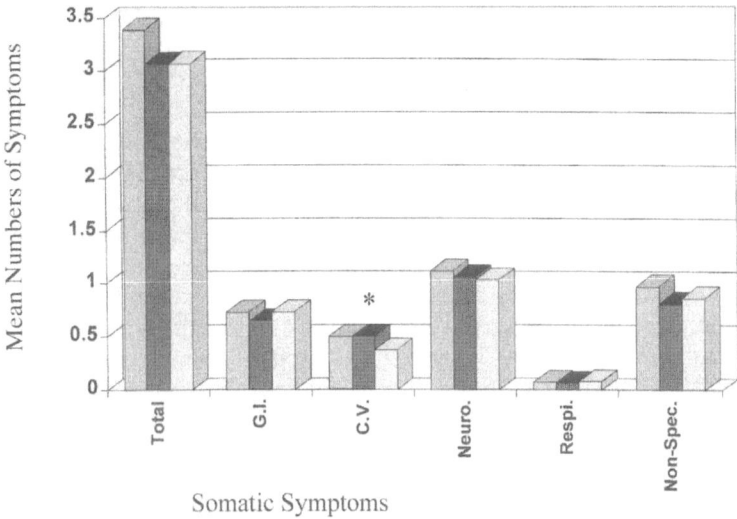

FIG. 1. Mean number of somatic symptoms associated with anxiety disorders in three ethnic groups. *G.I.*, gastrointestinal; *C.V.*, cardiovascular; *Neuro.*, neurological; *Respi.*, respiratory; *Non-Spec*, nonspecific. *Black bar*, Hispanic children; *gray bar*, African American children; *light-gray bar*, European American children. *$P \leq 0.05$

# Discussion

As with other studies reported in the literature, females had higher rates of somatic symptoms than males, and the most common symptoms reported were headaches and gastrointestinal problems, the latter ones being more common in younger age cohorts [3]. However, contrary to expected, significant differences by gender were also observed in the younger age cohort. This may be due to the fact that our cohort did not include children below age 9, and it may be that it is only in younger age cohorts that no difference in somatic symptoms by gender is observed.

Prior studies of adult populations [14] have reported higher rates of somatic symptoms in Hispanic samples. However, in this study, most somatic symptoms were equally prevalent in the three ethnic groups studied. Only cardiovascular symptoms were significantly more prevalent in children of Hispanic heritage, and a tendency for higher symptoms was observed for African American children as compared to European American children. This difference seemed to be mostly due to the higher prevalence of these symptoms in boys and in younger children belonging to these ethnic groups.

Prior studies of somatic symptoms in the general adult population of Puerto Rico had shown a higher prevalence in males [15]. However, further analyses of the data showed that this difference was accounted for the lower educational level of males as compared to females in the population of Puerto Rico. When analyses were performed controlling for the interaction of gender and education, somatic symptoms emerged as more prevalent in adult women. Similar analyses with this child population are not appropriate, since the educational level of the child itself is not relevant, given that children of different ages have attained naturally different educational levels. We thought of performing the analyses by examining the interaction between gender and school expulsion or desertion, which would be a more appropriate analysis. However, the proportion of children in the sample who had deserted or were expelled from school was too low to permit this type of analysis.

Prior analyses of this data set have shown differences in parental education and family income among the three ethnic groups studied, with Hispanic and African American families reporting lower educational and income levels as compared to European American families [25]. Because of this, the assessment of differences among groups was done with multiple regression analysis controlling for parental educational level, and age and gender when appropriate. Cardiovascular symptoms remained significantly more prevalent in Hispanic families even after accounting for these parental educational differences.

Differences among ethnic groups could also have been due to differences in the prevalence of anxiety disorders. As previously mentioned, somatic symptoms are common in children with anxiety disorders [9]. In fact, the prevalence of each of the 19 symptoms ascertained in this study was significantly higher in children who met criteria for any anxiety disorder as compared to those who did not meet criteria (data not shown). Given the fact that somatic symptoms in this sample could only be ascertained if the child endorsed an anxiety symptom, this finding is not surprising since the probabilities of having a high proportion of somatic symptoms would increase with higher prevalence of any anxiety disorder. Thus, the higher prevalence of cardiovascular symptoms in the Hispanic children could potentially be due to higher prevalence of anxiety disorders in this ethnic group as compared to European Americans. For this reason, multiple regression analyses were performed controlling for the prevalence of any anxiety disorder in the three ethnic groups. The results showed that cardiovascular symptoms remained significantly more prevalent in Hispanic children: the tendency among African Americans to have more symptoms remained as compared to European Americans (data not shown). However, it is important to mention that ethnicity accounted for less than 1% of the variance in explaining the prevalence of somatic symptoms in these groups. This suggests that there are other important variables that need to be examined in future studies that may be accounting for the differences observed. Differences in the ethnic groups in exposure to stressful and traumatic life events, parental psychopathology, familial history of somatization, physical illness, or disability in a parent, which have been found to be important predictors of somatic symptoms in children, could be accounting for the differences observed [9–12]. Future studies would need to be done where these variables are introduced into the model before we can conclude with certainty that cross-cultural differences exist in the expression of somatic symptoms in pediatric populations. In addition, future, cross-cultural studies should ascertain a wider range of somatic symptoms independently of any psychiatric disorder, and include children in a younger age range than the one studied in this sample.

# References

1. Apley J, Meadow R (1978) The child and its symptoms: a comprehensive approach, 3rd edn. Blackwell, Oxford
2. American Psychiatric Assciation (1994) Diagnostic and Statistical Manual of Mental Disorders—4th edn. American Psychiatric Associateion, University of Vermont
3. Beidel DC, Christ MAG, Long PJ (1991) Somatic complaints in anxious children. J Abnorm Child Psychol 19:659–670
4. Campo JV, Fritsch SL (1994) Somatization in children and adolescents. J Am Acad Child Adolesc Psychiatry 33:1223–1235
5. Eminson M, Benjamin S, Shortall A et al (1996) Physical symptoms and illness attitudes in adolescents: an epidemiological study J Child Psychol Psychiatry 35:519–528
6. Garber J, Zeman J, Walker LS (1990) Recurrent abdominal pain in children: psychiatric diagnoses and parental psychopathology. J Am Acad Child Adolesc Psychiatry 29:648–656
7. Walker LS, Garber, J, Greene JW (1991) Somatization symptoms in pediatric abdominal pain patients: relation to chronicity of abdominal pain and parent somatization. J Abnorm Child Psychol 19:379–394
8. Taylor D, Szatmari P, Boyle M et al (1996) Somatization and the vocabulary of everyday bodily experiences and concerns: a community study of adolescents. J Am Acad Child Adolesc Psychiatry 35:491–499
9. Bernstein GA, Massie ED, Thuras PD et al (1997) Somatic symptoms in anxiousdepressed school refusers. J Am Acad Child Adolesc Psychiatry 36:661–668
10. Jolly JB, Wherry JN, Wiesner DC et al (1994) The mediating role of anxiety in selfreported somatic complaints of depressed adolescents. J Abnorm Child Psychol 22:691–702
11. Garralda ME (1996) Somatization in children. J Child Psychol Psychiatry 37:13–33
12. Walker LS, Garber J, Greene JW (1994) Somatic complaints in pediatric patients: a prospective study of the role of negative life events, child social and academic competence, and parental somatic symptoms. J Consult Clin Psychol 62:1213–1221
13. Escobar J, Canino G (1989) Unexplained physical complaints; psychopathology and epidemiological correlates. Br J Psychiatry 155:24–47
14. Escobar J, Rubio-Stipec M, Canino G et al (1989) Somatic Symptom Index (SSI): a new and abridged somatization construct. Prevalence and epidemiological correlates in two large community samples. J Nerv Ment Dis 177:140–146
15. Canino I, Escobar J, Canino G et al (1992). Functional somatic symptoms: a crossethnic comparison. Am J Orthopsychiatry 62:605–612
16. Mezzich JE, Raab ES (1980) Depressive symptomatology across the Americas. Arch Gen Psychiatry 37:818–823
17. Rubio-Stipec M, Canino G, Robins LN et al (1993) The somatization schedule of the composite diagnostic interview: the use of the Probe Chart in 17 different countries. Intern J Methods Psychiatr Res 3:129–136
18. Lahey BB, Flagg EW, Bird HR et al (1996) The NIMH methods for the epidemiology of child and adolescent mental disorder (MECA) study: background and methodology. J Am Acad Child Adolesc Psychiatry 35:855–864
19. Shaffer D, Fisher P, Dulcan M et al (1996) The NIMH Diagnostic Interview Schedule for Children (DISC 2.3): Description, acceptability, prevalence, and performance in the MECA study. J Am Acad Child Adolesc Psychiatry 35:865–877
20. American Psychiatric Association (1987) Diagnostic and statistical manual of mental disorders—Third edn. American Psychiatric Association, Washington

21. Jensen P, Roper M, Fisher P et al (1995) Test-retest reliability of the Diagnostic Interview Schedule for Children (DISC 2.1). Arch Gen Psychiatry 52:61–71
22. Schwab-Stone M, Dulcan M, Bird H et al (1996) The NIMH methods for the epidemiology of child and adolescent mental disorders (MECA) study: criterion validity of the NIMH Diagnostic Interview Schedule for Children Version 2.3 (DISC 2.3). J Am Acad Child Adolesc Psychiatry 35:878–888
23. Ribera JC, Canino, GJ, Rubio-Stipec et al (1996) The Diagnostic Interview Schedule for Children (DISC 2.1) in Spanish: reliability in a Hispanic population. J Child Psychol Psychiatry 37:195–204
24. Bravo M, Woodbury-Fariña M, Canino G et al (1993). The Spanish translation and cultural adaptation of the Diagnostic Interview Schedule for Children (DISC) in Puerto Rico. Cult Med Psychiatry 17:329–344
25. Goodman SH, Hoven CW, Narrow WE et al (1998) Measurement of risk for mental disorders and competence in a psychiatric epidemiologic community survey: the NIMH methods for the epidemiology of child and adolescent mental disorders (MECA) study. Soc Psychiatry Psychiatr Epidemiol 33:162–173

# Hypochondriasis

Arthur J. Barsky

*Summary.* Hypochondriasis research has made significant gains recently, and we can now reexamine our understanding of the condition in light of three basic questions: (1) What is the fundamental nature of hypochondriasis? (2) What is its etiology? (3) Where should our future research efforts be directed? The fundamental nature of hypochondriasis remains perplexing. Because hypochondriacal symptoms are not categorical and exist along a continuum in the population, and most people are hypochondriacal to some degree at some times in their lives, hypochondriasis may not be understood best as an Axis I disorder. The distinction between normal and abnormal hypochondriasis is arbitrary and may not be very helpful in trying to conceptualize it. Hypochondriasis might alternatively be thought of as a nonspecific index of psychological distress, a personality characteristic, one of several alternative "somatic styles," or a form of illness behavior. What is the etiology of hypochondriasis? Some empirical data suggest that cognitive and perceptual mechanisms are important in causing hypochondriasis. Other work suggests hypochondriasis is a nonverbal, interpersonal communication, a form of coping and help-seeking in response to a stressful life crisis. It has also been thought of as an intrapsychic defense mechanism. A more sophisticated etiological model of hypochondriasis might take into account three different types of causation: predisposing factors (such as personality characteristics or salient childhood experiences); precipitants (e.g., stressful events, medical threats); and factors which perpetuate or maintain hypochondriacal symptoms (e.g., sick role reinforcers, family dynamics). Where should future investigations be directed? Although developmental and longitudinal studies pose many practical difficulties, they are the only way to definitively examine the role of childhood and family experiences, thought by many observers to be key. The importance of cognitive schema and behavioral patterns deserve continued investigation. This should include experimental laboratory work to distinguish interoceptive, discriminative ability from response bias.

*Key words.* Somatization, Hypochondriasis, Treatment, Etiology, Research

Division of Psychiatry, Harvard Medical School and Brigham and Women's Hospital, 75 Francis Street, Boston, MA 02115, USA

# Introduction

Significant advances have recently been made in our knowledge about, and understanding of, hypochondriasis. A substantial body of information about its phenomenology, epidemiology, natural history, and treatment has emerged. But many of the most fundamental questions about this perplexing condition remain. In light of the new, empirical findings that are accumulating, it seems worthwhile re-examining three basic questions about hypochondriasis: What is the fundamental nature of this condition? What is its etiology? Where should our research efforts be directed in the future?

# The Fundamental Nature of Hypochondriasis

The fundamental nature of hypochondriasis is complex and despite many recent research advances, remains somewhat unclear. In part, this derives from the fact that hypochondriasis is a dimensional rather than a categorical condition. That is, it exists along a smooth continuum throughout the population; almost everyone is a little bit hypochondriacal, at least under certain circumstances and at certain times. Hypochondriasis is thus unlike schizophrenia or cancer (to take but two examples), which are present in some individuals and completely absent in others.

At one end of the hypochondriacal continuum are individuals who do not have a psychiatric disorder but are experiencing mild, transient, hypochondriacal worry; for example, they note a mole and worry briefly that it might be a melanoma, or can't remember a name and suspect that this is the first sign of Alzheimer's disease. Such transient, "normal" hypochondriasis is especially likely to emerge at times of stress, in particular when individuals face a significant threat to health or have lost something or someone very important to them. Such hypochondriacal concerns promptly subside with the passage of time or of the precipitating stress, and respond well to appropriate reassurance from a physician and medical evidence that they are not in fact sick. At the other end of the hypochondriacal continuum are individuals with fears and beliefs that are more severe, persistent, pervasive, and disabling, and which do not decline with explanation, education, reassurance, or the failure of any serious medical condition to emerge over time. These individuals' hypochondriacal concerns are more abnormal or psychopathological, and constitute a psychiatric disorder.

However, it is very difficult to draw a precise boundary line between the abnormal and the normal, between health and disorder. Very little distinguishes two patients who fall just on either side of this boundary line, and the distinction between them is quite arbitrary. This problem of course is not unique to hypochondriasis, or even to psychiatry. Hypertension and diabetes are obvious examples of dimensional medical conditions—all patients have blood pressures and blood glucose levels and the difference between one individual who just exceeds the diagnostic threshold for hypertension or diabetes and another who falls at the high end of normal may be so small as to be meaningless. In the case of hypochondriasis, this problem is so substantial that some have suggested that it is not really a psychiatric disorder and is better thought of as a form of illness behavior, a personality characteristic or trait, or a nonspecific symptom of psychological distress and dysphoria [1–3].

If, however, we can agree that there are some individuals whose fears about their health, preoccupation with their symptoms, and unrealistic beliefs about sickness are so chronic, severe, and disabling that they are suffering from a psychiatric disorder, then just what sort of psychiatric disorder is it? Here, several subsidiary questions arise. First, should a distinction be made between primary and secondary hypochondriasis? Hypochondriasis is more commonly occurs in combination with another comorbid, psychiatric disorder (secondary hypochondriasis) than occurs by itself as the sole disorder present (primary hypochondriasis). When it co-occurs with another psychiatric disorder, it is often difficult to determine which is the more pervasive, fundamental, underlying condition, and which came first.

Even when hypochondriasis occurs without other comorbid psychiatric disorder, it may be better thought of as an Axis II rather than an Axis I condition. Since primary hypochondriasis seems often to begin early in life, to arise developmentally, to persist throughout much of adulthood, and to be characterized as a way of coping with distress, an abnormal pattern of help-seeking, and an intolerance of physical discomfort, then it has been argued that it might better be considered on Axis II than Axis I [1, 2]. It does appear that medically unexplained complaints, high rates of medical consultation, and pronounced sick role behavior are frequently found in patients with a variety of personality disorders, particularly the DSM cluster B disorders.

Finally, even though there are some hypochondriacal patients who do seem to be suffering from an Axis I disorder, there is debate about where to situate this primary form of hypochondriasis within the taxonomy. It currently resides within the somatoform disorder section. These disorders were grouped together for the first time in DSM-III. This was done for reasons of clinical utility rather than with a theoretical rationale or because of empirical evidence that the somatoform disorders all shared common characteristics. Subsequently, there have been suggestions that hypochondriasis is more closely related to the anxiety disorders, and to OCD (obsessive-compulsive disorder) in particular, and therefore that it would be better situated in the anxiety disorder section of the DSM. Although there are a number of similarities between hypochondriasis and OCD, there also are a number of significant differences [4]. Likewise similarities have been noted between illness phobias and hypochondriasis. Finally, in generalized anxiety disorder, health (both one's own and that of one's family members) is often a prominent area of concern and source of worry.

## The Etiology of Hypochondriasis

Historically, several different etiological models of hypochondriasis have been proposed [5]. The oldest is the psychodynamic model, in which hypochondriacal symptoms are thought to have unconscious gratification and meaning. In particular, themes of dependency, hostility, and narcissism have been pointed out as especially salient. More recent attention has turned to a cognitive and perceptual model of hypochondriasis [6–8] in which the disorder is thought to result from a self-validating and self-perpetuating cycle of cognition and perception; the belief that one is sick causes a perceptual amplification of normal bodily sensation and benign dysfunction. This altered medical perception of endemic bodily distress in turn further reinforces the belief that one is sick, and the cycle continues. Finally, hypochondriasis has been understood as an interpersonal communication, a response to a seemingly insoluble life dilemma or insurmountable obstacle that one is facing. Hypochondriacal individuals have learned to seek the sick role in such circumstances, since it is a nonverbal way of telling those around them that they are in need of special attention and assistance, in essence of calling "time-out."

The development, course, and natural history of hypochondriasis is not yet sufficiently known to identify all of its predisposing, precipitating, and perpetuating causes. However, evidence is accumulating to suggest a predisposing role for certain childhood experiences (exaggerated parental attention to health, abuse or trauma in childhood, or a figure of identity who modeled the sick role and exemplified illness behavior [9–11]); personality traits (such as negative affectivity, cluster B personality disorder and, possibly, alexithymia [2, 12, 13]); cognitive style (including catastrophizing, external locus of control, and attributional style); and perceptual characteristics (such as an amplifying style and private self-consciousness).

These trait-like characteristics put an individual at risk for somatization, but this vulnerability may remain latent until an acute precipitant causes it to become clinically manifest [14]. A number of such factors are known. Life stress commonly leads to medically unexplained complaints [15–17]. Two distinctly different types of stress cause somatization: major life events which are distressing and force the individual to change and adapt (in particular threats to health, such as a heart attack, or the death of someone close); and more minor stresses, recurrent frustrations and irritants, such as friction at work or commuting problems. The frequency of such daily "hassles" is highly correlated with the reporting of somatic symptoms. Psychiatric disorders often serve to precipitate medically unexplained somatic symptoms and hypochondriacal concerns as well. Anxiety disorders (especially panic disorder and generalized anxiety disorder) and depressive disorders are most important in this respect, since they are so prevalent and so often include prominent bodily distress and health worries. Finally, somatization can be triggered by relatively minor events which activate latent, health-related cognitive schema which are faulty, unduly pessimistic, or alarming. Once activated, these schema then influence the individual's experience and appraisal of his/her bodily symptoms. For example, the sudden cardiac death of a popular celebrity, or attaining the age of a parent who died of a myocardial infarction, may precipitate hypochondriasis in an individual who has always harbored a latent suspicion that he was especially vulnerable to heart disease because of a family history of premature cardiac death.

Once hypochondriasis has developed, in most instances it resolves and remits spontaneously with nothing more than the passage of time. Clinical experience in general medical practice suggests that there are large numbers of patients with such transient forms of hypochondriasis. Their somatic symptoms and health anxieties tend to subside with the passage of time, explanation and reassurance, and perhaps some palliative medical treatment. Indeed, this transient form of hypochondriasis appears to be the rule rather than the exception. In an appreciable fraction of cases, however, clinically manifest hypochondriasis is perpetuated or maintained by one of several factors. Among the most important of these perpetuating factors is secondary gain [16, 18, 19]. The presence of secondary gain does not differentially distinguish psychogenic from organically based symptoms (since all illness results in some positive compensatory gains), but its presence does tend to foster and perpetuate symptoms.

Likewise, illness and sick role behavior, and invalidism tend to perpetuate somatization as well [20, 21]. In addition, the medical care process itself tends to reinforce and perpetuate symptoms. Finally, somatization may be maintained and prolonged by a continuation of the stressful situation or events which initially precipitated it; the persistence of those stressors perpetuates the somatizing response.

## Future Directions

In the light of our current understanding and knowledge, where ought our future efforts best be directed? Three research avenues seem particularly promising.

First, there is a great need for longitudinal and prospective studies. We need to better understand the processes whereby hypochondriasis becomes clinically manifest, and then either resolves or becomes chronic. Longitudinal studies are difficult to conduct, require large samples, and are expensive, but no other design provides comparable data. Hypochondriacal individuals may be particularly disposed to retrospective bias, viewing their past and their childhoods as difficult, painful, and unfortunate. This makes retrospective studies problematical. Mood congruent recall may also play a role in their histories, so that their current difficulties and discomfort prompts them to selectively recall, focus upon, and emphasize similar occasions in the past. Two sorts of prospective studies are needed. First are long-term studies beginning in childhood, which examine the childhood events and family dynamics which place some individuals at increased risk for subsequently becoming hypochondriacal adults. Although most observers believe that early influences are crucial in the subsequent development of a hypochondriacal style, there are few empirical data about this. Second, we need longitudinal studies of the influence of family dynamics and family responses to the hypochondriacal patient on the disorder. Again, although it is widely held that the patient's family's responses and reactions are crucial in shaping the illness and influencing its course, almost no empirical study of this exists. This may partly be due to the fact that such studies of family dynamics and interpersonal interaction are difficult to conduct and pose many methodological problems. Nonetheless, this is one of the most promising, and most underexplored, areas of research.

Experimental investigation of symptom amplification is another priority area for future study. The hypochondriacal patient's somatic complaints may result from benign dysfunctions, mild infirmities, and normal physiology which he/she is more sensitive to and better able to perceive than is the nonhypochondriacal individual. This implies that hypochondriacs are able to make finer visceral and somatic discriminations, and to detect more subtle irregularities and infirmities than other people can. Alternatively, the hypochondriac's symptoms could result from a response bias, i.e., a general tendency to find bodily sensation unpleasant, uncomfortable, and noxious. This distinction between discriminative acuity on the one hand, and reporting style on the other, is crucial. It could be explored using experimental paradigms in which a measurable stimulus is administered and the patient's subjective experience of this stimulus is elicited and measured. If administered in a way which requires the subject to distinguish between two stimuli of slightly different magnitude, signal detection analysis can be applied to the resulting data. Signal detection analysis allows the investigator to derive two independent measures, one of discriminative ability and one of response bias. Ultimately, functional brain imaging might be used to determine the neural basis for the hypochondriacal patient's bodily experiences. While it may be a long time before hypochondriasis is studied with brain imaging, these techniques might be applied to somatoform pain disorder first. Recent work using positron emission tomography (PET) has been able to distinguish the site of nociception in the somatosensory cortex from the accompanying cognitive and emotional quality of noxiousness which results from activity in the anterior cingulate cortex [22].

Finally, because recent research lends support to a cognitive model of hypochondriasis and points to the salience of faulty cognitive schema about health and disease, further study of cognitive processing is indicated. Hypochondriacal patients appear to harbor a number of misconceptions and misunderstandings about health and disease, somatic sensation, and their bodies. These guide their processing of health-related information and their appraisal and assessment of their bodily experience. For example, they often evidence misconceptions about the symptom-free nature of good health, inaccurate appraisals of medical risk, faulty interpretations of laboratory test results, mistaken assumptions about medical diagnosis, and unrealistic expectations of treatment. Cognition is an important aspect of hypochondriasis to study further because it has immediate implications for therapy and can lead directly to the development of cognitive, behavioral, and educational therapies.

Valuable recent research has recently disclosed a great deal about this disturbing and disabling condition. Basic questions remain, however, about its fundamental nature; its origins, development, and natural history; and about the etiological mechanisms of symptom formation. One can confidently predict significant gains in these areas of ignorance in the near future. And with these advances will come further advances in our treatment of hypochondriasis.

## References

1. Bass C, Murphy M (1995) Somatoform and personality disorders: syndromal comorbidity and overlapping developmental pathways. J Psychosom Res 39:403–427
2. Kirmayer LJ, Robbins JM, Paris J (1994) Somatoform disorders: personality and the social matrix of distress. J Abnorm Psychol 3:125–136
3. Barsky AJ (1995) Somatoform disorders and personality traits. J Psychosom Res 39:399–402
4. Barsky AJ (1992) Hypochondriasis and obsessive compulsive disorder. Psychiatr Clin North Amer 15:791–801
5. Barsky AJ, Klerman GL (1983) Overview: hypochondriasis, bodily complaints, and somatic styles. Am J Psychiatry 140:273–283
6. Kirmayer L (1987) Somatization and the social construction of illness experience. In: McHugh S, Vallis M (eds) Illness behavior. Plenum, New York; pp 111–133
7. Kirmayer LJ (1984) Culture, affect and somatization part II. Transcult Psychiatr Res Rev 21:237–262
8. Barsky AJ, Wyshak G (1990) Hypochondriasis and somatosensory amplification. Br J Psychiatry 157:404–409
9. Benjamin S, Eminson DM (1992) Abnormal illness behaviour: childhood experiences and long-term consequences. Int Rev Psychiatry 4:55–70

10. Pribor EF, Dinwiddie SH (1992) Psychiatric correlates of incest in childhood. Am J Psychiatry 149:52–56
11. Whitehead WE, Crowell MD, Heller BR et al (1994) Modeling and reinforcement of the sick role during childhood predicts adult illness behavior. Psychosom Med 56:541–550
12. Kirmayer LJ, Taillefer S (1997) Somatoform Disorders. In: Herson M, Turner S (eds) Adult psychopathology, 3rd edn. Wiley, New York, pp 333–382
13. Pennebaker JW, Watson D (1991) The psychology of somatic symptoms. In: Kirmayer LJ, Robbins JM (eds) Current concepts of somatization: research and clinical perspectives. American Psychiatric Association Press, Washington, pp 24–35
14. Barsky AJ (1998) A comprehensive approach to the somatizing patient. J Psychosom Res 45:301–306
15. Ford CV (1983) The somatizing disorders illness as a way of life. Elsevier, New York
16. Kellner R (1990) Somatization: theories and research. J Nerv Ment Dis 178:150–160
17. Mechanic D (1978) Effects of psychological distress on perceptions of physical health and use of medical and psychiatric facilities. J Hum Stress 4:26–32
18. Kellner R (1986) Somatization and hypochondriasis. Praeger, New York
19. Kellner R (1991) Psychosomatic syndromes and somatic symptoms. American Psychiatric Press, Washington
20. Salkovskis PM, Warwick HMC (1986) Case histories and shorter communications. Behav Res Ther 24:597–602
21. Salkovskis PM (1989) Somatic problems. In: Hawton K, Salkovskis PM, Kirk JW et al (eds) Cognitive-behavioral approaches to adult psychiatric disorders: a practical guide. Oxford University Press, Oxford; pp 235–276
22. Rainville P, Duncan GH, Price DD et al (1997) Pain affect encoded in human anterior cingulate but not somatosensory cortex. Science 277:968–971

# Chronic Fatigue Syndrome

Simon Wessely

*Summary.* In this chapter contemporary views on the chronic fatigue syndrome (CFS) are discussed. The differences between a common syndrome encountered universally, which can be operationally defined and studied using the techniques of epidemiology, are contrasted with a belief-defined disorder, mainly found in the developed, Anglophone world. The former tells us much about the mechanisms of chronic fatigue and fatigability, and the interactions between physical and psychological factors in chronic illness. The latter informs us about views of illness and illness causation at the end of the twentieth century.

*Key words.* Chronic fatigue syndrome, Psychological factors, Fatigability, Epidemiology

## Definition

During the last decade a new term has entered the medical dictionary—that of chronic fatigue syndrome (CFS). Despite its media prominence, few are certain what it is, where it came from, how it should be defined, what causes it, what to do about it, and even what to call it. The relationship between CFS and somatisation, the subject of this book, is even more uncertain. Even to address this issue will cause offence in certain quarters, for reasons I shall elaborate. In this brief essay I shall address all these questions, but provide definitive answers to none. I have considered these topics elsewhere, and certainly cannot guarantee any fresh insights in this contribution [1–3].

What is the syndrome? Here are some extracts from a typical clinical description.

The symptoms in both the physical and psychical fields are equally prominent ... They are always languid, and tire easily upon waking or from slight muscular effort. The capacity for mental application diminishes rapidly ... they become forgetful with names and figures ...

Epidemiological and Liaison Psychiatry, Department of Psychological Medicine, King's College School of Medicine, King's College Hospital, Denmark Hill, London SE5 9RS, UK

depression is common ... but it rarely happens that the feeling of despair becomes intense enough to lead to suicidal attempts. It may appear suddenly, following an acute disease, especially influenza. In cases which resist treatment, the patients become chronic invalids of a most distressing kind. They go the rounds of physicians, pass from one sanatorium to another, taking all kinds of drugs.

Until the last sentence, with the mention of sanatoria, the above quotes could have come from any number of recent writings on CFS. The quotes are actually from Kraepelin writing about neurasthenia [4]. I and others have already drawn attention to the links between CFS and neurasthenia, arguing that the two conditions show remarkable similarities [5, 6]. It is indeed ironic, however, that as Lin points out, just as neurasthenia was abandoned by Western psychiatrists, and removed from the bible of orthodox psychiatry, the Diagnostic and Statistical Manual of the American Psychiatric Association, it became accepted in Chinese, Japanese, and other Asian psychiatric systems of thought. Hence when CFS burst onto the Western scene, few were around to point out its historical provenance, and many continue instead to regard CFS as a new condition and to look for its origins in some new feature of modern life, as many still do.

The rise of the label of CFS during the 1980s can be traced to the coincidence of new clinical and research observations, largely concerning possible links with infective agents and immune dysfunction (vide infra), the changing nature of the relationship of doctor and patient [7], and consumer pressure. The consequence was immediate confusion about its definition and nosological status. Most observers, usually working in specialist centres, noted certain characteristics of clinical samples. These included an over-representation of females, and of higher socio-economic groups. Strong physical attribution and intense disease conviction were the norm [8–10], whilst certain professions, such as doctors and teachers, seem to be particularly at risk.

A variety of names exist for this syndrome. Myalgic encephalomyelitis or ME is the commonest label in Britain, Australia, and South Africa, but is inappropriate for a number of reasons. The term post-viral fatigue syndrome sounds better, and is also used in the English-speaking world, but many problems exist with this term as well. Chronic fatigue syndrome, a label accurate, short, and free from unproven aetiological assumptions, is now the term of choice. However, although the introduction of an accepted operational definition is a major advance and a prerequisite for research, this should presuppose that we are dealing with a discrete disorder—indeed, the evidence suggests the opposite.

At present several operational case definitions have been presented. One started with the efforts of American infectious disease and immunology specialists [11], and has been refined on two occasions [12, 13]. Others come from Australia and the United Kingdom [14]. All require substantial functional impairment in addition to the complaint of severe fatigue after minimal exertion (although all are vague on how this should be measured). Differences are also apparent. For example, the American criteria attach particular significance to certain somatic symptoms such as sore throats, painful muscles, and lymph nodes, and, although the requirement for multiple symptoms has been modified in the latest revision, four symptoms chosen from a list of eight are still required [13]. The choice of symptoms reflects one school of thought that holds that an infective and/or immune process underlies CFS. In contrast, the

British definition does not emphasise somatic symptoms, instead insisting on both physical and mental fatigue and fatigability.

## Epidemiology

One of the key sources of confusion in this confused subject is the absence of sound epidemiological data [15, 16]. Chronic fatigue is one of the commonest symptoms encountered in the community. To take examples at random from a substantial literature, in one British community survey 38% of the sample reported substantial fatigue, which had been present for over 6 months in 18% [17]. In Germany 26.2% of a population survey in Mannheim complained of "states of fatigue and exhaustion" over a 7-day period [18]. Similar figures are encountered in other Western countries [19]. A point prevalence of 21% for fatigue of 6 months' duration, associated with other somatic symptoms such as sore throat, myalgia, and headache, was recorded in an American ambulatory care survey [20]. 32% of those attending an Israeli general practice reported at least one asthenic symptom [21]. Slightly lower prevalence are reported in British and Canadian primary care, where between 10% to 14% will admit to chronic fatigue [22, 23]. It was the principal reason for consultation in 7% of new attenders in primary care in France and Canada [23, 24].

So chronic fatigue is common, but what about chronic fatigue syndrome? Early estimates based on selected samples or key informant studies suggested it was rare, but these assumptions are now being challenged [16]. Recent studies with systematic case ascertainment report a different picture. Bates et al. [25] surveyed an American Ambulatory care clinic. In keeping with the literature 27% of those attending a primary care clinic had substantial fatigue lasting more than 6 months and interfering with daily life. The point prevalence of CFS according to the various definitions was 0.3% (CDC-1988), 0.4% (UK) and 1.0% (Australian), respectively. In a study of a Health Maintenance Organisation in Seattle, Buchwald and colleagues report a prevalence between 0.07% to 0.3%, depending on the assumptions made [26]. Similar findings will emerge from a random household survey carried out in San Francisco [27]. 1.6% of employees in a large office complex in California reported previous diagnoses of CFS [28], whilst 1% of a sample of US nurses satisfied criteria for CFS [29].

In a primary care study from the United Kingdom, CFS had prevalence ranging from 0.8% (CDC 1988) to 1.8% (CDC 1994) [30]. Many of these were comorbid with common psychiatric disorders, but even when these had been excluded the prevalence of CFS was 0.5% (CDC 1994) or 0.7% (Oxford criteria). In Scotland the prevalence was 0.6%, although the sample size was relatively small [31].

What can we conclude from these results? First, that estimates of prevalence based on selected samples (specialist centres or key informants) both underestimate prevalence, and, as we will see later, emphasise features of the disorder that turn out to be atypical. Nearly all those who fulfilled operational criteria for CFS were not labelled as such by either themselves or their general practitioners, and thus would not be identified in a key informant survey, or a tertiary setting [30]. Others might be reluctant, or unable, to access health care [32]. Among the vast numbers of subjects with excessive fatigue, only 1% believed themselves to be suffering from CFS [33]. This emphasises just how few of those who could be classified as CFS are labelled as CFS, or seek specialist help, and highlights the powerful role of selection bias in previous studies, which are almost all based on tertiary care samples of patients who have frequently made their own diagnosis before seeking specialist help, and are almost certainly an atypical and unrepresentative sample of CFS cases [34, 35].

Relevant prevalence data can also be obtained from studies using the ICD-10 criteria for neurasthenia, which has considerable overlap with CFS (see contribution from Lin). In the Zurich longitudinal survey, Merikangas and Angst reported prevalence of 6% for men and 10% for women [36]. The recent multinational WHO study of mental disorder in primary care reported a prevalence of ICD-10 neurasthenia of 5.5% [37].

It should be by now be clear that we are talking about two separate constructs here. The first is an operationally defined condition as it appears in either ICD-10 (under the label of either post-viral fatigue syndrome or neurasthenia) or in the definitions of CFS proposed by the Center for Disease Control. This is a construct that is susceptible to conventional epidemiological analysis. Such analyses are starting to suggest that CFS is more common than hittherto supposed, and that the stereotype so beloved of the anglophone media, of the high-achieving, female urban professional, is just that, a stereotype. On the other hand, we have the sociological concept of CFS, in this case better appreciated under its vernacular labels such as ME, CFIDS, low natural killer cell syndrome and the like. Now we are dealing with a belief—the belief that one is suffering from an illness of that name. Our studies have shown that many of those who fulfil criteria for CFS do not view themselves in that light—conversely many of those presenting to doctors saying "I have ME" do not fulfil criteria for CFS.

A failure to appreciate these distinctions can lead to numerous confusions. For example, the over-representation amongst those who consider themselves to have CFS of professions such as teachers or doctors have led to numerous speculations about the possible aetiological relevance of certain exposures, such as viral infections. Likewise, the dramatic over-representation of upper social classes has caused some to consider the aetiological relevance of differing standards of hygiene—such speculations being both unironic and in ignorance of similar observations made by their Victorian predecessors.

This division also raises many questions very relevant to the theme of this book. Perhaps the most tantalising relates to the epidemiology not of operationally defined CFS, but of the label of CFS. To date this is largely confined to the English-speaking world, and has achieved a remarkable prominence in the United States, Canada, Australia, New Zealand and Great Britain. It has also done well in the Netherlands, and to a lesser extent in Sweden and Norway. It has not prospered elsewhere. The events that triggered the spectacular rise of CFS in, for example, Britain and the United States, have happened elsewhere. There seems little doubt, for example, that the immediate trigger for the explosion of interest in Great Britain was an article ("An illness doctors don't recognise") by Sue Finlay in the *Observer* of June 1st 1986, relating her own experiences as a sufferer. Yet similar articles have emerged in similarly influential newspapers in France and Spain, and no doubt elsewhere, but without the same impact. Or, to take another example, I believe that CFS would not have caught the popular imagination in both Britain and the United States without the early appearance of professional validation in the form of scientific papers in the medical journals. But similar articles have also appeared in the German and Italian medical press, whilst anyway medical publication is now a global enterprise. There are indeed doctors in these countries who do subscribe to the CFS concept, and energetically pursue research and clinical activity in the field, but it is my impression these have not been accorded particular recognition. Likewise, if we judge professional interest by the pattern of reprint requests, and lay interest by the flow of letters, whether congratulatory or condemnatory, then CFS has not "caught on" in any of, for example, the countries of southern Europe.

I have no explanation for what I suspect is a key observation. Whereas I believe that CFS/neurasthenia is a universal form of human distress, the modern representation of CFS has only been accepted in certain societies. I suspect that the talents of other contributors to this volume are better able to explain this very striking discrepancy.

## Dimension Versus Category

The next role of epidemiology is to emphasise the arbitrary nature of case definitions of CFS. There is considerable evidence to support a dimensional, rather than a categorical, view, of the core symptom of fatigue. Population and primary care studies leave little doubt that fatigue and asthenia is best described along a continuous distribution [22, 33]. Not just fatigue, but all the symptoms and disabilities used to construct the diagnosis of CFS are dimensionally distributed in the community.

So far no one has provided sound evidence from a population-based study of a discrete syndrome of excessive fatigue, called CFS or anything else [16]. However, even if chronic fatigue is a dimensional variable that cannot be easily separated from the normal sensation and experience of tiredness, it still requires understanding and treatment. Because one cannot detect a clear-cut division between "normal" fatigue and the devastating illness so vividly detailed in the numerous first-person accounts of CFS sufferers, this no more invalidates the latter than the dimensional view of blood pressure invalidates the medical importance of severe hypertension. Cases of CFS, whether studied in primary care or specialist clinics, have levels of functional impairment greatly in excess of that found for all comparative chronic conditions such as ischaemic heart disease, arthritis, or chronic bronchitis, and have major occupational, personal, and recreational impairment [30, 38]. However, to a certain extent this is tautologous, since all definitions emphasise functional impairment as part of the CFS criteria.

# Aetiology

## CFS: An Infective Disorder?

At present the majority of those seen in specialist clinics trace their illness to the aftermath of a viral infection, with the curious exception of Japan, where most CFS patients do not recall such an association [39]. However, such factors as the frequency of common viral infections, recall bias and search after meaning suggest that more evidence is required before accepting that the cause of "post-viral fatigue" is an infective agent.

The example of the enteroviruses provides a cautionary tale. It has been strongly argued that a major cause of CFS is persistent infection by the Coxsackie virus. A sequence of reports have provided evidence of an association between infection and CFS, only for subsequent studies to fail to replicate each claim. A new method of diagnosis then appears, only for the sequence to be repeated. Other agents have also been proposed, such as retroviruses, HHV-6, and others, but none have been associated with convincing evidence (see Refs. [3, 40]).

At present the infective agent for which the best evidence exists for a post-infectious syndrome is the Epstein Barr virus (EBV), the virus that causes glandular fever. It was reports of an association between CFS and EBV that triggered the current revival of interest in CFS in the United States. These original studies are now seen as flawed [40], and there is no evidence for reactivation of EBV in CFS [41]. In the USA interest in the EBV virus has waned. However, researchers at St Bartholomew's Hospital lead by Peter White have completed the first prospective cohort study of the outcome of EBV. In a meticulously designed and executed study, they provided firm evidence that EBV is associated with a post-infection fatigue syndrome that is both more frequent than, and can be distinguished from, anxiety and depressive illnesses [42, 43]. Unlike depressive illnesses arising after EBV, the post-infectious syndrome was not associated with concurrent measures of life events [44]. Nevertheless, even after EBV prolonged fatigue is the exception rather than the rule. Of 337 cases presenting to a student health centre only 1.5% developed prolonged fatigue [45], and the median duration of fatigue is only 12 weeks [43]. As well as EBV, it also seems likely that Q fever should be added to the list of infections for which there is reasonable longitudinal evidence for a particular post-infectious syndrome [46].

So what can we say about the very common clinical situation in which people present to doctors with chronic fatigue, which they attribute to an otherwise unremarkable viral infection? Two studies from my institution have clarified matters. Cope and colleagues prospectively studied the outcome of viral infection in primary care [47]. They reported a modestly increased rate of fatigue in subjects 6 months after presenting to the GP with a symptomatic "viral" infection, but this is open to doubt because of the inadequate control group. We recruited over a thousand subjects attending general practice with symptomatic viral infections, and an equal number of controls attending for other reasons. Six months later there was no difference in chronic fatigue and CFS between those previously exposed to a virus, and those presenting with a range of other problems [48]. The same study also reported a strong association between measures of fatigue and psychological vulnerability completed before presenting to the general practitioner with a viral infection, and fatigue assessed 6 months later. Cope and colleagues also analysed the predictors of fatigue in their post-viral group. They found that somatic attributional style, less definite diagnosis by the GP, and the provision of sick note were the only significant predictors of chronic fatigue [47].

We can now bring these strands together. To date I believe that there are only five factors for which there is sufficient evidence from well conducted longitudinal factors to suggest a relationship with fatigue after infection. It will be seen that a variety of factors—infective, physiological and psychological—are involved.

- Epstein Barr virus infection
- Premorbid psychological disorder
- Somatic attributional style
- Encephalitis
- Physical deconditioning.

We have thus learnt to show more caution about overenthusiastic espousal of links between specific infection and CFS. Infective triggers for CFS do remain on the agenda, although the wealth of evidence reporting cases of CFS arising after a number of agents, viral, bacterial, and even protozoal, suggests that the condition is more likely to represent a non-specific response to a number of infective (and non-infective) agents, than solely attributable to any single agent [40]. Dividing cases into those that were apparently triggered by an infection and those that were not does not appear to identify a distinct subgroup [49, 50], although dividing subjects into those with acute or chronic onsets may have promise [51, 52].

## CFS and the Sense of Effort

Given that fatigue and myalgia are so central to CFS, it is understandable that several authors have suggested that a disorder of muscle function underlies the condition. The literature contains several papers with evidence of biochemical, functional, and structural abnormalities of muscle. However, the evidence for a neuromuscular origin to the symptoms of CFS is far from convincing. First, most agree that physical *and* mental fatigue and fatigability are at the heart of CFS, and cannot be accounted for by any known mechanism of muscular function. The neuropsychiatric symptoms of CFS, such as poor concentration, short-term memory impairment and so on, are not those of peripheral neuromuscular disorders [8, 53]. Some evidence has been presented of abnormalities in muscle structure, or on neurophysiological testing, such as single fibre EMG. However, these studies have largely either not been replicated, or could be explained as the consequences of inactivity, a sine qua non of the diagnosis of CFS. Meticulously conducted studies of dynamic muscle function have in general failed to show any evidence of peripheral neuromuscular dysfunction or delayed post-exertional muscle fatigability. Some, but not all, groups have also reported a disorder of the perception of effort—CFS patients rate themselves as more fatigued than they actually are, and thus cease work at an earlier stage than indicated by the state of their muscles.

The important message is that "On physiological and pathological grounds it is clear that CFS is not a myopathy" [54]. These observations are of direct clinical relevance, since the implication is that patients can be strongly reassured that physical activity is unlikely to be harmful, provided that it takes place within the limits of the subject's current physical status.

Sufferers from chronic fatigue report that not only is physical exercise associated with increased effort, so is mental activity. Pierre Janet recognised the same when he wrote that "Tiredness and a horrible sense of fatigue is caused in psychasthenics by the least sense of physical or psychological effort . . . fatigue rapidly affects sensations and perceptions, intellect and movement" [55]. A modern series of studies of neuropsychological function have yet to lead to any greater insights—in general the severity of subjective reports of difficulties in memory and concentration is not matched by evidence of equivalent deficits in neuropsychological testings, and although abnormalities of sustained attention, motor execution and information processing speed seem to be reproducible, the clinical significance of these findings is unclear. In some, but by no means all studies, adjustment for psychological distress removes these differences. Another explanation is that they may also be a relatively straightforward manifestation of acute fatigue caused by sleep deficits rather than evidence of underlying cerebral dysfunction [56].

Overall these findings are reminiscent of the results of formal studies of neuromuscular function in CFS, where evidence was found of a dissociation between subjective and objective reports of muscle dysfunction. One group has recently reported that not only are sufferers' subjective accounts of their physical activity not matched by the results of objective testings, actual recording of activity undertaken after an exercise challenge also does not reveal the substantial reductions in post-exercise activity so vividly described in the many first-person accounts of illness. What seems to be emerging is a picture of a mismatch between the subject's own perception of cognitive disturbance, and the level of actual decrements in performance determined on testing [57]. Although selective attention may be impaired, formal deficits in memory appear increasing unlikely [58]. This mismatch between subjective and objective dysfunction poses both challenges and difficulties.

The challenge is to find an underlying mechanism to link these observations. CFS may thus be associated with a disorder of effortful cognition, rather than any actual deficits in recall, just as it is associated with an increased sense of motor effort, rather than any objective deficits in neuromuscular function. It is this reviewer's opinion that studies of the sense of effort, and its neuropsychological basis, will be amongst the most profitable lines of future inquiry [59].

The difficulty is the one experienced by clinicians confronted with CFS patients. Clinicians, and presumably others as well, frequently report this conundrum. Most clinicians will, particularly if they are talking "off the record" express their bemusement when they encounter a patient whose principal complaint is of poor memory and concentration, yet maintains a lively interest during a prolonged consultation. A recent study of the "posts" made to Internet discussion groups for a variety of chronic illnesses found that those with CFS made the longest contributions, as well as the greatest self references [60]. Numerous similar anecdotes are the staple of medical conversations about CFS (although rarely given written form), and provide ammunition for sceptics, immense difficulties for sufferers, and a question for academics. Given that this author, who has an immense clinical experience with CFS sufferers, totally rejects the occasional allegation of deliberate misleading of clinicians or fabrication of disability by sufferers, it begs us to ask the question what exactly is the experience of disability in CFS, given that it is not simply a result of a disorder of neuromuscular or neuropsychological function.

## CFS: An Immunological or Allergic Disorder?

There is an influential school of thought that CFS is an immunological disorder, partly because the symptoms reported by sufferers (sore throats, swollen glands, allergies) seem reminiscent of immune dysfunction (although these symptoms are not specific to CFS). There has been a great deal of research using the tools of modern immunology, and, although evidence has been presented of alterations in various immune parameters, it is difficult to place these in perspective.

A number of abnormalities have been noted, chief amongst which are impairment of natural killer cell activity, and of T-cell subsets. In particular, three groups have noted a reduced ratio of CD4/CD45 RA T cells (see Ref. [61]). It has been argued that this represents the response of the immune system to chronic antigen stimulation. However, there is great deal of overlap between cases and controls, no relationship to clinical status, and even this finding has not been reported by all investigators. A similar finding has been reported in major depression [62], although there are also differences between the immune findings in CFS and in less severe depressive conditions [63]. Even if immune parameters are abnormal in a subgroup, no one has ever presented data of actual immune impairment.

The most recent reviews have concluded that it is currently impossible to determine the significance of the observed changes in immunological status in CFS. One authority suggests that these changes are those of a hyperactive immune system secondary to viral infection [64]. Levy argues that this chronically active immune system is thus reacting against the host as in autoimmune disorders. Recent research showing an increase in detectable autoantibodies supports this view [65]. As autoimmune diseases are commoner in women, Levy further argues that this provides one explanation for the increased prevalence of CFS in women [66]. Another group of experts see the immunological changes as primary leading to secondary evidence of viral reactivation—hence CFS is a disorder of immune regulation of viral activity, Yet scientists at NIH have written "the possibility that the immunological findings in CFS are also found in more classic psychological diseases remains very much alive . . . perhaps secondary to subtle endocrine changes, characteristic of certain abnormal psychological states" [67]. The next generation of studies of immune dysfunction and CFS must certainly consider the possibility that observed changes are secondary to the alterations in HPA function described elsewhere (vide infra).

## CFS: A Psychiatric Disorder?

### Prevalence of Psychiatric Disorder

Turning to CFS, numerous studies have been published concerning the role of psychiatric disorder [3]. A variety of instruments and operational criteria have been used, leading, not surprisingly, to considerable variety in the result. In one of the earliest studies approximately half of those seen in specialist care with a diagnosis of one or other form of CFS fulfilled criteria for affective disorder, even with fatigue removed from the criteria for mood disorder [8]. A further quarter fulfilled criteria for other psychiatric disorders, chief amongst which are anxiety and somatisation disorders. Between one quarter to one third did not fulfil any criteria. The figures for the comorbidity of neurasthenia and psychiatric disorders are also congruent with these findings—in the multinational WHO study of mental disorder in primary care [37], ICD-10 neurasthenia showed 71% psychiatric comorbidity.

Affective disorder is thus linked with CFS, but the association is not a simple one. First, the pattern of mood disorder is not always that with which psychiatrists are most familiar, and there is a suggestion that the atypical depressive disorders (in which there is increased sleep and appetite rather than the more customary decrease) may be more relevant. Assessing the phenomenology of depressive illness in CFS subjects is not always straightforward—difficulties can arise in distinguishing anhedonia from an inability to perform previously enjoyable activities.

Most studies and reviews on the subject of CFS and psychiatric disorder, including those by the current author, have tended to emphasise the role of depressive illness rather than anxiety disorders. However, this is probably unjustified. Anxiety disorders are also common [68], but often overlooked, partly because of the difficulties in determining whether or not avoidance is related to phobic processes, or neuromuscular weakness, whilst current behavioural formulations of CFS emphasise the key role played by fearful cognitions in determining avoidance behaviour and disability (vide infra). The neurobiology may also show closer overlaps with anxiety rather than depressive disorders. The emphasis on depression at the expense of anxiety may reflect both the hierarchial nature of psychiatric disorder, the demise of the rich historical tradition of neurocirculatory asthenia, effort syndrome, Soldier's heart and their close associations with anxiety disorders [69, 70], and the general shift of fashion and diagnostic preference from anxiety to depression [71]. Hyperventilation can play an important role in some patients. There have been claims that hyperventilation was found in all CFS patients [72]. Like any unitary explanation of CFS, this seems implausible, but a systematic study did suggest that between 10% and 25% of patients may have evidence of hyperventilation [73].

## Explanations

If psychiatric disorders are common, what are the possible explanations? One is artefactual—the criteria used to diagnose common psychological disorders overlap with those for the diagnosis of CFS. High rates of psychiatric disorders in CFS are thus inevitable, and do not themselves imply causality. As Kendell has written in the context of CFS, "the statement that someone has a depressive illness is merely a statement about their symptoms. It has no causal implications" [74].

The next explanation is that these are simply misdiagnosed cases of depression and anxiety (e.g., ref. [75]). This must be true for some, and there are many subjects for whom the standard psychiatric classification, explanations, and treatments are adequate to the situation. In its severe form the symptoms of CFS and those of major depression are hard to distinguish [76], and it is also known that depressive disorder alone is associated with severe functional impairment [77].

However, this unitary explanation flounders on the reasons outlined in the previous paragraph, since, with the occasional exception, it implies an implicit hierarchy of symptomatic classification. It also ignores the fact that in many there are insufficient grounds to justify a psychiatric diagnosis.

Could the observed psychological disorder simply be a reaction to physical illness? This explanation is the least appealing, since first there is as yet no definitive evidence of a specific physical pathology, and second at least seven studies that use medical controls find rates of psychiatric disorder in the CFS cases that are invariably in excess of those in the control, often substantially so. Alternatively, could it be due to selection bias? Again, this is unlikely, since a similar proportion seen in primary care with chronic fatigue or chronic fatigue syndrome also fulfil criteria for psychiatric disorder [78], although in many other ways the samples are different (vide supra).

The final explanation suggest that CFS and psychiatric disorder arises from a common pathology. This argument must therefore involve some common neurobiological dysfunction.

## CFS: A Neurobiological Disorder?

Models linking CFS with muscular dysfunction no longer find much favour. That interest has largely been transferred to studies of possible central nervous or neuroendocrine disorder. This is a welcome development, since, unlike muscular studies, this paradigm is closer to the clinical features of the condition. It is intriguing that a similar shift from peripheral to central models also occurred during the Victorian involvement with neurasthenia.

The first line of evidence comes from studies of neuroendocrine function. Several lines of inquiry have centred on neuroendocrine aspects of CFS. First, there is the relationship between mood disorder, with its well documented abnormalities in neuroendocrine function. Second, some have pointed out the similarities between CFS and glucocorticoid deficiency. Severe fatigue (including post-exertional fatigue), myalgia, arthralgia, mood and sleep disturbances occur in both. In a groundbreaking study, Demitrack and colleagues from the National Institutes of Health investigated hypothalamic-pituitary adrenal (HPA) activity in a series of 30 patients with CFS compared to 72 normal controls [79]. The patients had lower urinary excretion rates of free cortisol and reduced evening plasma cortisol concentrates in conjunction with an elevated plasma ACTH. The adrenal cortex was hypersensitive to low doses of ACTH, with a blunted ceiling response. ACTH responses to CRH were attenuated, despite low ambient cortisol levels (which therefore cannot be exerting an inhibitory feedback effect). The findings were compatible with impaired function at the level of the hypothalamus which is compromising CRH synthesis/secretion.

Subsequent studies have tended to support these findings, and have also reported similar, albeit not identical, findings in the sister condition of fibromyalgia [80, 81], discussed by Maes (this volume). The picture is by no means complete, and it is still unclear exactly at what level, or levels, lies the primary neuroendocrine dysfunction. However, what has become clear is that in a subgroup of CFS (those without evidence of major depression) a pattern can be discerned of an underactive HPA system, which should be contrasted with the overactive pattern classic of severe depression. Indeed, one can speculate that CFS and depression lie along a continuum of serotonin activity in the central nervous system, reflected in differing patterns of HPA activity, and finally in differing patterns of exhaustion versus agitation, insomnia versus hypersomnia and so on.

At the same time, studies using agents that act at the 5-HT receptor have shown that 5-HT neurotransmission is increased relative to not only normal, but also depressed controls [82, 83]. Our group measured the prolactin response to D-fenfluramine, a selective 5-HT releasing agent. The prolactin response was highest in the CFS patients, lowest in the depressed subjects (as expected), and intermediate in the controls [84]. The tentative conclusion is that those CFS patients without concurrent depression show evidence of reduced HPA axis activity and increased 5-HT function, the mirror image of major depression. This might either explain (or be the result of) the clinical observation that CFS is characterised by hypersomnia and preserved appetite, in contrast to classic major depression. What remains to be seen is whether such abnormalities have any primary significance, or whether, as has been argued elsewhere, both they and the neuropsychological symptoms already discussed are epiphemenona of other variables, such as sleep disorder [56, 85]. Perhaps more relevant for this contribution is that such findings suggest that although chronic fatigue syndrome is, in many instances, one of the many ways in which patients with major depression can present to medical services, and thus can be considered as a prime example of Kirmayer and Robbins first form of somatisation [86]—the physical presentation of psychiatric disorder—this relatively simple formulation will not suffice for all cases.

## Somatisation and CFS

So far I have trod carefully over the minefield of the links between CFS and psychiatric disorder, and in particular have avoided discussion of the most contentious area of all, the relationship between CFS and somatisation. Patients with long histories of multiple somatic symptoms, stretching back to adolescence, are common in CFS clinics, as they are across general medicine [87]. They may have previous episodes of unexplained abdominal pain, food allergies, chemical sensitivities, unresolved gynaecological problems, funny turns, and so on. Some may fulfil criteria for somatisation disorder (Briquet's syndrome).

To a certain extent this overlap between CFS and somatisation disorder is predictable, since the definitions of both CFS and somatisation disorder require multiple symptoms [88]. When Lane and colleagues compared those with CFS with chronically fatigued patients who did not fulfil the criteria for CFS, one of chief differences between them was that the former were more likely to fulfil criteria for somatisation disorder [89]. They concluded that the multiple symptom criteria for CFS actively select for somatisation disorder. When another group of researchers excluded those symptoms common to the definitions of CFS and SD, the prevalence of SD fell, but was still substantially elevated at 20% [90]. Remember that the expected prevalence of somatisation disorder in community samples is of the order of 0.03% to 0.3% [91].

This relationship was further extended by Katon and Russo in 1992, who showed that the greater the number of somatic symptoms in subjects with CFS, the greater the probability of all psychiatric disorder [92]. Our group has also confirmed this in a primary care sample [93]. These findings links CFS with the mainstream of psychiatric epidemiology, since it has been repeatedly demonstrated that a linear relationship exists between the number of somatic symptoms, and the risk of psychiatric disorder [16, 94].

Somatisation disorder is thus found in CFS clinics, but it is not the commonest diagnostic category. Somatisation disorder is also not unique to CFS clinics, and a similar situation exists in general medical clinics. The best survey to date [87] found a prevalence in all new medical outpatients of 8%, rising to 14% in those with doubtful medical diagnoses, not dramatically different from the prevalence in CFS clinics.

On the other hand, somatisation disorder is very uncommon in the community—the expected community prevalences range from 0.03% to 0.3% [91]. It is also very uncommon in samples of chronically fatigued patients identified in general practice—

with a prevalence of 0.6% in the ECA sample [95]. No cases were found in two UK community samples [30, 78].

## The Relevance of Somatisation Disorder to CFS

Somatisation disorder is a necessary, if unwelcome (to physicians, at least) part of medical life, rather than something intrinsic to CFS. Donna Stewart documented how one sample of patients with "twentieth century disease," also known as total allergy syndrome, had at various times also been labelled as candidiasis, hypoglycaemia, and now chronic fatigue syndromes [96]. Elsewhere I have discussed the links between CFS and such apparently diverse subjects as dental amalgam disease, food allergy, and multiple chemical sensitivity [2]. One thread is the theme of somatisation—indeed, many would have consistently fulfilled criteria for SD throughout their illness careers, even if their own disease attribution changed. A cadre of such patients now appears in the guise of chronic fatigue syndrome, and often appear in the self-help or media literature. Such patients may not shed much light on the nature of chronic fatigue syndrome as it exists in general practice, but illuminate our understanding of the sociology of illness and illness behaviour. This will be the theme of the second part of this essay.

Various groups have started to recognise this problem. An impressive multidisciplinary Australian research team have presented data showing that a minority (27%) of those seen in a CFS clinic can be differentiated from the majority by such variables as duration, prognosis, psychological morbidity, and disability, and also an index of immunological dysfunction [97]. They argue that the minority group should be classified under the somatoform disorders, reserving the label CFS for those with shorter duration, fewer more "typical" symptoms, and less disability. The UK consensus criteria [14] also suggest that CFS should not be diagnosed if the subject fulfils criteria for somatisation disorder (whereas depression or anxiety are still compatible with a diagnosis of CFS).

The irony is that the same subjects for whom there is a growing consensus that the label of CFS is inappropriate are often those who cling most firmly to the diagnosis. It is ill advised to challenge disease attributions anyway, but particularly in this group with strong convictions, if any therapeutic alliance is to be maintained. Management of somatisation disorder is already far from simple. Thus although excluded from most current case definitions, and hence excluded from the research effort in CFS (in theory anyway), excluding them from the label of CFS/ME serves little purpose except to ensure that the patients do not consult you again.

## *Chronic Fatigue, Somatisation, and the Fear of Mental Illness*

Why do patients some patients with chronic fatigue somatise, or more, accurately, why do some patients with any unexplained medical symptom prefer to be seen as having a physical than a psychological disorder?

The answer is not hard to find. Underneath the ME/CFIDS movement is a strong and passionate anti-psychiatry rhetoric. This has not arisen as a result of the interest shown by psychiatrists in the topic (few have much knowledge of, or contact with, sufferers). The first wave of publicity surrounding ME in this country already showed the suspicion of psychological medicine that may be among its hallmarks. This publicity lead to the formation of the most radical of the patient's organisations in this country, the ME Action Campaign. In its first newsletter Claire Francis, the President of the Campaign and probably the most famous sufferer in Britain, wrote "psychiatry is the dustbin of the medical profession" [98].

At the heart of the ME/CFIDS movement is the rejection of any form of psychological causation or treatment. Being referred to a psychiatrist is "being blackballed," being on trial or "imprisoned for a crime I didn't do" [99]. Courtroom analogies are apt, since the atmosphere surrounding the condition is now an adversarial one, accompanied by a rhetoric of struggle and injustice—a typical headline in one of our serious newspapers was "Justice for the neglected and maligned sufferers of ME." Paul Cheney, one of the most prominent doctors on the CFIDS scene in the United States, says that "we who believe that this is a real disease are almost in a death grip with those forces who would stifle debate, trivialize this problem, and banish patients who suffer from it beyond the edges of traditional medicine" [100]. A leading ME campaigner compared the plight of ME sufferers in Britain to the 27 years incarceration of Nelson Mandela and the ordeal of the Beirut hostages [101]. Such analogies run the risk of overstatement, but attest to the passions involved. Others speak of bitterness, anger, and hate. The accusation is not just that the sufferer is guilty of being depressed, or of having a psychiatric disorder, but of not being ill at all—of being a malingerer, of having an imaginary disease. It would be tedious to list the number of variations on the theme of "ME exists. It is not a psychological illness" that can be found in the media and popular literature. Curiously enough, such anti-psychiatry rhetoric does not seem to be prominent amongst the majority of sufferers, at least not those attending our service (Wood and Wessely, unpublished data).

External attribution, implicit in the process of somatisation, protects the patient from the stigma of being labelled psychiatrically disordered [102]. Viruses are the commonest attribution encountered in the specialist setting—partly because they are so common, partly because some infections are indeed associated with increased risk, but also because, with the possible exception of HIV, the victim of a viral infection is blameless [103]. In the context of CFS "to attribute the continuing symptoms to persistence of a "physical" disease is a mechanism that carries the least threat to a person's self esteem" [104]. The reviewer of one self-help book for a British newspaper wrote "an infection is respectable. It has none of the stigma of a psychologically induced illness, which implies weakness or lack of moral fibre" [105]. "Patients who suffer from unrelenting fatigue fear they have a serious, occult medical problem and worry that people will think they had a mental problem or a blameworthy characterological weakness of will" [75]. One sufferer put it at its simplest—"increasingly convinced that I had contracted some kind of 'bug' that was steadily destroying my health, I determined to identify and eliminate the evil foreign agent"[106].

In a previous paper I discussed how the popular literature on ME was suffused with the underlying message that psychological disorders in general, and depression in particular, were diagnoses to be avoided [99]. Sometimes such conditions are seen as unreal or non-existent—"all in the mind." At other times they are viewed as a moral judgement on the sufferer—something reflecting qualities such as lack of effort, poor motivation, and so on. Hence when a chronically fatigued patient is diagnosed as depressed, this can be equated with the message that the sufferer is not really ill, malingering, shirking their duties, and so on.

Regrettably, such impressions are by no means inaccurate. Such perceptions, which to a practising psychiatrist seem ill informed and naive, are all too often shared by the medical profession. Some doctors do equate psychological disorder with unreal disorder. A consultant physician who specialises in the disorder told a newspaper that "People with PVFS often have to put up with a lot of disbelief—there were many doctors who diagnosed this as a psychiatric disorder although on the whole it is taken much more seriously now" [107]. A doctor agreed that it is important that psychiatric patients are separated from ME because "some neurotic patients devalue the tales of genuine sufferers" [108]. Another is quoted as telling a medical conference that "ME is an imaginary disease ... for which the best treatment is psychiatric" [109].

Writing about the rise, and subsequent fall, of psychosomatic explanations for ulcerative colitis, Aronowitz and Spiro [110] note that an uncomfortable attribute of the psychosomatic concept is the potential it has for blaming the patient for the disease. According to anthropologist Norma Ware who has conducted a study of CFIDS patients in Boston, it "places the responsibility for illness on the shoulders of patients and, consequently, increases their suffering" [111]. A recent article on chronic Lyme disease talked about the difficulties faced by patients in their dealing with doctors—"some were even considered malingerers. Many were referred to psychiatrists when their medical physicians lost faith in the validity of their patients' complaints" [112]. Doctors thus share many of the prejudices of the ME/CFIDS sufferer—psychiatrists treat imaginary, malingered, or non-existent diseases.

The consequences of this lack of validation are many. There is little doubt that those who later receive a diagnosis of ME/CFIDS recall the previous lack of a diagnosis which they could accept as a source of distress, and react with relief when the label of ME is given [113, 114], even if they are also told that the disorder is untreatable. "The day Nomi Antelman learned she had an incurable disease, she rejoiced" [115]. Another sufferer was first told she had a virus that would go away. Later this optimistic prognosis was altered, as she learnt she had ME which would, in her own words, take away her independence, regress her to a being a baby and in which progress would be minimal. She "felt fantastic" [116].

Psychological diagnoses are unacceptable for a variety of reasons, both emotional and practical. One sufferer was refused sickness insurance benefit because his policy excluded depression, of which he had a past history. His claim to be now suffering from ME was rejected, although he was informed that this decision would be changed if a test for ME were to be developed and he tested positive [117]. Hence sufferers cannot afford to be depressed, both symbolically and literally.

## CFS as a Twentieth-Century Disease

At an early stage CFS was characterised as a new disease. One of the first papers on sporadic CFS began "A 'new disease' is spreading in the civilised world" [118]—incidentally also reinforcing the message that CFS is also restricted to Western settings. By 1987 "the diagnosis of the year" was chronic Epstein Barr virus [119]—the following year and across the Atlantic "there is no doubt that *the* illness of the year is ME" [120]. In order to maintain this "newness" it is necessary to update the period, so that from the "Malaise of the 80s" [121], CFS has become the "disease of the 90s" [122, 123] and even "disease of the fast paced 21st century" [124]. The single most common headline chosen for newspaper articles on ME is "The ME Generation."

If this is a new disease, then some new cause must be found to explain its sudden appearance. Another article entitled "the ME Generation" opened with the words "What is modern life doing to us?" [125]. The most frequent answer to that question invokes the concept of the immune system in trouble, weakening under the assault of late twentieth century life. "ME is very much a disease of our time—an attack on the immune system exacerbated by stress, pressure and the demands of twentieth century life" [126].

There is a body of scientific literature on immune dysfunction in CFS, but it is inconsistent and unclear, and there is little evidence of any relevant immune deficiency. In contrast the popular literature on ME/CFIDS makes much of the immune system, which provides a link with most of the other twentieth century diseases. "Weakening" of the immune system is at the heart of the popular models of CFIDS—this can be the result of viral infections, nutritional deficiencies, chemicals, candida, and so on [127]—indeed, one of the acceptable ways in the popular literature acknowledges a role for psychological factors and even depression is via their alleged effect on the immune system.

As a result of this onslaught ME is "an overload disease unique to this century" [109], since "the body can tolerate so much stress from whatever source, but at some point the bucket gets full" [128]. One frequently encountered contemporary source of this "overload" is the alleged over-prescription of antibiotics causing altered immunity. Another regular culprit is immunisation. Claire Francis, best selling author and former yachtswoman, traces her illness to childhood when she "was given her first polio vaccine injection" from which "she never really recovered" [129]. On another occasion she has labelled ME "an immune dysfunction disease, possibly caused by pollution" [130]. From whatever source the resulting strain on the immune system destroys the ability to resist infections such as viruses (hence post-viral fatigue) or candida, and also food allergies and intolerances that have previously been "hidden." Numerous popular books and magazines link this immune dysfunction with the air we breathe, the water we drink and the food we eat, all of them contributing to our "toxic lifestyle."

Such explanations are not mutually exclusive—indeed, the opposite is true. "Never in history have people been exposed to greater assaults on their bodies by environmental pollution. Food additives and drugs may also harm the body and adversely affect the immune system. Certain doctors even claim that long term antibiotics depress the immune system" [131].

What are the cultural sources of these explanations? HIV is one. "Who had heard of AIDS or ME . . . 10 years ago?" [132]. Some of the popular literature makes explicit a link between CFS and AIDS. CFS is "AIDS minor" or a "sister illness to AIDS" [133]. According to the President of the CFIDS Association in the USA "you would have to blind not to make the connection" (Marc Iverson, cited in ref. [133]). A complete issue of a New York magazine was devoted to making the links between AIDS and CFIDS—CFS was "the bottom of the AIDS iceberg." We are told that "Doctors at Harvard Medical School have gone so far as to question whether AIDS is actually a chronic and fatal form of ME" [134]. Thus when it was announced that researchers had identified a retrovirus in patients with CFS, the storm of publicity was not entirely unexpected. The subsequent failure of other researchers to confirm this finding went largely unnoticed.

I have already noted how the term CFIDS (chronic fatigue and immune deficiency syndrome) has been adopted by the largest patient's organisation in the United States. Some of the decision to adopt this name has been a conscious and stated attempt to draw upon the awareness, publicity, and political activism that surrounds AIDS. Another reason lies in the popular grasp of the HIV metaphor—the invisible but deadly virus destroying the immune system. Abbey and Garfinkel note that "CFS is built upon two of the most interesting themes in modern medicine, infectious disease and immunology" [5]. The result of the HIV epidemic is that the concept of a mysterious yet deadly virus that infects the immune system is now firmly in the popular consciousness, and provides an apparently scientific framework for what are other concerns.

Another source for the assault on the immune system comes from contemporary views on internal purity and pollution. These concerns appear in the literature linking candida infection of the gut, altered immunity, and CFIDS. The latter may be due to a "persistent and slight infection of intestines" [135]. In these formulations the candida infection itself, or the "toxins" it produces, or even simply the products of digestion, leak into the body and cause autointoxication, affecting, inevitably, the immune system. Thus "yeast toxins weaken your immune system" [127], but when your immune system is weak you develop yeast infections, illustrating the essential circularity of these models. For the ME patient candida is one more addition to the climate of fear—after all, the infection spreads to the "digestive tract, the lungs, the brain, the toenails. It was feasting on me" [136]. In consequence colonic lavage is now a common treatment for ME in the United Kingdom.

## CFS Is Not a Twentieth-Century Illness

The range of aetiologies visible in the popular literature on CFIDS and ME thus superficially reflect a variety of contemporary concerns—but just how contemporary are they? The answer is not very much. Even the claim to be modern is far from modern. The parent of CFS, neurasthenia, was also a "disease of our time." The phrase "disease of the century" was frequently used in the context of neurasthenia also described as "a bitter comment on 19th century life" [137]. Neurasthenia too was held to becoming more common, and to be a disease of civilisation, often expressed in racial tones that would be impossible today.

What about aetiologies? The modern popular explanations of "overload" from viruses, pollution, and stress all have strong resonances with the mechanisms and causes advanced for neurasthenia during the last century [1,5]. Neurasthenia was seen as an exhaustion of the supply of energy within the central nervous system, causing "cortical weakness" or "cortical irritability." The causes were either local to the brain—a failure of cerebral blood flow (claims of which currently dominate media coverage on ME one hundred years later) or a deficiency in energy sources, or arise from distant sources. The increased demands on the system could be the result of toxic, metabolic, or infective insults. The idea that neurasthenia was the result of acute or chronic infection was the subject of numerous papers (see ref. [6]).

Even the idea that we are slowly poisoning our bodies from our intestines is far from new. As Shorter has pointed out, thousands of women lost various intestinal organs during the vogue of autointoxication and focal infection. The former idea, that the products of the colon can leak into the blood stream causing toxic symptoms, was part of Victorian medical culture. Guy's Hospital surgeon Willie Lane made his reputation removing such colons at the start of this century, ending his career as a surgical Baronet.

Overload was thus the mechanism that the Victorians most commonly invoked to explain neurasthenia—but the cause of this overload was variously attributed to the deteriorating quality of life, to new organisms, new stresses, new ways of working, the decline of leisure, and the increasingly decadent and acquisitive nature of society.

I have shown how the concept of ME arising from overwork either at the start of illness, or alternatively excessive activity during illness, is central to the modern popular view of aetiology. But overwork, stress, and strain is not unique to our time either. The neurasthenia experts were equally preoccupied with the deleterious consequences of overwork, which they too blamed on a variety of contemporary changes in society. Medical authorities viewed emotional strain and overwork, the agent by which the nervous system became exhausted (which could be purely physical, mental or a mixture of both), as the inevitable consequence of a host of new social ills. Even before the introduction of neurasthenia, a variety of medical authorities were writing about the dangers of overwork [138]. George Beard, the father of neurasthenia, with his facility for similes, joined together a number of discontents into an explanatory model for his disease. For example, Beard, and many others, ascribed neurasthenia to the new, acquisitive nature of society, singling out, in a famous phrase, wireless telegraphy, science, steam power, newspapers, and the education of women, summed up as "modern civilisation" [139]. Much of this was conveyed by similes drawn from business life (the exhausted businessman overdrawn on his nervous capital, overspent nervous resources and others) or from technology (the flat battery, the battery that could not give its charge). Mental strain was similarly implicated—in France public inquiries and commissions considered the problem of neurasthenic children, blamed on the alleged excessive mental demands ("surménage") made by the new education system [138]—and similar views could be found on the other side of the Atlantic.

The dramatic rise of neurasthenia seemed to confirm its status as a disease of modern civilisation. Just as CFS today is the price paid for pollution, exhaust fumes, food additives, aerosols, antibiotics, and so on, neurasthenia was the price to be paid for industrialisation, the rise of capitalism, and the consequent strains to which the business and professional classes were exposed [140].

## CFS and Other Modern Illnesses

The illness models that surface in the popular conceptualisation of CFS are far from unique to that condition. Professional studies frequently refer to the symptomatic overlap between CFS and sick building syndrome [28, 141], candida [142], multiple chemical sensitivity [143], irritable bowel syndrome [144], premenstrual syndrome [145], and between each other. If one ignores the scientific aridity of consensus conferences and operational criteria and moves into the world of patient literature, then the similarities are overwhelming. The list of symptoms held to be typical of CFS reappears in texts on yeast infections, food allergies, electromagnetic sensitivity, hypo-glycaemia, sick building syndrome, dental amalgam, chemical sensitivity, and others. The explanations are similar, and overlap. CFS causes candida, candida is a cause of CFS. William Crook sold nearly a million copies of his book "The Yeast Connection" [146]. In 1992 he then published "Chronic Fatigue Syndrome and the Yeast Connection" [127]. Candidiasis is both a cause of CFS, and the result of CFS, a her-metic system of which any psychoanalyst would be proud. Similarly, dental amalgam disease, a very popular concept in Scandinavia, is a syndrome once again consisting of multiple physical symptoms, this time due to the mysterious toxic properties of mercury amalgam, leaking into our bodies and poisoning our immune system. It is another cause of CFS—some of my patients have had all their dental fillings removed at considerable pain and expense but for little benefit. Shorter has traced the history of multiple chemical sensitivity, which depends upon the concept of immune system dysfunction, as does food allergy [147]. Of the 30 self-help books that I possess on CFS, few fail to include some mention of themes such as food allergy, environmental sensitivity, hypoglycaemia, candida, and so on. These are seen partly as aetiological factors for CFS, partly as overlapping diagnoses, and partly as complications.

Nowhere is this clearer than in the overlap between ME/CFIDS and allergy. ME is a form of severe allergy for many, and most self-help books include large sections on allergy. One sufferer from ME relates how he became a total allergic—"this is a slightly dramatic state because if anyone walked into our house wearing after-shave, bang, I'd pass out" [101]. A doctor with ME proved to be allergic to over 100 different foods [148]. A young farmer with ME was tested by a clinical ecologist, and found to be "seri-ously allergic" to every one of 120 different substances. He subsequently committed suicide. Some media conceptions of the illnesses suffered by soldiers returning from the Persian Gulf War also reflect some of the same themes. One tragic soldier has appeared in many British newspapers—we are told that his "immune system has van-ished. He lives in a room lagged with tin foil against the risk of infection with a blue plastic tube inserted into his nostrils" [149].

The logical conclusion of such explanatory models is to combine them into what might almost be called a "General Theory." The New York magazine *Christopher Street* has published a series of articles under the banner "The Age of Chronic Immune Dysfunction." CFS, AIDS, and multiple chemical sensitivity are part of a "unified syn-drome of immune dysregulation" [150]. This article takes the familiar line that these new illnesses are "being noted in ever greater numbers around the world, but partic-ularly so in the 'civilised' First World." From this the author describes a syndrome in which the immune system is both "up" and "down" regulated. The key elements responsible include the Western diet, which consists of too many additives and not enough vitamins, the use of antibiotics leading to Candida overgrowth, virtually any infective agent, metal toxicity from pesticides, pollution and insecticides, mercury amalgam in our teeth, immunisation, radiation including electromagnetic emissions from power lines but also computers, word processors and hair dryers, and the ubiq-uitous stress [150]. A popular magazine echoed this risk factor, as well as introducing many more, in a recent feature on the hazards of daily life [151], and included over 40 different suggestions about how to reduce this risk, such as placing the television against an outside wall, avoiding barbecues, not walking near the kerb, avoiding canned food, and not talking for hours on your mobile phone. In another typical article the author explains how viruses alter the immune system making the body susceptible to the effects of bacteria, toxins, candida, chemicals, stress, and so on [152]. The logical conclusion of this general theory is to see ME or CFIDS as a "signal of the sickness of the planet" [153]—hence the solution can be nothing less than "improving the total environment" [154].

I conclude this section by observing that ME/CFS/CFIDS can be understood on many levels. On the one hand it is an operationally defined concept susceptible to epidemiological analysis. It is also a neurobiological disturbance, and hence we can expect that future neuroendocrine investigation will reveal further insights. It is also a socially determined construct which can tell us much about modern concepts of illness at the end of the twentieth century. Its modernity can best be understood as another manifestation of the perennial theme linking changes in society with unwelcome illness—the fervent claims made linking various contemporary factors with CFS are thus better understood in metaphorical rather than literal terms.

## Prognosis

The prognosis for chronic fatigue, even in primary care, is unsatisfactory. At 1 year follow-up only a third of fatigued patients seen in American ambulatory care (something which probably lies half way between UK primary and specialist care) had improved [155]. The prognosis for patients who reach specialist care is particularly worrying. The neurologist who has played a crucial role in establishing the legitimacy of CFS in the United Kingdom wrote that "most cases do not improve, give up their work and become permanent invalids, incapacitated by excessive fatigue and myalgia" [156]. 60% of those seen in a Seattle clinic were the same or worse 2 years later. Only 18% of those referred to a Belfast clinic improved, and only 13% of those seen in an infectious disease clinic in Oxford considered themselves fully recovered 2 years later, although more had improved. Only 6% of subjects who had taken part in treatment studies in Australia had fully recovered at 3 years (see Ref. [157]). Despite its poor prognosis, CFS is not associated with an increase in mortality, with the exception of suicide.

## Management

Many doctors are understandably bewildered by the controversy surrounding CFS. There are those who claim, with passion, that it is an organic condition due to a virus for which there is regrettably no treatment. For others it is a form of depression, treated by antidepressants, whilst some state it doesn't exist at all. It is thus not surprising that confusion exists surrounding appropriate management.

CFS patients have an illness. What, if any, disease underlies that illness remains to be seen. At present management is focused on the illness, and not any putative underlying disease. Perhaps this will change, and a future generation will obtain convincing evidence of an underlying disease process, and establish the means to reverse it. Until then, the mainstay of treatment for CFS revolves around management and rehabilitation. We have taken a pragmatic approach to rehabilitation that is derived from the literature in chronic pain.

In our unit and that run by our colleagues in Oxford we have developed treatment approaches based on cognitive behavioural principles [3, 158, 159]. We argue that whatever triggers CFS may not perpetuate it. For example, an ordinary viral infection may *precipitate* fatigue which, for the majority of the population, is resolved when a normal recovery is made. However, on rare occasions the presence of *perpetuating* factors (such as psychosocial stressors, rapid deconditioning, failure to rest adequately, or concurrent depression) may delay or impede recovery. Fatigue then becomes chronic, persisting long after the departure of the original trigger and maintained by new variables.

In summary, unitary models of CFS are an inadequate reflection of clinical reality, and instead than CFS may be better understood (and hence treated) by focusing on possible perpetuating factors, and the many ways in which they interact in self-perpetuating vicious circles of fatigue, behaviour, beliefs, and disability [3, 159].

How might treatment proceed in practice? The process of excluding other causes for chronic fatigue rarely takes much time. In contrast engaging the sufferer in treatment can be a time-consuming process, but no part of the treatment process is as crucial [160]. Any active intervention, be it graded activity, cognitive therapy or anti-depressants may be viewed with trepidation: either a rigid exercise programme which will worsen the sufferer's condition, or, conversely, as little more than a thinly veiled way of telling them the problem is "psychological" (and therefore not "real") after all. Most will have had other, unsatisfactory encounters with health care practitioners, and therefore it is important that they feel listened to and taken seriously. The doctor should be explicit in conveying belief in the reality of both physical symptoms and psychological distress. The patient's own views on the nature of their illness and its management should be sought and discussed. Becoming enmeshed in a dichotomous "psychological" versus "physical" debate is to be avoided, and there is no point in simply replacing one set of explanations (organic) with another (psychological). Schultz issued a pertinent warning; "attributing a symptom to a psychosocial cause depends not just on recognising that a significant emotional event preceded the onset of a physical symptoms, but on having a model of how a psychosocial event could generate the observed symptom. In the absence of such models, it may be easier to explain a physical symptom by a corresponding physical problem" [161]. Such models might include hyperventilation, inactivity, muscle tension, poor sleep, and so on [162]. The role of the doctor is to open the discussion to a wider range of possibilities, and help the patient understand the multiple factors that contribute to ill health [160].

The principal intention of treatment is to reduce functional disability, and hence increase activity. All treatments have the same intention, but in conventional approaches this is assumed to occur as the consequence of symptom relief. However, we have argued that in CFS, as in chronic pain, it is necessary to increase activity first, without waiting for symptoms to alleviate, since it is lack of activity that perpetuates the symptoms. Treatment enables increases in activity to be undertaken by allowing patients to reconsider any beliefs that might impede such progress, and then providing a safe framework for the activity increase to occur.

Planning activity and choosing behavioural targets is the next step. Simply prescribing exercise can be counterproductive, and, if carried out to excess, may well cause precisely the type of myalgic symptoms that must be avoided. Targets may avoid virtually no exercise at all—such as getting out of bed for a certain length of time, or going to the toilet unaided. The initial level of activity must be set sufficiently low to be attainable. It is often important to actually restrict activity, since many patients have become caught in a cycle of excessive rest followed by excessive activity on the few "good days" that result—the "boom and bust" pattern already mentioned.

As important as activity is the planning of rest. Immediate reductions in the amount of rest taken are rarely advised in the early stages. Instead the current pattern of rest is determined, and built into the timetable. As with activity, the consequence is to make rest predetermined, and not in response to symptoms. The patient can be reassured that as the amount of rest remains the same, no physiological consequences will result. Instead, the goal of the early stages of treatment is to combat the experience of unpredictability of symptoms [160].

Increasing activity can cause a temporary increase in symptoms, both by physiological mechanisms outlined above, and by understandable anxiety when carrying out a programme which others have said may be harmful, and appears contrary to previous experience. It is essential to emphasise that *gradual* increase in activity is not associated with harm, and that habituation will occur in time. A gradually increased level of activity over several weeks causes a transient (inactivity associated), rather than a persistent, increase in muscle fatigue and pain. The aim of treatment is to avoid the handicapping stimulus-driven cycle of CFS, in which symptoms are always a signal to rest, and replace previous sensitisation by tolerance.

## Does It Work?

A doctor searching the literature for randomised controlled trials relating to the management of CFS will not be overwhelmed by the size of the literature, largely because the category of CFS is a relatively recent addition to the Medline index. However, plenty of evidence can be found from other sources. For example, as already pointed out, there are considerable similarities between CFS and fibromyalgia. Controlled trials of increased activity in fibromyalgia have shown that exercise retraining is beneficial on overall symptom scores, sleep, and pain [163], although ideas of a simple relationship between fitness level and symptom severity are simplistic [164]. In fibromyalgia, unlike CFS, there seems to be no dissenting voice from the view that patients should be encouraged to cautiously interrupt the "cycle of inactivity, fatigue, pain and inactivity" [165].

Most clinicians are now using similar approaches for the management of CFS, usually in a pragmatic common-sense fashion, based on a dislike of the therapeutic nihilism that can be associated with the diagnosis. Only a few continue to advocate rest as the basis of management. Nevertheless, although these measures represent a common sense approach that will probably be endorsed by most general practitioners, firm evidence has yet to be presented. We carried out an uncontrolled evaluation of cognitive behaviour therapy in 50 patients seen in a specialist setting with high levels of disability. The results were encouraging, although problems were encountered with refusal [158]. Gains were maintained 4 years later [166].

However, in the first randomised controlled trial of CBT, active treatment was no better than simple clinic attendance and reassurance [167]. Lloyd and colleagues conclude that active treatment was helpful, but no more than non-specific clinic attendance and reassurance. It is plausible that just as others have noted a high placebo response to physical treatments (see Refs. [168, 169]), intensive psychologically based treatments have a similar placebo effect. On the other hand, the control treatment received was far more than the "treatment as usual" that CFS sufferers often receive, a thinly veiled euphemism for nothing at all. This was not the case in this trial, and the non-specific effects of good clinical care may have been considerable [170]. Two further randomised controlled trials have been more encouraging. The Oxford trial, which had a cognitive flavour, used a waiting list/"usual treatment" control group. Active treatment was effective [171]. We have used a more behavioural approach, and also taken account of the non-specific effects of treatment, since the control group received an equal number of sessions (12) of relaxation therapy. Again, active treatment proved successful [172]. In both studies it was noticeable that although differences between CBT and the control groups were present at the end of treatment, these did not become substantial until the end of the 6-month follow-up period, suggesting that patients continued to practice the principles of rehabilitation with benefit after the end of active treatment. A third controlled trial of graded exercise per se also showed that active treatment was effective [173].

If CBT and/or graded activity are indeed effective for some patients with CFS, why? The answers have relevance to the entire subject matter of this book. It is not simply due to overcoming the effects of physical deconditioning, since measures of muscle strength, cardiac function and the like do not correlate with clinical improvement— patients do not have to get fit to get better, which is hardly surprising since many patients were not fit before getting ill. It is also not due to a direct change in attribution, and in particular to a switch from a physical attribution to a psychological one. Again, this is perhaps not surprising, since achieving such a shift is not the aim of CBT, although some think it is. Replacing one set of assumptions with another equally arbitrary set would neither be intellectually nor empirically desirable, and would contradict the oft quoted desires by people who write on medically unexplained syndromes to avoid tedious mind body dualism. Instead for patients to improve whilst receiving CBT it is merely necessary that they alter their views about the most effective way of coping with symptoms, and shift from a short-term view, that rest is the only treatment, to a longer term view which views rest as less helpful and exercise as less harmful than previously thought [171, 174]. We believe this to be generalisable beyond the narrow confines of CFS—challenging illness beliefs is both unprofitable and unnecessary. Instead our clinical efforts should be concentrated on the modifying some of the maladaptive consequences of such beliefs—one might say that "yes, we agree that your illness may well have a physical cause—but are you sure that rest is the best option for getting better?"

## Pharmacological Approaches to CFS

There is no single established pharmacological management for CFS. There are a number of compelling reasons why antidepressants should be effective [170], and indeed there is plenty of evidence to suggest that tricyclic antidepressants prescribed in doses lower than those used in conventional psychiatric settings, are effective in the short-term management of fibromyalgia [163]. However, evidence for the effectiveness of any antidepressant in CFS is presently not compelling. Several uncontrolled or open studies have suggested benefit, but the first controlled trial in CFS, of fluoxetine, was resoundingly negative [175], and a second trial provided evidence of only modest efficacy [176]. On the other hand, a new trial of a reversible monoamine oxidase inhibitors (MAOI) was more successful [177], which is perhaps understandable given the links between the symptoms of CFS and those of atypical depression.

Moving away from antidepressants a number of specific treatments have been proposed to deal with the presumed underlying "cause" of the abnormal fatigability, principally involving either antiviral drugs or agents acting on the immune system. None have been convincing [3].

Perhaps the most common treatment modality used by patients who believe they have CFS are those encountered in the world of alternative medicine. In my country it is the exceptional patient seeking treatment who has not tried some combination of vitamins, diets, nutritional supplements and the like. There are several reasons. First, as in any chronic disease, regression to the mean or the physician's friend, ensures that some will benefit. Second, these approaches are in keeping with the contemporary *zeitgeist* surrounding CFS. Most self-help books effortlessly promote illness models involving external environmental agents (allergy, amalgam, candida, electromagnetic radiation, pollution, poor diet, viruses, and so on) that owe more to "green" ideas of health than any observable evidence. In turn these can lead to environmental and nutritional interventions that probably owe their success to the congruence of the illness model of patient and therapist. Third, these approaches are based on a model of illness (vitamin deficiency, virus, allergy, and so on), in which the patient avoids any stigma for his or her predicament. Most of these approaches have not been systematically evaluated, whilst the results of those that have are not been encouraging.

I have already drawn attention to the historical continuities that exist linking the various fatigue syndromes over the years. This is particularly true of treatment. When Charles Dana wrote that "it is notorious the number of 'cures' that exist for the neurasthenic" [178] he could equally well be writing about CFS.

## Conclusions

Understanding the legacy and consequences of somatisation in the late twentieth century is relevant not only to the many clinicians who work in this area (and there are few general physicians who do not), but to all those who are interested in the social and cultural history of medicine. In this essay I have attempted to use the example of CFS in its popular idiom of ME and CFIDS, to draw attention to several relevant themes. These have included the modern preoccupation with the immune system, itself linked to the appearance of HIV, the belief that this system is being compromised by various features of contemporary life, the concept of "overload," the themes of toxicity and purity, the general increasing fascination with medicine, the increased promise of medical science but also the reaction against modern medical science, and the rise in medical consumerism. I have also shown how the fear and stigma of mental illness, and the need for explanations that are both protective of self esteem and in keeping with modern views on sickness and health are also important. Of course, CFS is much more than this, and some will argue that any such cultural or social analysis is demeaning to those with the affliction. I do not accept this, any more than an analysis of the cultural representations of cancer was demeaning to those with the disease [179]. Instead I will conclude that it is ambiguity of CFS, and in particular its position midway between the worlds of psychiatry and medicine that offers an opportunity to explore these areas, one not afforded by better defined and characterised illnesses. Anyone interested in mind-body medicine should take note.

## References

1. Wessely S (1990) Old wine in new bottles: neurasthenia and "ME". Psychol Med 20:35–53
2. Wessely S (1997) Chronic fatigue syndrome: a twentieth century illness? Scand J Work Environ Health 23(Suppl 3):7–16
3. Wessely S, Hotopf M, Sharpe M (1998) Chronic fatigue and its syndromes. Oxford University Press, Oxford
4. Kraepelin E (1902) Clinical psychiatry. MacMillan, London
5. Abbey S, Garfinkel P (1991) Neurasthenia and chronic fatigue syndrome: the role of culture in the making of a diagnosis. Am J Psychiatry 148:1638–1646
6. Wessely S (1991) History of the Postviral Fatigue Syndrome. British Medical Bulletin 47:919–941
7. Shorter E (1992) From paralysis to fatigue: a history of psychosomatic illness in the modern era. Free Press, New York
8. Wessely S, Powell R (1989) Fatigue syndromes: a comparison of chronic "postviral" fatigue with neuromuscular and affective disorder. J Neurol Neurosurg Psychiatry 52:940–948
9. Hickie I, Lloyd A, Wakefield D, Parker G (1990) The psychiatric status of patients with chronic fatigue syndrome. Br J Psychiatry 156:534–540
10. Schweitzer R, Robertson D, Kelly B, Whiting J (1994) Illness behaviour of patients with chronic fatigue syndrome. J Psychosom Res 38:41–50
11. Holmes G, Kaplan J, Gantz N et al (1988) Chronic fatigue syndrome: a working case definition. Ann Intern Med 108:387–389
12. Schluederberg A, Straus S, Peterson P et al (1992) Chronic fatigue syndrome research: definition and medical outcome assessment. Ann Intern Med 117:325–331
13. Fukuda K, Straus S, Hickie I, Sharpe M, Dobbins J, Komaroff A (1994) The chronic fatigue syndrome: a comprehensive approach to its definition and study. Ann Intern Med 121:953–959
14. Sharpe M, Archard L, Banatvala J et al (1991) Chronic fatigue syndrome: guidelines for research. J R Soc Med 84:118–121
15. David A, Wessely S, Pelosi A (1988) Post-viral fatigue: time for a new approach. Br Med J 296:696–699
16. Wessely S (1995) The epidemiology of chronic fatigue syndrome. Epidemiol Rev 17:139–151
17. Cox B, Blaxter M, Buckle A et al (1987) The health and lifestyle survey. Health Promotion Research Trust, London
18. Schepank H (1987) Epidemiology of psychogenic disorders; the Mannheim study. Springer, Berlin
19. Lewis G, Wessely S (1992) The epidemiology of fatigue: more questions than answers. J Epidemiol Comm Health 46:92–97
20. Buchwald D, Sullivan J, Komaroff A (1987) Frequency of "chronic active Epstein-Barr virus infection" in a general medical practice. J Am Med Assoc 257:2303–2307
21. Shahar E, Lederer J (1990) Asthenic symptoms in a rural family practice: epidemiologic characteristics and a proposed classification. J Fam Pract 31:257–262

22. David A, Pelosi A, McDonald E et al (1990) Tired, weak or in need of rest: fatigue among general practice attenders. Br Med J 301:1199–1122

23. Cathebras P, Robbins J, Kirmayer L, Hayton B (1992) Fatigue in primary care: prevalence, psychiatric comorbidity, illness behaviour and outcome. J Gen Intern Med 7:276–286

24. Fuhrer R, Wessely S (1995) Fatigue in French primary care. Psychol Med 25:895–905

25. Bates D, Schmitt W, Lee J, Kornish R, Komaroff A (1993) Prevalence of fatigue and chronic fatigue syndrome in a primary care practice. Arch Intern Med 153:2759–2765

26. Buchwald D, Umali P, Umali J, Kith P, Pearlman T, Komaroff A (1995) Chronic fatigue and the chronic fatigue syndrome: prevalence in a Pacific Northwest Health Care System. Ann Intern Med 123:81–88

27. Steele L, Dobbins J, Fukuda K et al (1998) The epidemiology of chronic fatigue in San Francisco. Am J Med (in press)

28. Shefer A, Dobbins J, Fukuda K et al (1997) Fatiguing illness among employees in three large state office buildings, California, 1993: was there an outbreak? J Psychiatr Res 31:31–43

29. Jason L, Wagner L, Rosenthal S et al (1998) Estimating the prevalence of chronic fatigue syndrome among nurses. Am J Medicine 105(3A):915–935

30. Wessely S, Chalder T, Hirsch S, Wallace P, Wright D (1997) The prevalence and morbidity of chronic fatigue and chronic fatigue syndrome: a prospective primary care study. Am J Publ Health 87:1449–1455

31. Lawrie S, Pelosi A (1995) Chronic fatigue syndrome in the community: prevalence and associations. Br J Psychiatry 166:793–797

32. Jason L, Taylor R, Wagner L et al (1995) Estimating rates of chronic fatigue syndrome from a communit y-based sample: a pilot study. Am J Comm Psychol 23:557–568

33. Pawlikowska T, Chalder T, Hirsch S, Wallace P, Wright D, Wessely S (1994) A population based study of fatigue and psychological distress. Br Med J 308:743–746

34. Richman J, Flaherty J, Rospenda K (1994) Chronic fatigue syndrome: have flawed assumptions been derived from treatment-based studies? Am J Publ Health 84:282–284

35. Euba R, Chalder T, Deale A, Wessely S (1996) A comparison of the characteristics of chronic fatigue syndrome in primary and tertiary care. Br J Psychiatry 168:121–126

36. Merikangas K, Angst J (1994) Neurasthenia in a longitidunal cohort study of young adults. Psychol Med 24:1013–1024

37. Ormel J, VonKorff M, Ustun B, Pini S, Korten A, Oldehinkel T (1994) Common mental disorders and disabilities across cultures: results from the WHO collaborative study on psychological problems in general health care. J Am Med Assoc 272:1741–1748

38. Komaroff A, Fagioli L, Doolittle T et al (1996) Health status in patients with chronic fatigue syndrome and in general population and disease comparison groups. Am J Med 101:281–290

39. Minowa M, Jiamo M (1996) Descriptive epidemiology of chronic fatigue syndrome based on a nationwide survey in Japan. J Epidemiol 6:75–80

40. Fekety R (1994) Infection and chronic fatigue syndrome. In: Straus S (ed) Chronic fatigue syndrome. Marcel Dekker, New York, pp 101–180

41. Swanink C, Melchers W, van der Meer J et al (1994) Enteroviruses and the chronic fatigue syndrome. Clin Infect Dis 19:860–864

42. White P, Thomas J, Amess J, Grover S, Kangro H, Clare A (1995) The existence of a fatigue syndrome after glandular fever. Psychol Med 25:907–916

43. White P, Thomas J, Amess J, Crawford D, Grover S, Kangro H (1998) The incidence, prevalence and prognosis of the fatigue syndrome which follows Epstein-Barr virus infection. Br J Psychiatry 173:475–481

44. Bruce-Jones W, White P, Thomas J, Clare A (1994) The effect of social disadvantage on the fatigue syndrome, psychiatric disorders and physical recovery, following glandular fever. Psychol Med 24:651–659

45. Chang R, Bittner W (1991) Chronic fatigue syndrome. J Am Med Assoc 265:337
46. Marmion B, Shannon M, Maddocks I, Strom P, Penttila I (1996) Protracted fatigue and debility after acute Q fever. Lancet 347:977-978
47. Cope H, David A, Pelosi A, Mann A (1994) Predictors of chronic "post viral" fatigue. Lancet 344:864-868
48. Wessely S, Chalder T, Hirsch S, Pawlikowska T, Wallace P, Wright D (1995) Post infectious fatigue: a prospective study in primary care. Lancet 345:1333-1338
49. Wood P (1941) Da Costa's syndrome (or effort syndrome). Br Med J i:767-772; 805-811; 845-851
50. Buchwald D, Umali J, Pearlman T, Kith P, Ashley R, Wener M (1996) Post infectious chronic fatigue: a distinct syndrome? Clin Infect Dis 23:385-387
51. Deluca J, Johnson S, Ellis S, Natelson B (1997) Sudden vs gradual onset of chronic fatigue syndrome differentiates individuals on cognitive and psychiatric measures. J Psychiatr Res 31:83-90
52. Mawle A, Nisenbaum R, Dobbins J et al (1997) Immune responses associated with chronic fatigue syndrome: a case-control study. J Infect Dis 175:136-141
53. Wood G, Bentall R, Gopfert M, Edwards R (1991) A comparative psychiatric assessment of patients with chronic fatigue syndrome and muscle disease. Psychol Med 21:619-628
54. Edwards R, Gibson H, Clague J, Helliwell T (1993) Muscle physiology and histopathology in chronic fatigue syndrome. In: Kleinman A, Straus S (eds) Chronic fatigue syndrome, vol 173. John Wiley, Chichester, pp 101-131
55. Janet P (1919) Les obsessions et la psychasthénie, vol 1. Alcan, Paris
56. Smith A, Pollock J, Thomas M, Llewelyn M, Borysiewicz L (1996) The relationship between subjective ratings of sleep and mental functioning in healthy subjects and patients with chronic fatigue syndrome. Hum Psychopharmacol 11:161-167
57. Schmaling K, DiClementi J, Cullum M, Jones J (1994) Cognitive functioning in chronic fatigue syndrome and depression: A preliminary comparison. Psychosom Med 56:383-388
58. Wearden A, Appleby L (1996) Research on cognitive complaints and cognitive functioning in patients with chronic fatigue syndrome (CFS): what conclusions can we draw? J Psychosom Res 41:197-211
59. Lawrie S, MacHale S, Power M, Goodwin G (1997) Is the chronic fatigue syndrome best understood as a primary disturbance of the sense of effort? Psychol Med 27:995-999
60. Davison K, Pennebaker J (1997) Virtual Narratives: Illness representations in online support groups. In: Petrie K, Weinman J (eds) Perceptions of health and illness: current research and applications. Harwood, London, pp 463-486
61. Straus S, Fritz S, Dale J, Gould B, Strober W (1993) Lymphocyte phenotype and function in the chronic fatigue syndrome. J Clin Immunol 13:30-40
62. Maes M, Jacobs J, Lambreckhts J (1992) Evidence for a systemic immune activation during depression; results of leucocyte enumeration by flow cytometry in conjunction with antibody staining. Psychol Med 22:45-53
63. Lloyd A, Hickie I, Wilson A, Wakefield D (1994) Immune function in chronic fatigue syndrome and depression; implications for understanding these disorders and for therapy. Clin Immunother 2:84-88
64. Levy J (1994) Introduction; viral studies of chronic fatigue syndrome. Clin Infect Dis 18(suppl 1):S117-120
65. Konstantinov K, von Mikecz A, Buchwald D, Jones J, Gerace L, Tan E (1996) Autoantibodies to nuclear envelope antigens in chronic fatigue syndrome. J Clin Invest 98:1888-1896
66. Levy J, Landay A, Jessop C, Lennette E (1993) Chronic fatigue syndrome; is it a state of chronic immune activation against an infectious virus? Contemp Issues Infect Dis 10:127-145

67. Strober W (1994) Immunological function in chronic fatigue syndrome. In: Straus S (ed) Chronic fatigue syndrome. Marcel Dekker, New York, pp 207–240
68. Fischler B, Cluydts R, De Gucht V, Kaufman L, DeMeirleir K (1997) Generalised anxiety disorder in chronic fatigue syndrome. Acta Psychiatr Scand 95:405–413
69. Paul O (1987) Da Costa's syndrome or neurocirculatory asthenia. Br Heart J 58: 306–315
70. Fava G, Magelli C, Savron G et al (1994) Neurocirculatory asthenia: a reassessment using modern psychosomatic criteria. Acta Psychiatr Scand 89:314–319
71. Young D (1989) Neurasthenia and related problems. Culture Med Psychiatry 13: 131–138
72. Rosen SD, King JC, Wilkinson JB, Nixon PGF (1990) Is chronic fatigue syndrome synonymous with effort syndrome. J R Soc Med 83:761–764
73. Saisch S, Deale A, Gardner W, Wessely S (1994) Hyperventilation and chronic fatigue syndrome. Q J Med 87:63–67
74. Kendell R (1991) Chronic fatigue, viruses and depression. Lancet 337:160–162
75. Greenberg D (1990) Neurasthenia in the 1980s: chronic mononucleosis, chronic fatigue syndrome, and anxiety and depressive disorders. Psychosomatics 31:129–137
76. Levine P, Kreuger G, Straus S (1989) Postviral chronic fatigue syndrome: a round table. J Infect Dis 160:722–724
77. Wells K, Stewart A, Hays R et al (1989) The functioning and well-being of depressed patients: results from the Medical Outcomes Study. J Am Med Assoc 262:914–919
78. McDonald E, David A, Pelosi A, Mann A (1993) Chronic fatigue in general practice attenders. Psychol Med 23:987–998
79. Demitrack M, Dale J, Straus S et al (1991) Evidence for impaired activation of the hypothalamic-pituitary-adrenal axis in patients with chronic fatigue syndrome. J Clin Endocrinol Metab 73:1224–1234
80. Crofford L, Pillemer S, Kalogeras K et al (1994) Hypothalamic-pituitary-adrenal axis perturbations in patients with fibromyalgia. Arthritis Rheum 37:1583–1592
81. Pillemer S, Bradley L, Crofford L, Moldofsky H, Chrousos G (1997) The neuroscience and endocrinology of fibromyalgia. Arthritis Rheum 40:1928–1939
82. Bakheit A, Behan P, Dinan T, Gray C, O'Keane V (1992) Possible upregulation of hypothalamic 5-hydroxytryptamine receptors in patients with postviral fatigue syndrome. Br Med J 304:1010–1012
83. Sharpe M, Hawton K, Clements A, Cowen P (1997) Increased brain serotonin function in men with chronic fatigue syndrome. Br Med J 315:164–165
84. Cleare A, Bearn J, Allain T et al (1995) Contrasting neuroendocrine responses in depression and chronic fatigue syndrome. J Affect Disord 35:283–289
85. Leese G, Chattington P, Fraser W, Vora J, Edwards R, Williams G (1996) Short-term night-shift working mimics the pituitary-adrenocortical dysfunction of chronic fatigue syndrome. J Clin Endocrinol Metab 81:1867–1870
86. Kirmayer L, Robbins J (1991) Three forms of somatization in primary care: prevalence, co-occurence and sociodemographic characteristics. J Nerv Ment Dis 179: 647–655
87. Van Hemert A, Hengeveld M, Bolk J, Rooijmans H, Vandenbroucke J (1993) Psychiatric disorder in relation to medical illness among patients of a general medical out-patient clinic. Psychol Med 23:167–173
88. Johnson S, Deluca J, Natelson B (1996) Assessing somatization disorder in the chronic fatigue syndrome. Psychosom Med 58:50–57
89. Lane T, Manu P, Matthews D (1991) Depression and somatization in the chronic fatigue syndrome. Am J Med 91:335–344
90. Katon W, Buchwald D, Simon G, Russo J, Mease P (1991) Psychiatric illness in patients with chronic fatigue and rheumatoid arthritis. J Gen Intern Med 6:277–285
91. Escobar J, Burnam A, Karno M, Forsythe A, Golding J (1987) Somatization in the community. Arch Gen Psychiatry 44:713–718

92. Katon W, Russo J (1992) Chronic fatigue syndrome criteria: a critique of the requirement for multiple physical complaints. Arch Intern Med 152:1604–1609
93. Wessely S, Chalder T, Hirsch S, Wallace P, Wright D (1996) Psychological symptoms, somatic symptoms and psychiatric disorder in chronic fatigue and chronic fatigue syndrome: a prospective study in primary care. Am J Psychiatry 153:1050–1059
94. Simon G, VonKorff M (1991) Somatization and psychiatric disorder in the NIMH epidemiologic catchment area study. Am J Psychiatry 148:1494–1500
95. Walker E, Katon W, Jemelka R (1993) Psychiatric disorders and medical care utilisation among people who report fatigue in the general population. J Gen Intern Med 8:436–440
96. Stewart D (1990) The changing face of somatisation. Psychosomatics 31:153–158
97. Hickie I, Lloyd A, Hadzi-Pavlovic D, Parker G, Bird K, Wakefield D (1995) Can the chronic fatigue syndrome be defined by distinct clinical features? Psychol Med 25:925–935
98. Francis C (1988) A Beginning. Interaction, vol 1
99. Wessely S (1994) Neurasthenia and chronic fatigue: theory and practice in Britain and America. Transcult Psychiatry Res Rev 31:173–209
100. Ostrom N (1989) It's a dirty little war: proponents of a "psychoneurotic" cause of CFIDS try again. Christopher Street 1:32–33
101. Masefield P (1994) Link to life. M.E. Boxtree, London, pp 1–29
102. Abbey S (1993) Somatization, illness attribution and the sociocultural psychiatry of chronic fatigue syndrome. In: Kleinman A, Straus S (eds) Chronic fatigue syndrome, vol 173. Wiley, Chichester, pp 238–261
103. Helman C (1978) Feed a cold and starve a fever. Cult Med Psychiatry 7:107–137
104. Katz B, Andiman W (1988) Chronic fatigue Syndrome. J Paediatr 113:944–947
105. Seagrove J (1989) The ME Generation. Guardian, 19 May
106. Miller P (1992) My healing journey through chronic fatigue. Yoga J 61–124
107. Anon. (1994) Watchdog to look into ME resources. Dundee Courier and Advertiser, 11 November
108. Timbs O (1987) Postviral puzzle. Observer, 2 August
109. Steincamp J (1989) Overload: beating M.E. Fontana, London
110. Aronowitz R, Spiro H (1988) The rise and fall of the psychosomatic hypothesis in ulcerative colitis. J Clin Gastroenterol 10:298–305
111. Ware N (1993) Society, mind and body in chronic fatigue syndrome: an anthropological view. In: Kleinman A, Straus S (eds) Chronic fatigue syndrome, vol 173. Wiley, Chichester, pp 62–82
112. Burrascano J (1993) The overdiagnosis of Lyme disease. J Am Med Assoc 270:2682
113. Woodward R, Broom D, Legge D (1995) Diagnosis in chronic illness: disabling or enabling—the case of chronic fatigue syndrome. J R Soc Med 88:325–329
114. Cooper L (1997) Myalgic encephalomyelitis and the medical encounter. Sociol Health Illness 19:17–37
115. Ames M (1985) Learning to live with incurable virus. Chicago Tribune, 9 June, Section 5, p 3
116. Forna A (1987) A real pain. Girl About Town, 21 May
117. Stopp C (1993) ME sufferers forced to battle with insurers. Independent on Sunday, 27 June
118. Holt G (1965) Epidemic neuromyasthenia: the sporadic form. Am J Med Sci 124–138
119. Hales D (1987) The fatigue diseases: why are you so tired? Am Health, 54–57
120. Hodgkinson L (1988) ME: the mystery disease. Woman's Journal, November
121. Anon (1986) Malaise of the 80s. Newsweek, 27 October
122. Willsher K (1990) I beat the disease of the 90s. Daily Express, 11 April
123. Cowley G, Hager M, Joseph N (1990) Chronic fatigue syndrome: a medical mystery. Newsweek, 12 November

124. Anon (1989) Craig faces two year battle to beat 21st-Century disease. Today, 13 March
125. Askwith R (1989) The ME Generation. Sunday Telegraph Magazine, 22 January
126. Flett K (1990) Why M.E? Arena, March
127. Crook W (1992) Chronic fatigue syndrome and the yeast connection. Professional Books, Jackson
128. Jacobs G (1990) Candida albicans: yeast and your health. Optima, London
129. Francis C (1992) Bad Cow Disease. Evening Standard, 3 April
130. Fletcher M, Francis C (1992) Why I have to fight this living death. Sun, 17 February
131. Anon (1992) In search of a cause. Awake, 22 August
132. Bradford N (1992) How to beat the new bugs. Good Housekeeping, March
133. Regush N (1990) AIDS: Words from the front. Spin 6:69–70, 79–80
134. Chaitow L (1988) Postviral fatigue syndrome: fact or fantasy. Women's Journal, March
135. Garrison J (1991) Chronic fatigue: an ancient ill? San Francisco Examiner, 17 March
136. Cleave M (1993) The ME Generation. Evening Standard, 1 September
137. Paul C (1894) The treatment of neurasthenia. J Ment Sci 40:134–135
138. Rabinbach A (1990) The human motor: Energy, fatigue and the origins of modernity. Basic Books, New York
139. Beard G (1881) American nervousness. Putnam's, New York
140. Haller J (1970) Neurasthenia: the medical profession and urban "blahs". N Y State J Med 70:2489–2497
141. Chester A, Levine P (1994) Concurrent sick building syndrome and chronic fatigue syndrome: epidemic neuromyasthenia revisited. Clin Infect Dis 18(Suppl 1):S43–48
142. Renfro L, Feder H, Lane T, Manu P, Matthews D (1989) Yeast connection among 100 patients with chronic fatigue. Am J Med 86:165–168
143. Buchwald D, Garrity D (1994) Comparison of patients with chronic fatigue syndrome, fibromyalgia, and multiple chemical sensitivities. Arch Intern Med 154:2049–2053
144. Gomborone J, Gorard D, Dewsnap P, Libby G, Farthing M (1996) Prevalence of irritable bowel syndrome in chronic fatigue. J R Coll Physicians Lond 30:512–513
145. King C (1989) Parallels between neurasthenia and premenstrual syndrome. Women and Health 15:1–23
146. Crook W (1989) The yeast connection, 3rd edn. Professional Books, Jackson
147. Shorter E (1997) Multiple chemical sensitivity: pseudodisease in historical perspective. Scand J Work Environ Health 23(Suppl 3):35–42
148. Fairley J (1995) Will my life ever be normal again? Woman's Journal March 116–117
149. Norman M (1993) Soldier of misfortune. Evening Standard 29th October 1993
150. Culbert M (1994) Chronic and acute elements of a syndrome of immune dysregulation—Part 1. Int J Altern Complem Med 25–32
151. Dickson J (1995) Beating your toxic lifestyle. Options June 1995
152. Allen J (1992) Myalgic encephalomyelitis. Homeopathy 42:152–154
153. Griffin S (1992) The internal athlete. Ms., vol II, 37–38
154. Steincamp J (1984) M.E. mystery epidemic. NZ Listener 19 May 1984
155. Kroenke K, Wood D, Mangelsdorff D, Meier N, Powell J (1988) Chronic fatigue in primary care: Prevalence, patient characteristics and outcome. J Am Med Assoc 260:929–934
156. Behan P, Behan W (1988) Postviral fatigue syndrome. Crit Rev Neurobiol 4:157–179
157. Joyce J, Hotopf M, Wessely S (1997) The prognosis of chronic fatigue and chronic fatigue syndrome: a systematic review. Q J Med 90:223–233
158. Butler S, Chalder T, Ron M, Wessely S (1991) Cognitive behaviour therapy in chronic fatigue syndrome. J Neurol Neurosurg Psychiatry 54:153–158
159. Surawy C, Hackmann A, Hawton K, Sharpe M (1995) Chronic fatigue syndrome: a cognitive approach. Behav Res Ther 33:535–544
160. Sharpe M, Chalder T, Palmer I, Wessely S (1997) Chronic fatigue syndrome: a practical guide to assessment and management. Gen Hosp Psychiatry 19:195–199
161. Schultz T (1982) Rules of causal attribution. Monogr Soc Res Child Dev 47:1–51

162. Sharpe M, Bass C (1992) Pathophysiological mechanisms in somatization. Int Rev Psychiatry 4:81–97
163. Carrette S (1995) What have clinical trials taught us about the treatment of fibromyalgia? J Musculoskel Pain 3:133–140
164. Klug G, McAuley E, Clark S (1989) Factors influencing the development and maintenance of aerobic fitness: lessons applicable to the fibrositis syndrome. J Rheumatol 16(suppl 19):30–39
165. Bennett R (1989) Physical fitness and muscle metabolism in fibromyalgia syndrome: an overview. J Rheumatol 16(suppl 19):28–29
166. Bonner D, Butler S, Chalder T, Ron M, Wessely S (1994) A follow-up study of chronic fatigue syndrome. J Neurol Neurosurg Psychiatry 57:617–621
167. Lloyd A, Hickie I, Brockman A et al (1993) Immunologic and psychological therapy for patients with chronic fatigue syndrome. Am J Med 94:197–203
168. Gantz N, Holmes G (1989) Treatment of patients with chronic fatigue syndrome. Drugs 38:855–862
169. Kaslow J, Rucker L, Onishi R (1989) Liver extract-folic acid-cyanocobalamin vs placebo for chronic fatigue syndrome. Arch Intern Med 149:2501–2503
170. Wilson A, Hickie I, Lloyd A, Wakefield D (1994) The treatment of chronic fatigue syndrome; science and speculation. Am J Med 96:544–549
171. Sharpe M, Hawton K, Simkin S et al (1996) Cognitive behaviour therapy for chronic fatigue syndrome; a randomized controlled trial. Br Med J 312:22–26
172. Deale A, Chalder T, Marks I, Wessely S (1997) A randomised controlled trial of cognitive behaviour versus relaxation therapy for chronic fatigue syndrome. Am J Psychiatry 154:408–414
173. Fulcher K, White P (1997) Randomised controlled trial of graded exercise in patients with chronic fatigue syndrome. Br Med J 314:1647–1652
174. Deale A, Chalder T, Wessely S (1998) Illness beliefs and outcome in chronic fatigue syndrome: is change in causal attribution necessary for clinical improvement? J Psychosom Res 45:77–83
175. Vercoulen J, Swanink C, Zitman F et al (1996) Fluoxetine in chronic fatigue syndrome; a randomized, double-blind, placebo-controlled study. Lancet 347:858–861
176. Wearden A, Morriss R, Mullis R et al (1998) A double-blind, placebo controlled treatment trial of fluoxetine and a graded exercise programme for chronic fatigue syndrome. Br J Psychiatry 172:485–490
177. Hickie I, Wilson A, Wright J, Bennett B, Wakefield D, Lloyd A (1998) A randomised, double-blind, placebo controlled trial of moclobemide in patients with chronic fatigue syndrome. Br J Psychiatry (in press)
178. Dana C (1904) The partial passing of neurasthenia. Boston Med Surg J 60:339–344
179. Sontag S (1986) Illness as metaphor. Penguin, London

# Biological Markers of Fibromyalgia

Michael Maes

*Summary.* Fibromyalgia is a chronic condition characterized by widespread mus-culoskeletal pain and pressure hyperalgesia at characteristic sites, i.e., soft tissue tender points. The biophysiology of fibromyalgia, however, has remained elusive. This paper reviews recent biological research on the role of the neuroendocrine and immune systems in the biophysiology of fibromyalgia. It is suggested that fibromyalgia is determined by a combination of different pathophysiological mechanisms, which reside in the catecholaminergic and immune systems and in peptidase activities. Subsensitive platelet α2-adrenoceptors suggest a lowered affinity of presynaptic receptors and thus could indicate a lower autoinhibitory activity on the catecho-laminergic neuron. The results do not corroborate the hypotheses that fibromyalgia is accompanied by a deficiency in serotonergic metabolism or in disturbances in the hypothalamic-pituitary-adrenal axis. It is hypothesized that aberrant pain perception and depressive symptoms in fibromyalgia may result from decreases in prolyl endopeptidase (PEP, EC 3.4.21.26), a cytosolic endopeptidase which inactivates algesic (e.g., bradykinin, substance P) and depression-related peptides. Most results show no significant signs of inflammation in fibromyalgia, but show indications of immunosuppression.

*Key words.* Catecholamines, Peptidases, Fibromyalgia, Serotonin, Immunology

## Introduction

Fibromyalgia is a chronic condition characterized by widespread musculoskeletal pain, pressure hyperalgesia at characteristic sites, i.e., soft tissue tender points, and morning stiffness [1]. More variable characteristics are subjective swelling, fatigue, a variety of bodily complaints, sleep disturbances, vegetative signs, and psychological

Clinical Research Center for Mental Health (CRC-MH), University Department of Psychiatry, AZ Stuivenberg, Lange Beeldekensstraat 267, 2060 Antwerp, Belgium
The research reported was supported in part by the Staglin Investigator Award to Dr. M. Maes (NARSAD); the Funds for Scientific Research, Vlaanderen, Belgium (FWO); and the CRC-MH, Antwerp, Belgium. The secretarial assistance of Mrs. M. Maes is greatly appreciated.

disturbances, such as depression and anxiety [2]. Community studies show a prevalence of 2%–4% with more than 90% of cases occurring in women [2, 3].

There is a strong comorbidity between major depression and fibromyalgia and an increased incidence of depressive symptoms in fibromyalgia patients [4]. Patients with fibromyalgia score higher than normal controls on psychiatric rating scales for depression [5]. Hudson et al. [6] found a higher incidence rate of depression amongst fibromyalgia patients and their first-degree relatives than among patients with rheumatoid arthritis. Hawley and Wolfe [7] found that depressive symptoms may be secondary to fibromyalgia. There are some other phenomenological similarities between fibromyalgia and major depression. Major depression and fibromyalgia are conditions associated with increased stress and stressor perception [8]. Antidepressants have not only efficacy in the treatment of major depression, but also in fibromyalgia [9]. Indeed, there are reports that tricyclic (TCA) antidepressants as well as selective serotonin reuptake inhibitors (SSRIs) have some efficacy in fibromyalgia, and improve pressure hyperalgesia, pain symptoms, sleep disturbances, and depressive symptoms in fibromyalgia patients [9].

The biophysiology of fibromyalgia, however, has remained elusive [10]. Some current etiologic hypotheses which have been forwarded are: (i) fibromyalgia is related to muscle abnormalities or abnormal muscular repair; (ii) it is a psychiatric disorder related to major depression; (iii) it results from mechanical abnormalities of the cervical or lumbar spine; (iv) it results from aberrant central pain mechanisms with peripheral modulation; (v) it is a disorder of the sleep-wake system; (vi) it is psychoneuroendocrine disorder; and (vii) it is an inflammatory disorder [2, 11, 12].

This chapter will review some highlights of biological research in fibromyalgia, with the aim of elucidating the role of the neuroendocrine and immune systems in the pathogenesis or pathophysiology of that illness.

# The Neuroendocrine Pathophysiology of Fibromyalgia

## Fibromyalgia and Catecholamines

It has long been suggested that changes in sympathetic activity may occur in fibromyalgia. Russell [13] found significantly lower 3-methoxy-4-hydroxyphenylglycol (MHPG) and homovanillic acid (HVA) concentrations in CSF of fibromyalgia patients than in normal controls. Bennett et al. [14] found that the increased sympathetic tone in fibromyalgia was correlated with an increased density of platelet $\alpha$2-adrenoceptor ($\alpha$2-AR) binding sites. Elam et al. [15] reported decreased sympathetic activity in fibromyalgia. Yunus et al. [16], however, found no significant differences in plasma and urinary catecholamine levels, such as epinephrine, norepinephrine, and dopamine, between patients and controls.

We have examined platelet $\alpha$2-AR binding characteristics in fibromyalgia patients as compared with normal controls. Platelet $\alpha$2-ARs have similar kinetic and pharmacologic properties as brain $\alpha$2-ARs, suggesting that platelet $\alpha$2-ARs can be used as a model for the brain receptors [17]. Adrenoceptors of the $\alpha$2A subtype are expressed on platelets and presynaptically on noradrenergic neurons, where they show an autoinhibitory activity [18, 19]. $\alpha$2-ARs may play a role in the biophysiology of fibromyalgia because: (i) central (e.g., locus coeruleus and pontospinal noradrenergic A7 neurons) as well as peripheral (e.g., dorsal horn neurons of the spinal cord) $\alpha$2-ARs mediate nociception, analgesia, causalgia, and tactile hyperesthesia [20, 21]; (ii) the A subtype of the $\alpha$2-AR ($\alpha$2A-AR) mediates antinociception [22]; (iii) noradrenaline can produce hyperalgesia via $\alpha$2-AR-related mechanisms [23]; (iv) intrathecal or epidural administration of $\alpha$2-AR agonists, such as clonidine, may diminish tactile hyperalgesia in rats and sympathetically maintain pain in humans [24–27].

We measured the number of platelet binding sites ($B_{max}$) and their affinity ($K_d$) for [$^3$H]rauwolscine, a selective $\alpha$2-AR antagonist, in 13 normal volunteers and 22 fibromyalgia patients. The fibromyalgia diagnosis was made according to the American College of Rheumatology (ACR) criteria [1]. These include a history of widespread pain for at least 3 months in the following sites: left side of the body, right side of the body, above and below the waist, axial skeletal pain; and pressure hyperalgesia using digital palpation with an approximate force of 4*T*kg in 11 of the following tender points: occiput left and right (L and R), low cervical LR, trapezius LR, supraspinatus LR, second rib LR, lateral epicondyle LR, gluteal LR, knee LR. We excluded fibromyalgia patients with any use of anti-inflammatory drugs within 4 weeks before this study; use of any other medication for the symptoms of fibromyalgia (except paracetamol); and a present and past history of axis-I diagnoses, according to DSM-III-R criteria [28] made with the aid of the Semistructured Clinical Interview for the DSM-III-R (SCID) [29].

We found that [$^3$H]rauwolscine binding $K_d$ values were significantly increased in fibromyalgia. Moreover, [$^3$H]rauwolscine binding $K_d$ values were significantly increased in fibromyalgia patients in an early phase of illness (less than three years) than in fibromyalgia patients with a protracted illness (more than three years). Subsensitive platelet $\alpha$2-ARs suggest a lowered affinity of presynaptic $\alpha$2-ARs in the periphery and maybe the brain, and thus could indicate a lower auto-inhibitory activity on the catecholaminergic neuron. These findings may suggest that changes in $\alpha$2-ARs and, consequently, in sympathetic turnover may occur in the early phase of fibromyalgia with a normalization later on. Previous research in fibromyalgia did not take into account these possible effects of duration of illness, and this could explain the contradictory results in the literature.

## Serotonin and Fibromyalgia

There is a vast body of literature which states that the pathophysiology of fibromyalgia may be related to a deficiency in serotonergic neuronal functioning [30–33]. This evidence includes the following: (i) total plasma tryptophan, the precursor of serotonin, and the ratio of plasma tryptophan to amino acids known to compete for the same cerebral uptake mechanisms (i.e., the competing amino acids (CAA) tyrosine, valine, leucine, isoleucine, and phenylalanine) are significantly reduced in fibromyalgia [31, 32]; (ii) lowered serum serotonin concentrations are frequently reported in fibromyalgia patients [34–37]; (iii) the serotonin metabolites in CSF are significantly lower in patients with fibromyalgia than in normal volunteers [37]; and (iv) the number of platelet [$^3$H]imipramine binding sites is significantly decreased in fibromyalgia [38]. Moreover, significant relationships have been found between severity measures of fibromyalgia and serotonergic markers: (i) plasma free tryptophan, another indicator of the availability of tryptophan to the brain, is inversely related to severity of pain in fibromyalgia [33]; and (ii) a significant correlation between serum serotonin and hyperalgesia is found in fibromyalgia [36].

We examined the following serotonergic markers in fibromyalgia, i.e., platelet [³H]paroxetine binding characteristics ($B_{max}$ and $K_d$) and plasma total tryptophan, as well as the tryptophan/CAA ratio. Blood platelets are able to take up, store, and release 5-HT via mechanisms that are very similar to those of central 5-HT neurons. [³H]Paroxetine binds with high affinity to a specific population of binding sites located on platelets and neuronal membranes associated with 5-HT uptake mechanisms. It is reported that the cloned 5-HT transporter on human platelets is identical to the 5-HT transporter in human brain. The 5-HT transporter plays a critical role in 5-HT neurotransmission by reclaiming synaptic 5-HT.

We determined the above serotonergic variables in 13 and 21 fibromyalgia patients, respectively, and in 33 normal controls. We were unable to find any significant differences in [³H]paroxetine binding $B_{max}$ and $K_d$ values, plasma tryptophan, or the tryptophan/CAA ratio between fibromyalgia patients and normal controls. We did not find any significant correlations between the [³H]paroxetine binding characteristics, or the availability of tryptophan and myalgic or depressive symptoms. Thus, there are no major alterations in the metabolism of peripheral serotonin in fibromyalgia. Our results do not corroborate the hypothesis that fibromyalgia is accompanied by a deficiency in serotonergic metabolism, as indicated by lower [³H]paroxetine binding $B_{max}$ values, an indicator of the serotonergic transporter system, and lower plasma tryptophan availability to the brain.

## Hypothalamic-Pituitary-Adrenal (HPA) Axis and Fibromyalgia

There are some reports that fibromyalgia may be accompanied by disorders in HPA-axis function. For example, it is reported that 35% of the fibromyalgia patients have abnormal results of the dexamethasone suppression test (DST). A considerable number of patients with fibromyalgia show a loss of the diurnal variation in plasma cortisol [39]. Other groups, however, described indicators of low 24-h urinary cortisol (UC) excretion in fibromyalgia patients [40, 41] or a lowered rate of DST nonsuppression in patients with fibromyalgia than in normal controls [42].

We measured 24 UC in 17 normal volunteers and 14 fibromyalgia patients. The 24-h urine collections started at 11 p.m. and subjects were instructed to rest during the urine collections. The urine collections were considered to be complete if the creatinine excretion exceeded 0.7*T*g/day and urine volume 0.7*T*l/day. Cortisol was assayed by means of an enzyme-linked immunosorbent assay method (Cortisol Diagnostic Kit, Eurogenetics, Tessenderlo, Belgium). We found that there were no significant differences in 24-h UC excretion between fibromyalgia patients and controls. In fibromyalgia, there were no significant correlations between 24-h UC excretion and the Hamilton Depression Rating Scale score, the total myalgic score, and the measurements on a visual analog scale, i.e., global myalgic symptoms, anergy, stiffness and pain, and duration of illness. As pointed out above, previous research on the function of the HPA-axis in fibromyalgia had produced conflicting results. Chronic fatigue syndrome is another condition which shows a strong comorbidity with major depression and fibromyalgia, and may be accompanied by lowered activity of the HPA-axis [43].

Taken together, the data on HPA-axis function in fibromyalgia do not provide firm evidence that there are major dysfunctions in the HPA-axis in that condition.

## Peptidases and Fibromyalgia

We have examined the activity of serum prolyl endopeptidase (PEP) in fibromyalgia because of the following. Depression, which often accompanies fibromyalgia, is characterized by lower serum PEP [44, 45]. Lower PEP activity may deactivate the catabolism of neuropeptides, which modulate nociception, allodynia, and hyperalgesia. Two of these neuropeptides are bradykinin and substance P [46, 47]. Very high PEP activities are detected in skeletal muscles, where PEP functions degrade substance P [48, 49]. PEP also degrades many other behaviorally active neuropeptides or hormones, such as arginine vasopressin (AVP), luteinizing hormone-releasing hormone (LH-RH), thyrotropin releasing hormone (TRH), oxytocin, neurotensin, and angiotensin [50].

We measured serum PEP activity in 21 fibromyalgia patients and 28 normal controls. Serum PEP activity was significantly lower in fibromyalgia than in normal controls. In fibromyalgia, there were significant and positive correlations between serum PEP activity and the total myalgic scores. The results showed that serum PEP activity was significantly lower in fibromyalgia patients with severe pressure hyperalgesia as compared with those without severe pressure hyparalgesia. Moreover, in this study we found highly significant inverse relationships between serum PEP activity and the severity of the cognitive symptoms of depression. Thus, the findings suggest that lower PEP activity may be related to the pressure hyperalgesia and the cognitive depressive symptoms in fibromyalgia.

As explained above, PEP degrades peptides with potent algesic properties, i.e., substance P and bradykinin. The latter has an important role in the generation of pain, and hyperalgesia associated with tissue damage and inflammation [51–53]. It is known that PEP degrades bradykinin [51]. Substance P, on the other hand, mediates pain transmission and sensation [54–56]. Substance P may be cleaved by PEP into biologically active fragments which are subsequently removed by reuptake or degradation by exopeptidases [57]. Therefore, one hypothesis is that lower serum PEP may have caused a diminished degradation of bradykinin and substance P. This, in turn, could have induced tenderness, chronic pain, and hyperalgesia in fibromyalgia. The results of our study also show that lowered serum PEP activity may be related to the depressive symptoms in fibromyalgia. PEP may cleave many neuropeptides or hormones that have been shown to be involved in the pathophysiology of depression, e.g., TRH and AVP (see Introduction) and possibly corticotropin releasing hormone (CRH) [44, 50]. The results of our studies suggest that disturbances in PEP may play a role in the pathophysiology of fibromyalgia. Future research should focus on measurements of PEP activity in skeletal muscles and joints.

# The Inflammatory Response System (IRS) and Fibromyalgia

There are some reports that some fibromyalgia patients suffer from a low-grade inflammatory process [58] or from exaggerated neurogenic inflammatory responses [59]. Skin biopsies of fibromyalgia patients showed some indications of inflammatory responses [60]. Furthermore, there is now evidence that major depression, which shows a high degree of comorbidity with fibromyalgia, is accompanied by an activation of the IRS with an increased production of proinflammatory cytokines, such as interleukin-1 (IL-1) and IL-6 [61]. Interestingly, these cytokines may induce hyperalgesia by directly influencing the responsiveness of nociceptive neurons [62–67]. Moreover, both cytokines can induce fatigue, sleep disorders, and depression-like symptoms, which are other symptoms of fibromyalgia [68, 69]. Since fibromyalgia may be an inflammatory disorder and since IL-1 and IL-6 may induce the characteristic symptoms of fibromyalgia, we anticipated finding signs of IRS activation in fibromyalgia.

We examined the following IRS variables in 33 healthy controls and 21 fibromyalgia patients: serum IL-6, IL-6 receptor (IL-6R), IL-1R antagonist (IL-1RA), gp130, and sCD8 concentrations. Gp130 is the signal transducer protein for IL-6 and serum sgp130 may inhibit IL-6 signals through membrane-anchored gp130 [70, 71]. Serum gp130 may, like the sIL-6R, be generated by proteolysis (shedding) of the membrane receptor components [72]. We found no significant differences in serum IL-6, sIL-6R, and sIL-1RA between fibromyalgia patients and healthy controls. Serum gp130 concentrations were significantly higher in fibromyalgia patients. The area under the ROC curve for serum gp130 was 92.8%. At the optimal cutoff point, i.e., serum gp130 $\geqslant$ 1370*T*ng/ml, the sensitivity was 80.9%; specificity 93.9%; predictive value (PV) for a positive test result 89.4%; and the PV for a negative test result 88.6%. Serum CD8 concentrations were significantly lower in fibromyalgia patients than in healthy volunteers. Phrased differently, no significant signs of IRS activation, such as increased IL-6, IL-6R, and IL-1RA concentrations, could be found in fibromyalgia. On the contrary, fibromyalgia patients showed indications of immunosuppression, such as lower serum CD8 and increased serum gp130. Indeed, lower serum CD8 may indicate a defect in the early stages of $CD8^+$ T lymphocyte activation [73]. Second, serum gp130 competes with its membrane-bound counterpart and, consequently, may interfere with the signaling of a number of cytokines, such as IL-6, IL-11, leukemia inhibitory factor (LIF), oncostatin M (OSM), and ciliary neurotrophic factor (CNTF) [70, 71]. These results do not confirm those of previous studies showing signs of inflammation in fibromyalgia. Our results are in agreement with previous reports which were unable to detect IRS activation in fibromyalgia. For example, Hader et al. [74] found reduced mitogen-induced IL-2 secretion in patients with fibromyalgia. No significant differences in antinuclear antibodies could be found between fibromyalgia patients and normal controls [75]. The numbers of activated T cells expressing the activation markers CD25 and CD69 were found to be decreased in fibromyalgia patients [76]. The same authors did not detect any significant differences in lymphocyte subpopulations, such as the number of B lymphocytes (CD19), T lymphocytes (CD3), natural killer cells (NK), T-cytotoxic/T-suppressor lymphocytes (CD8), and T-helper/T-inducer lymphocytes (CD4) between patients with primary fibromyalgia and controls. There are also investigators who were unable to find evidence for inflammation in muscle biopsies [77, 78].

One hypothesis is that the changes in serum sgp130 may play a role in the etiology of fibromyalgia. Indeed, neurotrophic cytokines or neurokines, such as IL-6, IL-11, OSM, CNTF, and LIF have important effects on neuromuscular functioning. First, LIF and CNTF play an important role in (1) functions, such as the development, differentiation, survival, and neurotransmission of sensory, sympathetic, and motorneurons, and skeletal muscle cells; (2) the viability and vitality of muscle cells; and (3) the cholinergic phenotyping of sympathetic neurons [79, 82]. IL-6 modulates sympathetic nervous functions and plays a role in nerve regeneration [83]. IL-11 regulates neurogeneration [84]. IL-6, IL-11, and OSM regulate the cholinergic phenotype of sympathetic neurons [85]. In this respect, it has been shown that IL-6-deficient mice are hyperalgesic [86] and that local IL-6 administration elicits antinociception [87]. Thus, decreased gp130 signaling may be related to fibromyalgia symptoms through decreased signaling of the above neurokines.

# Conclusions

In conclusion, fibromyalgia may be a condition determined by different pathophysiological mechanisms, such as disorders in catecholaminergic metabolism, PEP activity, and decreased IL-6 signaling through increased serum concentrations of gp130 [88, 89]. The results of our studies suggest that future research should focus on the role of α2-ARs, peptidases, and decreased IL-6 signaling in fibromyalgia. This research should include, for example, measurements of α2-ARs, IL-6Rs, the signaling of IL-6, and other neurokines and PEP activity in skeletal muscles, the joints, and motoneurons.

## References

1. Wolfe F, Smythe HA, Yunus MB, Bennett RM, Bombardier C, Goldenberg DL, Tugwell P, Campbell SM, Abeles M, Clark P et al (1990) The American College of Rheumatology 1990 Criteria for the Classification of Fibromyalgia. Report of the Multicenter Criteria Committee. Arthritis Rheum 33:160–172
2. Schochat T, Croft P, Raspe H (1994) The epidemiology of fibromyalgia. Workshop of the Standing Committee on Epidemiology European League Against Rheumatism, Bad Säckingen, 19–21 November, 1992. Br J Rheumatol 33:783–786
3. Reiffenberger DH, Amundson LH (1996) Fibromyalgia syndrome: a review. Am Fam Physician 53:1698–1712
4. Hudson JI, Goldenberg DL, Pope HG, Keck PE, Schlesinger L (1992) Comorbidity of fibromyalgia with medical and psychiatric disorders. Am J Med 92:363–367
5. Krag NJ, Norregaard J, Larsen JK, Danneskiold-Samsoe B (1994) A blinded controlled evaluation of anxiety and depressive symptoms in patients with fibromyalgia, as measured by standardized psychometric interview scales. Acta Psychiatr Scand 89:370–375
6. Hudson JI, Hudson MS, Pliner LF, Goldenberg DL, Pope HG Jr (1985) Fibromyalgia and major affective disorder: a controlled phenomenology and family history study. Am J Psychiatry 142:441–446
7. Hawley DJ, Wolfe F (1993) Depression is not more common in rheumatoid arthritis: a 10-year longitudinal study of 6153 patients with rheumatic disease. J Rheumatol 20:2025–2031
8. Wilke WS (1996) Fibromyalgia. Recognizing and addressing the multiple interrelated factors. Postgrad Med 100:153–156
9. Gruber AJ, Hudson JI, Pope HG (1996) The management of treatment-resistant depression in disorders on the interface of psychiatry and medicine. Fibromyalgia, chronic fatigue syndrome, migraine, irritable bowel syndrome, atypical facial pain, and premenstrual dysphoric disorder. Psychiatr Clin North Am 19:351–369

10. Granges G, Zilko P, Littlejohn GO (1994) Fibromyalgia syndrome: assessment of the severity of the condition 2 years after diagnosis. J Rheumatol 21:523–529
11. Hudson JI, Pope HG (1989) Fibromyalgia and psychopathology: is fibromyalgia a form of affective spectrum disorder? J Rheumatol (suppl) 19:15–22
12. Moldofsky H (1995) Sleep, neuroimmune and neuroendocrine functions in fibromyalgia and chronic fatigue syndrome. Adv Neuroimmunol 5:39–56
13. Russell IJ (1989) Neurohormonal aspects of fibromyalgia syndrome. Rheum Dis Clin North Am 15:149–165
14. Bennett RM, Clark SR, Campbell SM, Ingram SB, Burckhardt CS, Nelson DL, Porter JM (1991) Symptoms of Raynaud's syndrome in patients with fibromyalgia. A study utilizing the Nielsen test, digital photoplethysmography, and measurements of platelet alpha 2-adrenergic receptors. Arthritis Rheum 34:264–269
15. Elam M, Johansson G, Wallin BG (1992) Do patients with primary fibromyalgia have an altered muscle sympatetic nerve activity? Pain 48:371–375
16. Yunus MB, Daily JW, Aldag JC, Masi AT, Jobe PC (1992) Plasma and urinary catecholamines in primary fibromyalgia: a controlled study. J Rheumatol 19:95–97
17. Stahl SM (1985) Peripheral models for the study of neurotransmitter receptors in man. Psychopharmacol Bull 21:663–671
18. Hieble JP, Bondinell WE, Ruffolo RR (1995) $\alpha$1- and $\alpha$2-adrenoceptors: from the gene to the clinic. 1. Molecular biology and adrenoceptor classification. J Med Chem 38:3415–3444
19. Limberger N, Funk L, Trendelenburg AU, Starke K (1995) Subclassification of presynaptic $\alpha$2-adrenoceptors: $\alpha$2-autoreceptors in rabbit atria and kidney. Naunyn-Schmiedeberg's Arch Pharmacol 352:31–42
20. Sato J, Perl ER (1991) Adrenergic excitation of cutaneous pain receptors induced by peripheral nerve injury. Science 251:1608–1610
21. Yeomans DC, Clark FM, Paice JA, Proudfit HK (1992) Antinociception induced by electrical stimulation of spinally projecting noradrenergic neurons in the A7 catecholamine cell group of the rat. Pain 48:449–461
22. Millan MJ (1992) Evidence that an alpha 2A-adrenoceptor subtype mediates antinociception in mice. Eur J Pharmacol 14:355–356
23. Khasar SG, Green PG, Chou B, Levine JD (1995) Peripheral nociceptive effects of alpha 2-adrenergic receptor agonists in the rat. Neuroscience 66:427–432
24. McQuay HJ (1988) Pharmacological treatment of neuralgic and neuropathic pain. Cancer Surv 7:141–159
25. Rauck RL, Eisenach JC, Jackson K, Young LD, Southern J (1993) Epidural clonidine treatment for refractory reflex sympathetic dystrophy. Anesthesiology 79:1163–1169
26. Lee Y-W, Yaksh TL (1995) Analysis of drug interaction between intrathecal clonidine and MK-801 in peripheral neuropathic pain rat model. Anesthesiology 82:741–748
27. Glynn C, O'Sullivan K (1995) A double-blind randomized comparison of the effects of epidural clonidine, lignocaine and the combination of clonidine and lignocaine in patients with chronic pain. Pain 64:337–343
28. American Psychiatric Association (1987) Diagnostic and statistical manual of mental disorders (3rd edn., revised). American Psychiatric Association, Washington
29. Spitzer RL, Williams JBW, Gibbon MSW, First MB (1990) Structured Clinical Interview according to DSM-III-R. American Psychiatric Press, Washington
30. Neeck G, Riedel W (1994) Neuromediator and hormonal perturbations in fibromyalgia syndrome: results of chronic stress? Baillieres Clin Rheumatol 8:763–775
31. Yunus MB, Dailey JW, Aldag JC, Masi AT, Jobe PC (1992) Plasma tryptophan and other amino acids in primary fibromyalgia: a controlled study. J Rheumatol 19:90–94
32. Russell IJ, Michalek JE, Vipraio GA, Fletcher EM, Wall K (1989) Serum amino acids in fibrositis/fibromyalgia syndrome. J Rheumatol Suppl 19:158–163
33. Moldofsky H, Warsh JJ (1978) Plasma tryptophan and musculoskeletal pain in non-articular rheumatism ("fibrositis syndrome"). Pain 5:65–71

34. Wolfe F, Russell IJ, Vipraio G, Ross K, Anderson J (1997) Serotonin levels, pain thresh-old, and fibromyalgia symptoms in the general population. J Rheumatol 24:555–559
35. Samborski W, Stratz T, Schochat T, Mennet P, Muller W (1996) Biochemical changes in fibromyalgia. Z Rheumatol 55:168–173
36. Stratz T, Samborski W, Hrycaj P, Pap T, Mackiewicz S, Mennet P, Muller W (1993) Serotonin concentration in serum of patients with generalized tendomyopathy (fibromyalgia) and chronic polyarthritis. Med Klin 88:458–462
37. Russell IJ, Vaeroy H, Javors M, Nyberg F (1992) Cerebrospinal fluid biogenic amine metabolites in fibromyalgia/fibrositis syndrome and rheumatoid arthritis. Arthritis Rheum 35:550–556
38. Russell IJ, Michalek JE, Vipraio GA, Fletcher EM, Javors MA, Bowden CA (1992) Platelet $^3$H-imipramine uptake receptor density and serum serotonin levels in patients with fibromyalgia/fibrositis syndrome. J Rheumatol 19:104–109
39. McCain GA, Tilbe KS (1989) Diurnal variation in fibromyalgia syndrome: a compari-son with rheumatoid arthritis. J Rheumatol (Suppl) 19:154–157
40. Crofford LJ, Pillemer SR, Kalogeras KT, Cash JM, Michelson D, Kling MA, Sternberg EM, Gold PW, Chrousos GP, Wilder RL (1994) Hypothalamic-pituitary-adrenal axis perturbations in patients with fibromyalgia. Arthritis Rheum 37:1583–1592
41. Van Denderen JC, Boersma JW, Zeinstra P, Hollander AP, Van Neerbos BR (1992) Physiological effects of exhaustive physical exercise in primary fibromyalgia syndrome (PFS): is PFS a disorder of neuroendocrine reactivity? Scand J Rheumatol 21:35–37
42. Hudson JI, Pliner LF, Hudson MS, Goldenberg DL, Melby JC (1984) The dexametha-sone suppression test in fibrositis. Biol Psychiatry 19:1489–1493
43. Cleare AJ, Bearn J, Alaain T, McGregor A, Wessely S, Murray RM, O'Keane V (1995) Contrasting neuroendocrine responses in depression and chronic fatigue syndrome. J Affect Disord 18:283–289
44. Maes M, Goossens F, Scharpe S, Meltzer HY, D'Hondt P, Cosyns P (1994) Lower serum prolyl endopeptidase enzyme activity in major depression: further evidence that pep-tidases play a role in the pathophysiology of depression. Biol Psychiatry 35:545–552
45. Maes M, Scharpe S, Meltzer HY, Calabrese J (1995) Plasma prolyl endopeptidase enzyme activity in major depression, schizophrenia and mania: effects of antidepres-sive drugs, neuroleptics and valproate. Psychiatr Res 58:217–225
46. Lotz M, Vaughan JH, Carson DA (1988) Effect of neuropeptides on production of inflammatory cytokines by human monocytes. Science 241:1218–1221
47. Watkins LR, Maier SF, Goehler LE (1995) Immune activation: the role of pro-inflammatory cytokines in inflammation, illness responses and pathological pain states. Pain 63:289–302
48. Kato T, Okada M, Nagatsu T (1980) Distribution of post-proline cleaving enzyme in human brain and the peripheral tissues. Mol Cell Biochem 32:117–121
49. Moriyama A, Nakanishi M, Sasaki M (1988) Porcine muscle endopeptidase and its endogenous substrates. J Biochem 104:112–117
50. Welches WR, Brosnihan KB, Ferrario CM (1993) A comparison of the properties and enzymatic activities of three angiotensin processing enzymes: angiotensin converting enzyme, prolyl endopeptidase and neutral endopeptidase 24.11. Life Sci 52:1461–1480
51. Bhoola KD, Figueroa CD, Worthy K (1992) Bioregulation of kinins: kallikreins, kilino-gens, and kininases. Pharmacol Rev 44:1–80
52. Dray A, Perkins M (1993) Bradykinin and inflammatory pain. Trends Neurosci 16:99–104
53. Tracey DJ, Walker JS (1995) Review: Pain due to nerve damage: are inflammatory medi-ators involved? Inflamm Res 44:407–411
54. Pernow B (1983) Substance P. Pharmacol Rev 35:85–141
55. Piercey MF, Moon MW, Blinn JR, Dobry-Schreur PJK (1986) Analgesic activities of spinal cord substance P antagonists implicate substance P as a neurotransmitter of pain sensation. Brain Res 385:74–85

56. Saria A (1987) The role of substance P and other neuropeptides in transmission of pain. Acta Neurochirurg 38 (Suppl):33–35
57. Sandberg BEB, Iversen LL (1982) Substance P. J Med Chem 25:1009–1015
58. Caro XJ (1989) Is there an immunologic component to the fibrositis syndrome? Rheum Disease Clin North Am 15:169–186
59. Littlejohn GO, Weinstein C, Helme RD (1987) Increased neurogenic inflammation in fibrositis syndrome. J Rheumatol 14:1022–1025
60. Enestrom S, Bengtsson A, Frodin T (1997) Dermal IgG deposits and increase of mast cells in patients with fibromyalgia—relevant findings or epiphenomena? Scand J Rheumatol 26:308–313
61. Maes M (1997) The immune pathophysiology of major depression. In: Honig A, van Praag HM (eds) Depression, neurobiological, psychopathological and therapeutic advances. Wiley, Chichester, pp 197–215
62. Cunha FQ, Poole S, Lorenzetti BB, Ferreira SH (1992) The pivotal role of tumour necrosis factor alpha in the development of inflammatory hyperalgesia. Br J Pharmacol 107:660–664
63. DeLeo JA, Colburn RW, Nichols M, Malhotra A (1996) Interleukin-6-mediated hyperalgesia/allodynia and increased spinal IL-6 expression in a rat mononeuropathy model. J Interf Cytokine Res 16:695–700
64. Ferreira SH, Lorenzetti BB, Bristow AF, Poole S (1988) Interleukin-1 beta as a potent hyperalgesic agent antagonized by a tripeptide analogue. Nature 25:698–700
65. Oka T, Aou S, Hori T (1994) Intracerebroventricular injection of interleukin-1 beta enhances nociceptive neuronal responses of the trigeminal nucleus caudalis in rats. Brain Res 656:236–244
66. Oka T, Oka K, Hosoi M, Hori T (1995) Intracerebroventricular injection of interleukin-6 induces thermal hyperalgesia in rats. Brain Res 692:123–128
67. Watkins LR, Wiertelak EP, Goehler LE, Smith KP, Martin D, Maier SF (1994) Characterization of cytokine-induced hyperalgesia. Brain Res 654:15–26
68. Bluthé RM, Crestani F, Kelley KW, Dantzer R (1992) Mechanisms of the behavioral effects of interleukin 1. Ann NY Acad Sci 650:268–275
69. Spath-Schwalbe E, Hansen K, Schmidt F, Schrezenmeier H, Marshall L, Burger K, Fehm HL, Born J (1998) Acute effects of recombinant human interleukin-6 on endocrine and central nervous sleep functions in healthy men. J Clin Endocrinol Metabol 83: 1573–1579
70. Murakami-Mori K, Taga T, Kishimoto T, Nakamura S (1996) The soluble form of the IL-6 receptor (sIL-6R) is a potent growth factor for AIDS-associated Kaposi's sarcoma (KS) cells; the soluble form of gp130 is antagonistic for IL-6Rα-induced AIDS-KS cell growth. Int Immunol 8:595–602
71. Narazaki M, Yasukawa K, Saito T, Ohsugi Y, Fukui H, Koishihara Y, Yancopoulos GD, Taga T, Kishimoto T (1993) Soluble forms of the interleukin-6 signal-transducing receptor component gp130 in human serum possessing a potential to inhibit signals through membrane-anchored gp130. Blood 82:1120–1126
72. Peters M, Jacobs S, Ehlers M, Vollmer P, Mullberg J, Wolf E, Brem G, Meyerzum-Buschenfelde KH, Rose-John S (1996) The function of the soluble interleukin-6 (IL-6) receptor in vivo: sensitization of human soluble IL-6 receptor transgenic mice towards IL-6 and prolongation of the plasma half-life of IL-6. J Exp Med 183:1399–1406
73. Kim HS, Degiannis D, Raskova J, Raska K (1991) Cyclosporine A and prednisolone inhibit lectin- and alloantigen-induced release of sCD8: correlation with proliferative responses. Clin Immunol Immunopathol 60:27–39
74. Hader N, Rimon D, Kinarty A, Lahat N (1991) Altered interleukin-2 secretion in patients with primary fibromyalgia syndrome. Arthritis Rheum 34:866–872
75. Yunus MB, Hussey FX, Aldag JC (1993) Antinuclear antibodies and connective tissue

disease features in fibromyalgia syndrome: a controlled study. J Rheumatol 20: 1557–1560

76. Hernanz W, Valenzuela A, Quijada J, Garcia A, De La Iglesia JL, Gutierrez A, Povedano J, Moreno I, Sanchez B (1994) Lymphocyte subpopulations in patients with primary fibromyalgia. J Rheumatol 21:2122–2124

77. Kalyan-Raman UP, Kalyan-Raman K, Yunus MB, Masi AT (1984) Muscle pathology in primary fibromyalgia syndrome: a light microscopic, histochemical and ultrastructural study. J Rheumatol 11:808–813

78. Yunus MB, Kalyan-Raman UP, Kalyan-Raman K, Masi AT (1986) Pathologic changes in muscle in primary fibromyalgia syndrome. Am J Med 29:38–42

79. Cannon JG (1995) Cytokines in aging and muscle homeostasis. J Gerontol 50:120–123

80. Li M, Sendtner M, Smith A (1995) Essential function of LIF receptor in motor neurons. Nature 378:724–727

81. Sendtner M, Carroll P, Holtmann B, Hughes RA, Thoenen H (1994) Ciliary neurotrophic factor. J Neurobiol 25:1436–1453

82. Vakakis N, Bower J, Austin L (1995) In vitro myoblast to myotube transformations in the presence of leukemia inhibitory factor. Neurochem Int 27:329–335

83. Hirota H, Kiyama H, Kishimoto T, Taga T (1996) Accelerated nerve regeneration in mice by upregulated expression of interleukin (IL) 6 and IL-6 receptor after trauma. J Exp Med 183:2627–2634

84. Quesniaux VFJ (1996) Interleukin-11. In: Cavaillon J-M (ed) Les cytokines. Masson, Paris, pp 253–266

85. Fann MJ, Patterson PH (1994) Neuropoietic cytokines and activin A differently regulate the phenotype of cultured sympathetic neurons. Proc Natl Acad Sci USA 91:43–47

86. Xu XJ, Hao JX, Andell-Jonsson S, Poli V, Bartfai T, Wiesenfeld-Hallin Z (1997) Nociceptive responses in interleukin-6-deficient mice to peripheral inflammation and peripheral nerve section. Cytokine 9:1028–1033

87. Czlonkowski A, Stein C, Herz A (1993) Peripheral mechanisms of opioid antinociception in inflammation: involvement of cytokines. Eur J Pharmacol 242:229–235

88. Maes M, Libbrecht I, VanHunsel F, Lin A, Bonaccorso S, Goossens F, DeMeester I, DeClerck L, Biondi M, Scharpe S, Janca A (1998) Lower serum peptidase activity in fibromyalgia is related to myalgic pain and cognitive symptoms of depression. Psychol Med 28:957–965

89. Maes M, Libbrecht I, van Hunsel F, Lin A, DeClerck L, Stevens W, Kenis G, DeJong R, Bosmans E, Neels H, Scharpe S (1999) Alterations in the immune-inflammatory response system in fibromyalgia: increased serum soluble gp130, the common signal tranducer protein for various neurotrophic cytokines. Psychoneuroendocrinology, in press

# Part 2
# Studies on Somatoform Disorders in Different Cultures

# WHO International Study of Somatoform Disorders: An Overview of Methods and Preliminary Results

Aleksandar Janca[1], Gianluigi Tacchini[2], and Mohan Isaac[3]

*Summary.* This chapter summarises methods and preliminary results of the International Study of Somatoform Disorders—one of the most recent multi-site research projects coordinated by the World Health Organisation (WHO). The project has been carried out in 11 countries representing different regions, cultures and socio-economic settings of the world. Both qualitative and quantitative research methods have been employed in different stages of the project, which comprises: an expert review of published literature on somatisation; a mail questionnaire survey of cross-cultural applicability of diagnostic definitions and criteria for somatoform disorders; development and testing of instruments for the assessment of somatoform disorders; assessment of rates and culture-specific characteristics of somatoform disorders in different parts of the world; and development of educational materials and management guidelines for somatoform disorders, for use in primary care, general medical and psychiatric settings.

*Key words.* Somatization, Somatoform disorders, Trans-cultural psychiatry, Psychiatric assessment, World Health Organization

## Introduction

Research projects carried out by WHO follow public health principles and are focused on problems and disorders that are frequent, disabling and represent a burden on health systems, communities and societies all over the world [1]. Somatoform disorders are characterised by multiple, persistent and medically unexplained somatic symptoms which cause significant distress to the patients. Such patients are often preoccupied with their symptoms and, in spite of repeated negative findings

[1] Department of Psychiatry and Behavioural Science, University of Western Australia, 50 Murray Street, Perth, WA 6000, Australia
[2] Psychiatric Clinic, University of Milan, Via Francesco Sforza 35, 20122 Milan, Italy
[3] Department of Psychiatry, National Institute of Mental Health and Neurosciences, Bangalore 560029, India

and reassurances by doctors that the symptoms have no physical basis, are persistent in their requests for further medical investigations. Because of their high rate of help-seeking behaviour and refusal to accept psychological explanation of their illness, patients with somatoform disorders represent an important part of the burden in primary care and general medical practice all over the world [2–4].

In response to this burden, a multi-site international study of somatoform disorders was launched in 1993 by WHO with the following objectives: (i) to explore the cross-cultural applicability of latest diagnostic definitions and criteria for somatoform disorders; (ii) to develop a set of diagnostic instruments for the assessment of somatoform disorders and test their acceptability and reliability in different cultures and settings; (iii) to assess the rates and culture-specific characteristics of somatoform disorders in different parts of the world; and (iv) to produce an educational program, training materials and management guidelines for somatoform disorders intended for use in primary care, general medical and psychiatric settings [5]. The project, which is still under way, consists of several components and they are described hereafter.

## Expert Review of Recent Literature on Somatisation

As a preliminary step in developing protocols and instruments for WHO International Study of Somatoform Disorders, a large body of existing data and published literature was reviewed, so as to obtain information on currently available knowledge and issues that require further research in the field of somatoform disorders. The expert review pointed out: (i) a need to study the nature of somatoform disorders with specific reference to symptom patterns, consulting behaviour, attribution, course, disability and response to treatment; (ii) necessity to develop assessment tools for somatoform disorders which would enhance comprehensive collection of comparable and reliable data in different cultures and settings; (iii) a need for research on cross-cultural aspects of somatoform disorders involving large samples of clinical and non-clinical populations to understand the complex interplay of social and cultural factors and somatisation; and (iv) a need to develop and evaluate cost-effective intervention strategies for patients with somatoform disorders [6].

## Mail Questionnaire Survey

Also prior to the beginning of the project, a mail questionnaire survey was organised to obtain expert opinion on the cross-cultural applicability of, at that time just published, ICD-10 [7] definitions of somatoform disorders. In addition, experts were asked to rate cultural relevance of specific characteristics of the medically unexplained somatic symptoms according to ICD-10 criteria, including their frequency, suggestiveness of somatisation, and patients' refusal to accept psychological explanation.

A somatic symptom questionnaire which consisted of ICD-10 definitions of somatoform disorders and an extensive list of more than 60 somatic symptoms was mailed to 80 experts including a number of members of WHO Expert Panel on Mental Health (known for their interest in ICD-10) and other professionals working in the fields of cross-cultural psychiatry, psychology, sociology, epidemiology and anthropology. The response was obtained from 42 experts in 23 countries representing all five continents. The results of the survey showed that the ICD-10 concept of somatoform disorders was generally acceptable for use across cultures. However, many experts pointed out the relative restrictiveness of ICD-10 criteria for Somatisation Disorder and emphasised the usefulness of having the more inclusive category of Undifferentiated Somatoform Disorder in the Classification. Some experts also listed a number of culture-specific symptoms, characteristics and terms that do not appear in ICD-10, but were found to be common and important for diagnosis of somatoform disorders in their particular cultures (e.g., in India: loss of semen while urinating; in Japan: body odour) [8].

# Development and Testing of Instruments

In Phase I of the project, the following standardised instruments for the assessment of somatoform disorders were produced:

(i) Somatoform Disorders Schedule (SDS) [9]—a highly structured diagnostic instrument based on the Composite International Diagnostic Interview (CIDI) [10] and intended for the assessment of: Somatisation Disorder, Dissociative (Conversion) Disorder, Somatoform Autonomic Dysfunction, Undifferentiated Somatoform Disorder, Persistent Somatoform Pain Disorder, Hypochondriasis and Neurasthenia. The symptom questions in the SDS are fully standardised and the respondent's positive answers are explored by a clearly specified probing system (i.e., a set of predetermined follow-up questions). Such a high degree of standardisation allows the administration of the SDS not only by clinicians but also by trained lay-interviewers.

(ii) Somatoform Disorders Symptom Checklist [11]—a semi-structured diagnostic instrument designed for use by clinicians and intended for the assessment of symptoms of all those diagnostic categories of somatoform disorders covered by SDS. The Checklist provides an extensive listing of both ICD-10 and DSM-IV [12] symptoms of somatoform disorders, and clinician interviewers are required to phrase symptom questions and explore clinical relevance of positive answers as in routine clinical interview. Brief diagnostic scoring algorithms are provided at the end of the Checklist so as to enable clinicians to make quick diagnostic statements according to the ICD-10 criteria.

(iii) Screener for Somatoform Disorders [13]—a 12-item screening instrument that can be self-or interviewer administered. Three or more positive somatic symptoms during the period 6 months or one or more positive somatic symptoms of at least 1 month duration represent the screening threshold of this instrument.

The instruments were tested for their cross-cultural applicability and reliability in the following centres: Bangalore (India), São Paulo (Brazil), Milan and Cagliari (Italy), Harare (Zimbabwe) and Temple (Texas, USA). A sample of 180 patients from general psychiatry, primary care and general medical settings were interviewed with the instruments within a 3-day interval by non-clinician and clinician interviewers. The agreement between the two interviews was tested using the Intraclass Correlation Coefficients (ICC) and Kappa statistic. The test-retest reliability of the SDS was found to be very good (the ICC for all the centres was 0.76; overall Kappa value for SDS questions was 0.58; one-third of SDS questions had a Kappa value of 0.60 or higher). The content analysis of collaborating investigators' reports showed that the SDS was found to be easy to learn and use by both clinician and non-clinician interviewers. The reports also indicated that the SDS was cross-culturally applicable and well accepted by professionals belonging to different psychiatric schools and clinical traditions [14].

# Frequency and Cultural Connotations of Somatic Symptoms

The earlier described mail questionnaire survey showed that the frequency and cultural aspects of medically unexplained somatic symptoms differ across cultures and that some of the somatic symptoms that are considered frequent or indicative of somatisation are scarce or atypical in other cultures [8]. The frequency and culture-specific characteristics of medically unexplained somatic symptoms covered by the SDS were further explored using the data obtained during the field testing of the instrument. The analysis of such collaterally obtained information showed that various aches and pains in different parts of the body represented cross-culturally the most frequent symptoms for which there was no medical explanation. Since such symptoms may indicate the presence of an underlying mental disorder, this finding bears particular significance for health professionals in primary and general medical care who are most likely to encounter patients presenting with multiple, persistent and medically unexplained somatic symptoms [15].

The content analysis of participating investigators' reports showed that certain symptoms of somatoform disorders were found to be dependent on specific cultures and settings. For example, symptoms such as blotchiness or discolouration of the skin were not relevant in India and Zimbabwe, while symptoms such as belching or hiccough were infrequently reported in the United States. Some of the symptoms posed translation difficulties: for patients in India it was difficult to distinguish between fainting, seizures and unconsciousness; in the Kannada language, the translated word for amnesia was mistaken by many patients for forgetfulness or loss of memory. The Indian centre also reported that patients from rural areas tended to attribute their somatic symptoms to a variety of reasons that included displacement of abdominal organs from their normal positions, non-observance of post-partum rituals, consumption of "hot" or "cold" food items, sorcery, etc.

A number of centres reported a temporal relationship between frequently seen somatic symptoms and some significant or stressful life event. Exposure to numerous socioeconomic problems and consequent demoralisation was reported as a possible contributing factor to the frequently seen medically unexplained somatic symptoms in Brazil [15].

# Rates of Somatoform Disorders in Different Cultures

Phase II of the project was focused on the assessment of rates and culture-specific characteristics of somatoform disorders in primary care and general medical settings in different regions of the world, and was carried out in the following centres: Bangalore (India), São Paulo (Brazil), Temple (Texas, USA), Milan and Cagliari (Italy), Tartu (Estonia), Harare (Zimbabwe), Sofia (Bulgaria), Mainz (Germany), Stoke-on-Trent (UK) and Beijing (China). The study instruments used in this phase of the project included SDS, Screener for Somatoform Disorders and anxiety, depression and alcohol use sections of the CIDI. Instruments were translated into local languages and training courses were organised for research teams by WHO. The assessment procedure also included reviews of medical records, laboratory and other test reports as well as clinician's detailed examinations of complex cases.

About 1200 randomly chosen attendants of the primary care and general medical settings were examined and their mean and median age was 40; 65% of the patients were females. The majority of the patients (67%) entered the detailed assessment by having been screened for three or more positive medically unexplained symptoms present in the period of six months prior to the examination.

The overall prevalence rates of specific somatoform disorders were as follows: Somatisation Disorder 1%: Undifferentiated Somatoform Disorder 7%; Hypochondriacal Disorder 1%; Somatoform Autonomic Dysfunction 4%; Persistent Somatoform Pain Disorder 15%; and Neurasthenia 4%. The analysis also showed that more than 24% of assessed patients fulfilled criteria for more than one somatoform disorder, thus indicating insufficiently clear boundaries between specific diagnostic categories of somatoform disorders. A detailed report on this phase of the project is being prepared.

# Comment

It has been traditionally believed that somatic expression of psychological disorders is predominant in non-Western and developing countries and among ethnic groups in the West. However, there has been growing evidence that suggests that somatisation is a universal phenomenon and that somatoform disorders represent an important burden created by psychological illness in general practice in Western cultures too [16].

In response to this significant public health problem, the WHO has recently launched an international study of somatoform disorders, the objectives, methods and preliminary results of which have been described in this chapter. Phase III of this project is under way and is aimed at developing an educational program and set of management guidelines for use in primary care, general medical and psychiatric settings. The overall results of the project will eventually be used in refining the diagnostic criteria and instruments for the assessment of somatoform disorders. It is hoped that this WHO project will enhance the recognition and management of somatoform disorders in different cultures and settings.

*Acknowledgements.* The WHO International Study of Somatoform Disorders study has been coordinated by Dr. A. Janca, formerly Medical Officer, Division of Mental Health and Prevention of Substance Abuse, WHO, currently Associate Professor, Department of Psychiatry and Behavioural Science, University of Western Australia, Perth, Australia (responsible WHO officer at present is Dr. J.M. Bertolote). The plans have been developed in collaboration with Dr. A.C. Altamura, Institute of Psychiatry, Cagliari, Italy; Dr. L.A. Bennett, Department of Anthropology, University of Memphis, TN, USA; Dr. J.D. Burke Jr., Department of Psychiatry, Texas A & M University, Temple, TX, USA; Dr. A. Forgione, Ravizza Farmaceutici Spa., Muggio, Italy; Dr. L.N. Robins, Department of Psychiatry, Washington University School of Medicine, St. Louis, MO, USA; and Dr. G. Tacchini, Department of Psychiatry, University of Milan, Milan, Italy. Dr. N. Sartorius, former Director of the Division of Mental Health, WHO, inspired the development of this project from its inception and has provided valuable advice in all its stages.

Phase I participants: Dr. C. Torres de Miranda, Department of Psychiatry, Escola Paulista de Medicina, Sao Paulo, Brazil; Dr. C.R. Chandrashekar, National Institute of Mental Health and Neurosciences, Bangalore, India, Dr. C.A. Altamura and Dr. M. Carta, Institute of Psychiatry, Cagliari, Italy; Dr. G. Tacchini, Department of Psychiatry, University of Milan, Milan, Italy; Dr. J.D. Burke Jr. and Mrs. K. Burke, Department of Psychiatry, and Dr. G. Couchman, Department of Family Medicine, Texas-A & M University, Temple, TX, USA; and Dr. S.W. Acuda and Dr. C.M. Winston, Department of Psychiatry, University of Zimbabwe, Harare, Zimbabwe.

Phase II participants: participants in Phase I and: Dr. B. Ivanov, Psychiatric Clinic, VMI Medical Faculty, Sofia, Bulgaria; Dr. Meng Fanqiang, Institute of Mental Health, Beijing Medical University, Beijing, China; Dr. W. Maier and Dr. O. Weiffenbach, Psychiatrische Klinik und Poliklinik, Johannes Gutenberg Universität Mainz Klinikum, Mainz, Germany; Dr. M. Asai and Dr. Y. Ono, Department of Neuropsychiatry, Keio University School of Medicine, Tokyo, Japan; Dr. J.L. Cox and Dr. A.P. Boardman, Department of Psychiatry, School of Postgraduate Medicine, Keele University, Stoke-on-Trent, UK.

The WHO International Study of Somatoform Disorders is supported by a donation received from Ravizza Farmaceutici Spa., BASF Group, Muggio, Italy.

# References

1. Sartorius N (1993) WHO's work on the epidemiology of mental disorders. Soc Psychiatry Psychiatr Epidemiol 28:147–155
2. Harding TW, de Arango MV, Baltazar J, Climent CE, Ibrahim HHA, Ladrido-Ignacio L, Srinivasa Murthy R, Wig NN (1980) Mental disorders in primary health care: a study of their frequency and diagnosis in developing countries. Psychol Med 10:231–241
3. Bridges K, Goldberg D, Evans B, Sharpe T (1987) Determinants of somatisation in primary care. Psychol Med 21:473–483
4. Escobar JI, Golding JM, Hough RL, Kamo M, Burnam MA, Wells KB (1987) Somatisation in the community: relationship to disability and use of services. Am J Publ Health 77(7):337–340
5. World Health Organisation (1993) WHO international study of somatoform disorders: study protocol and instruments. WHO, Geneva

6. Janca A, Isaac M, Costa e Silva JA (1995) A World Health Organisation international study of somatoform disorders—background and rationale. Eur J Psychiatry 9(2):100–110

7. World Health Organisation (1992) ICD-10 classification of mental and behavioural disorders. WHO, Geneva

8. Janca A, Isaac M, Bennett LA, Tacchini G (1995) Somatoform disorders in different cultures—a mail questionnaire survey. Soc Psychiatry Psychiatr Epidemiol 30:44–48

9. World Health Organisation (1993) Somatoform disorders schedule (SDS). WHO, Geneva

10. World Health Organisation (1993) Composite international diagnostic interview (CIDI). APPI, Washington, DC

11. Janca A, Isaac M, Tacchini G (1993) Somatoform disorders symptom checklist. WHO, Geneva

12. American Psychiatric Association (1994) Diagnostic and statistical manual of mental disorders, fourth edition (DSM-IV). APA, Washington, DC

13. Isaac M, Tacchini G, Janca A (1993) Screener for somatoform disorders. WHO, Geneva

14. Janca A, Burke JD, Isaac M, Burke KC, Costa e Silva JA, Acuda SW, Altamura AC, Chandrashekar CR, Miranda CT, Tacchini G (1995) The World Health Organisation somatoform disorders schedule: a preliminary report on design and reliability. Eur Psychiatry 10:373–378

15. Isaac M, Janca A, Burke KC, Costa e Silva JA, Acuda SW, Altamura AC, Burke JD, Chandrashekar CR, Miranda CT, Tacchini G (1995) Medically unexplained somatic symptoms in different cultures. Psychother Psychosom 64:88–93

16. Isaac M, Janca A, Orley J (1996) Somatisation—a culture-bound or universal syndrome? J Ment Health 5(3):219–222

# Help-Seeking Behavior Across Different Age and Culture Groups

Yutaka Ono[1], Nobuo Araki[2], Mitsue Mitani[3],
and Kimio Yoshimura[4]

*Summary.* The present study investigates and discusses the help-seeking behavior of patients who exhibited somatic symptoms that have not been clearly defined clinically. These patients consisted of those who participated in the WHO International Study of Somatoform Disorders conducted at nine centers internationally. Most of the patients had consulted a psychiatrist on multiple occasions prior to visiting the test center. The pattern of consultation differed among the various groups, suggesting that the help-seeking behavior and attitudes these patients have towards their somatic symptoms exhibit cultural differences. Most of the patients in this study consulted other professionals despite an apparent improvement. These findings suggest that the patients' perception of their somatic symptoms must be modified in accordance with their cultural background.

*Key words.* Help-seeking behavior, Somatoform disorders, Cultural differences

## Introduction

Somatic symptoms that have not been clearly defined clinically were listed in the official nomenclature as somatoform disorders for the first time in the DSM-III [1]. These symptoms have since been commonly seen among patients in primary care settings as well as among the general population. The health care utilization patterns of these patients are affected by societal as well as individual factors [2]. For example, these patterns may be influenced by a patient's experience with such somatic symptoms as affected by various socio-cultural factors [3]. Cognitive health anxiety, which was described in another section of this book, could also affect such experiences. Clinically, medical specialists need to identify the underlying perception of patients

---

[1] Keio University School of Medicine
[2] Nippon Kokan Hospital
[3] PHP Research Institute
[4] Cancer Information and Epidemiology Division, National Cancer Center Research Institute

with poorly defined somatic symptoms in order to improve health care. Thus, these sociocultural factors are important considerations in the proper diagnosis and treatment of such patients.

No systematic research has been conducted in which the cultural differences among such patients examined. Thus, the present study investigates the help-seeking behavior of patients with poorly defined somatic symptoms in several different countries, and discusses the treatment implications based on the findings of the WHO International Study of Somatoform Disorders.

## Subjects and Methods

The present study was conducted internationally by the World Health Organization. The details of the study will be described in chapter the chapter by Janca et al., this volume. The following centers participated in this project: India, United States, Brazil, Japan, Italy, China, Zimbabwe, Estonia, and Bulgaria.

Patients for the study were recruited from the following medical centers: primary care clinics, family/general practices and polyclinics in most of the countries, from general hospitals in China and Japan, and from a special unit for neurotic disorders in Estonia.

A total of 8399 outpatients who agreed to participate in this WHO international project were assessed by a Screener for Somatoform Disorders and by a physical examination done by a physician. Seven hundred fifty-nine patients who were diagnosed as being medically ill or as having poorly defined symptoms based on the above mentioned tests were subsequently evaluated by the Composite International Diagnostic Interview (CIDI) [4] and by the Somatoform Disorders Schedule (SDS) [5]. The latter contains a section for assessing the patient's help-seeking behavior.

Table 1 shows the demographics of the subjects. The number of female subjects was three times that of the male subjects. The average age for all patients was 39 years (SD14).

TABLE 1. Demographic data

|  | Total (%) | Sex | | Age | | | |
|  |  | Male | Female | Min. | Max. | Mean | SD |
|---|---|---|---|---|---|---|---|
| India | 120 (15.8) | 30 | 90 | 18 | 60 | 40.3 | 11.6 |
| USA | 94 (12.4) | 6 | 88 | 19 | 64 | 42.4 | 9.8 |
| Brazil | 60 (7.9) | 11 | 49 | 18 | 65 | 41.8 | 14.4 |
| Japan | 72 (9.5) | 29 | 43 | 18 | 60 | 41 | 13.4 |
| Italy | 17 (2.2) | 5 | 12 | 20 | 70 | 44.8 | 15.4 |
| China | 140 (18.4) | 61 | 79 | 18· | 66 | 36.2 | 10 |
| Zimbabwe | 128 (16.9) | 28 | 100 | 18 | 62 | 28.5 | 9.4 |
| Estonia | 41 (5.4) | 5 | 36 | 20 | 54 | 34.7 | 9 |
| Bulgaria | 87 (11.5) | 16 | 71 | 19 | 86 | 53 | 18.1 |
| Total | 759 (100) | 191 | 568 | 18 | 86 | 39.3 | 13.9 |

# Results

Table 2 shows the ratio of prior consultations to nonconsultations within each country. Among the 714 participants with poorly defined somatic symptoms, 666 (93.3%) had consulted some professional before they visited one of the centers participating in the present study. In contrast, only 48 (6.7%) patients had not consulted any professional. Table 3 shows the frequency of consultations. The percentage of patients who consulted professionals more than three times prior to joining the study was 78.1%.

Table 4 shows a profile of the professionals whom the patients consulted. Multiple answers were allowed in this section. Eighty-seven percent of the patients consulted a general practitioner, whereas only 18% consulted a psychiatrist, except for in Estonia where the rate of consultations with a psychiatrist was much higher (95.1%). The center in Estonia specializes in the treatment of neuroses. There were some cross-cultural differences. For example, in Zimbabwe, all 119 patients consulted a nurse. In contrast, 39.0%, 21.0%, and 18.8% respectively, of patients in Estonia, Zimbabwe, and China consulted traditional healers and/or religious healers prior to joining the study.

TABLE 2. Prior consultation

|  | Consulted | Not consulted |
|---|---|---|
| India ($n = 111$) | 110 (99.1%) | 1 (0.9%) |
| USA ($n = 84$) | 70 (83.3%) | 14 (16.7%) |
| Brazil ($n = 60$) | 50 (83.3%) | 10 (16.7%) |
| Japan ($n = 60$) | 52 (86.7%) | 8 (13.3%) |
| Italy ($n = 15$) | 15 (100.0%) | 0 (0.0%) |
| China ($n = 138$) | 130 (94.2%) | 8 (5.8%) |
| Zimbabwe ($n = 119$) | 119 (100.0%) | 0 (0.0%) |
| Estonia ($n = 41$) | 41 (100.0%) | 0 (0.0%) |
| Bulgaria ($n = 86$) | 79 (91.9%) | 7 (8.1%) |
| Total ($n = 714$) | 666 (93.3%) | 48 (6.7%) |

TABLE 3. Frequency of consultation

|  | Once | Twice | Three times or more |
|---|---|---|---|
| India ($n = 213$) | 15 (7.3%) | 29 (14.1%) | 162 (78.6%) |
| USA ($n = 53$) | 19 (28.4%) | 11 (16.4%) | 37 (55.2%) |
| Brazil ($n = 60$) | 7 (14.0%) | 10 (20.0%) | 33 (66.0%) |
| Japan ($n = 81$) | 15 (22.1%) | 9 (13.2%) | 44 (64.9%) |
| Italy ($n = 22$) | 1 (4.8 %) | 1 (4.8%) | 19 (90.5%) |
| China ($n = 22$) | 13 (11.0%) | 9 (7.6%) | 96 (81.4%) |
| Zimbabwe ($n = 133$) | 4 (3.1%) | 9 (6.9%) | 117 (90.0%) |
| Estonia ($n = 41$) | 3 (7.3%) | 3 (7.3%) | 35 (85.4%) |
| Bulgaria ($n = 88$) | 3 (3.8%) | 10 (12.7%) | 66 (83.5%) |
| Total ($n = 780$) | 80 (10.3%) | 91 (11.7%) | 609 (78.1%) |

TABLE 4. Consulted professionals

| | Nurse | General | Psychiat | Spec | Psychol | Pharm | Healer | Relig | Other |
|---|---|---|---|---|---|---|---|---|---|
| India (n = 111) | 1 (0.9) | 109 (98.2) | 9 (8.1) | 11 (9.9) | 0 (0.0) | 0 (0.0) | 12 (10.8) | 10 (9.0) | 1 (0.9) |
| USA (n = 84) | 3 (3.6) | 55 (65.5) | 5 (6.0) | 5 (6.0) | 5 (6.0) | 2 (2.4) | 0 (0.0) | 1 (1.2) | 12 (14.3) |
| Brazil (n = 60) | 2 (3.3) | 49 (81.7) | 4 (6.7) | 26 (43.3) | 5 (8.3) | 6 (10.0) | 3 (5.0) | 3 (5.0) | 3 (5.0) |
| Japan (n = 60) | 1 (1.7) | 48 (80.0) | 1 (1.7) | 2 (3.3) | 0 (0.0) | 8 (13.3) | 3 (5.0) | 0 (0.0) | 7 (11.7) |
| Italy (n = 15) | 0 (0.0) | 15 (100.0) | 4 (26.7) | 11 (73.3) | 3 (20.0) | 2 (13.3) | 0 (0.0) | 0 (0.0) | 0 (0.0) |
| China (n = 138) | 7 (12.3) | 124 (89.9) | 45 (32.6) | 11 (8.0) | 15 (10.9) | 3 (2.2) | 26 (18.8) | 7 (5.1) | 14 (10.1) |
| Zimbabwe (n = 119) | 119 (100) | 114 (95.8) | 0 (0.0) | 2 (1.7) | 0 (0.0) | 2 (1.7) | 25 (21.0) | 22 (18.5) | 0 (0.0) |
| Estonia (n = 41) | 10 (24.4) | 32 (78.0) | 39 (95.1) | 34 (82.9) | 18 (43.9) | 4 (9.8) | 16 (39.0) | 1 (2.4) | 8 (19.5) |
| Bulgaria (n = 86) | 5 (5.8) | 75 (87.2) | 26 (30.2) | 51 (59.3) | 0 (0.0) | 3 (3.5) | 6 (7.0) | 0 (0.0) | 5 (5.8) |
| Total (n = 714) | 158 (22.1) | 621 (87.0) | 133 (18.6) | 153 (21.4) | 46 (6.4) | 30 (4.2) | 91 (12.7) | 44 (6.2) | 50 (7.0) |

General, general practitioner; Psychiat, psychiatrist; Spec, other specialist; Psychol, psychologist; Pharm, pharmacologist; Healer, traditional healer; Relig, religious healer.

Table 5 shows the mean age of patients who had consulted a professional. The average age of the patients who consulted traditional healers or/and religious healers was not different from that of patients who consulted other professionals.

Table 6 shows the treatment methods provided for these patients. Fifty-eight percent of patients were treated with drugs, while a number underwent surgery. This was especially true in Brazil. Seven percent of the patients received some sort of psychotherapy or counseling. In China, 18% of the patients received acupuncture. A number of patients in Bulgaria, Zimbabwe, China, and Estonia were treated with traditional healing practices, while some in Zimbabwe and China received ritual cures such as talismans.

Table 7 shows the mean age of patients who received some sort of medical treatment. There was very little difference in the average age of patients amongst the various treatment modalities.

Table 8 shows the reported outcome of consulting a professional. Approximately 56% of patients reported an improvement in their condition after their visit. Eighty-two percent of patients who visited nurses reported an improvement, while those who consulted psychologists reported an improvement in 63% of the cases. Of the patients in the other groups, 50%–60% reported an improvement.

Table 9 shows the reported outcome of each treatment modality. Excluding the patients who were treated by acupuncture (37%) and other alternative treatment (43%), more than half of the patients reported an improvement in their somatic symptoms after treatment (56%).

## Discussion

Patients with somatic symptoms that have not been clearly defined clinically frequently consult professionals. A majority of patients from all the countries participating in the study consulted a professional prior to visiting one of the test centers and 78% of them did so more than three times, suggesting that this is a worldwide phenomenon. Such frequent visits would create a burden on the patients themselves as well as on society. Most of the patients with poorly defined physical symptoms consulted professionals on multiple occasions despite an apparent improvement. This finding suggests that these patients visit different professionals even though they are satisfied to a certain degree with the treatment. In the study of Kirmayer et al. [6], the presence of a negative affect was associated with a high level of both somatic as well as emotional distress, suggesting that the patients in the present study may have been anxiously seeking a complete release from physical distress. This would explain their compulsive help-seeking behavior. To counteract this, a clinician should focus on each patient's perception of their symptoms as well as the assumptions they have about their own illness [7].

Although most patients with somatoform symptoms visited a general practitioner, the rate varied from 100% to 65.5% among the centers participating in the present study. The type of specialist consulted and the treatment received also varied among the centers. In some countries such as Bulgaria, Zimbabwe, China, and Estonia, a considerable number of patients were treated with traditional healing methods and most reported being satisfied with it. The tendency to choose a traditional approach rather

TABLE 5. Mean age of patients who consulted a professional

| | Nurse | General | Psychiat | Spec | Psychol | Pharm | Healer | Relig | Other |
|---|---|---|---|---|---|---|---|---|---|
| India | – | 40.7 | 40.3 | 33.8 | – | – | 40.2 | 37.8 | 29.0 |
| USA | 49.7 | 43.4 | 34.0 | 46.6 | 36.5 | 46.0 | – | 41.0 | 41.9 |
| Brazil | 23.5 | 39.7 | 51.3 | 39.0 | 36.8 | 44.5 | 33.3 | 37.0 | 52.3 |
| Japan | 60.0 | 43.3 | 26.0 | 55.0 | – | 37.6 | 46.3 | – | 40.6 |
| Italy | – | 43.9 | 42.0 | 43.1 | 39.7 | 49.5 | – | – | – |
| China | 41.6 | 36.3 | 36.1 | 44.8 | 36.3 | 32.7 | 37.9 | 34.6 | 30.7 |
| Zimbabwe | 28.9 | 29.0 | – | 42.5 | – | 31.5 | 30.1 | 31.5 | – |
| Estonia | 32.4 | 34.1 | 35.1 | 33.9 | 33.0 | 38.3 | 33.6 | 31.0 | 40 |
| Bulgaria | 62.6 | 55.1 | 57.0 | 51.1 | – | 44.7 | 52.0 | – | 50.0 |
| Total | 32.0 | 39.5 | 40.7 | 42.8 | 35.3 | 40.2 | 36.4 | 34.0 | 39.9 |

TABLE 6. Treatment provided

| | Med | Surg | Counsel | Acu | Alter | Ritual | Trad | Other | Norx |
|---|---|---|---|---|---|---|---|---|---|
| India ($n = 133$) | 110 (82.7) | 2 (1.5) | 1 (0.8) | 0 (0.0) | 1 (0.8) | 2 (1.5) | 15 (11.3) | 2 (1.5) | 0 (0.0) |
| USA ($n = 99$) | 44 (44.4) | 2 (2.0) | 14 (14.1) | 0 (0.0) | 1 (1.0) | 0 (0.0) | 0 (0.0) | 7 (7.1) | 31 (31.3) |
| Brazil ($n = 91$) | 51 (56.0) | 19 (20.9) | 6 (6.6) | 2 (2.2) | 1 (1.1) | 1 (1.1) | 2 (2.2) | 3 (3.3) | 6 (6.6) |
| Japan ($n = 61$) | 46 (75.4) | 4 (6.6) | 0 (0.0) | 1 (1.6) | 3 (4.9) | 0 (0.0) | 0 (0.0) | 6 (9.8) | 1 (1.6) |
| Italy ($n = 15$) | 9 (60.0) | 0 (0.0) | 4 (26.7) | 0 (0.0) | 1 (6.7) | 0 (0.0) | 0 (0.0) | 0 (0.0) | 1 (6.7) |
| China ($n = 220$) | 84 (38.2) | 4 (1.8) | 27 (12.3) | 39 (17.7) | 26 (11.8) | 11 (5.0) | 22 (10.0) | 1 (0.5) | 6 (2.7) |
| Zimbabwe ($n = 158$) | 119 (75.3) | 1 (0.6) | 2 (1.3) | 0 (0.0) | 0 (0.0) | 17 (10.8) | 19 (12.0) | 0 (0.0) | 0 (0.0) |
| Estonia ($n = 77$) | 39 (50.6) | 3 (3.9) | 7 (9.1) | 6 (7.8) | 6 (7.8) | 0 (0.0) | 6 (7.8) | 9 (11.7) | 1 (1.3) |
| Bulgaria ($n = 126$) | 74 (58.7) | 1 (0.8) | 8 (6.3) | 4 (3.2) | 5 (4.0) | 2 (1.6) | 19 (15.1) | 4 (3.2) | 9 (7.1) |
| Total ($n = 1001$) | 576 (58) | 35 (3) | 70 (7) | 53 (5) | 47 (5) | 33 (3.3) | 87 (8.7) | 40 (4.0) | 60 (6.0%) |

Percentage in parentheses.
Med, medicine; Surg, surgery; Counsel, psychotherapy or counseling; Acu, acupuncture; Alter, other alternative treatment; Ritual, ritual cure; Trad, traditional healing; Other, other treatment; Norx, No treatment, does not know.

TABLE 7. Mean age of patients receiving some type of treatment

|  | Med | Surg | Counsel | Acu | Alter | Ritual | Trad | Other | Norx |
|---|---|---|---|---|---|---|---|---|---|
| India | 40.6 | 59.5 | 56.0 | – | 32.0 | 36.5 | 39.3 | 36.5 | – |
| USA | 43.8 | 41.5 | 37.9 | – | 37.0 | – | – | 47.0 | 41.8 |
| Brazil | 43.7 | 49.2 | 40.3 | 43.0 | 24.0 | 24.0 | 48.0 | 52.0 | 28.3 |
| Japan | 43.8 | 39.0 | – | 40.0 | 43.3 | – | – | 40.5 | 41.0 |
| Italy | 38.8 | – | 34.8 | – | 33.0 | – | – | – | 59.0 |
| China | 36.7 | 46.3 | 39.4 | 37.8 | 37.9 | 32.3 | 36.1 | 30.4 | 32.0 |
| Africa | 28.9 | 38.0 | 34.0 | – | – | 34.2 | 29.9 | – | – |
| Estonia | 35.0 | 42.7 | 35.0 | 36.0 | 30.0 | – | 30.7 | 37.8 | 25.0 |
| Bulgaria | 56.4 | 65.0 | 48.6 | 52.8 | 57.6 | 51.5 | 57.9 | 53.0 | 27.7 |
| Total | 40.0 | 47.5 | 39.6 | 39.0 | 38.9 | 34.4 | 40.1 | 40.9 | 37.0 |

TABLE 8. Reported outcome of consultation

|  | Improvement | Worsening | No change |
|---|---|---|---|
| Nurse ($n = 158$) | 130 (82.3%) | 1 (0.6%) | 26 (16.5%) |
| General ($n = 621$) | 325 (52.3%) | 17 (2.7%) | 238 (38.3%) |
| Psychiat ($n = 134$) | 68 (50.7%) | 10 (7.5%) | 52 (38.8%) |
| Spec ($n = 153$) | 86 (56.2%) | 7 (4.6%) | 48 (31.4%) |
| Psychol ($n = 47$) | 30 (63.8%) | 3 (6.4%) | 13 (27.7%) |
| Pharm ($n = 30$) | 15 (50.0%) | 2 (6.7%) | 13 (43.3%) |
| Healer ($n = 91$) | 46 (50.5%) | 5 (5.5%) | 39 (42.9%) |
| Relig ($n = 44$) | 25 (56.8%) | 1 (2.3%) | 18 (40.9%) |
| Other ($n = 56$) | 20 (35.7%) | 2 (3.6%) | 20 (35.7%) |
| Total ($n = 1334$) | 745 (55.8%) | 48 (3.6%) | 467 (35.0%) |

TABLE 9. Reported outcome of treatment

|  | Improvement | Worsening | No change |
|---|---|---|---|
| Med ($n = 576$) | 336 (58.3%) | 16 (2.8%) | 212 (36.8%) |
| Surg ($n = 36$) | 21 (58.3%) | 2 (5.6%) | 11 (30.6%) |
| Counsel ($n = 69$) | 38 (55.1%) | 4 (5.8%) | 26 (37.7%) |
| Acu ($n = 52$) | 19 (36.5%) | 4 (7.7%) | 27 (51.9%) |
| Alter ($n = 44$) | 19 (43.2%) | 1 (2.3%) | 23 (52.3%) |
| Ritual ($n = 33$) | 21 (63.6%) | 0 (0.0%) | 12 (36.4%) |
| Trad ($n = 83$) | 42 (50.6%) | 5 (6.0%) | 34 (41.0%) |
| Oth ($n = 39$) | 16 (41.0%) | 1 (2.6%) | 14 (35.9%) |
| Norx ($n = 55$) | 2 (3.6%) | 0 (0.0%) | 12 (21.8%) |
| Total ($n = 957$) | 540 (56.4%) | 33 (3.4%) | 371 (38.8%) |

than a more modern clinical approach did not differ among the different age groups, suggesting that the help-seeking behavior determined by sociocultural factors has not changed to any great degree.

The difference in this help-seeking behavior could be explained by the different ways patients from different cultures interpret somatic symptoms. This different interpretation may have been determined by their beliefs and assumptions about health and illness [7–9]. If a patient with a certain underlying assumption about illness interprets an innocuous somatic sensation as being noxious [10], he or she will become anxious and start seeking professional help. Their choice of professional is also affected by their culturally determined beliefs. This is one reason for the variation in the choice of specialists.

Such assumptions could also influence treatment outcome. If a specialist chooses a treatment approach with which a patient is familiar, the patient tends to be satisfied with the outcome. This is suggested by the lack of a difference among the treatment modalities.

Our findings, however, should be interpreted with caution. As this study was done at only one center per country, the patients are not necessarily representative of the entire country. For example, Tokyo is the most westernized city in Japan, and the lifestyle of the people living in Tokyo may well be different from that of people living in other areas.

Despite such limitations, our findings still have the following important implications for healthcare. Most of the patients in the present study who exhibited somatic symptoms that were poorly defined clinically visited other professionals on multiple occasions despite an apparent improvement in their condition. The difference in help-seeking behavior among countries suggests a cultural difference in the way patients interpret somatic symptoms. These findings suggest that a patient's perception of their somatic symptoms must be modified in accordance with his or her cultural background.

*Acknowledgement.* We are indebted to the members of the WHO International Study of Somatoform Disorders who collaborated in this project: Dr. A. Janca, Dr. S. W. Acuda, Dr. C. A. Altamura, Dr. L. Bennett, Dr. J. D. Burke, Ms. K. C. Burke, Dr. C. R. Chandrashekar, Dr. J. Cox, Dr. A. Forgione, Dr. M. Isaac, Dr. B. Ivanov, Dr. W. Maier, Dr. Meng Fanqiang, Dr. C. T. Miranda, Dr. L. Robins, Dr. N. Sartorius, Dr. J. Shlik, and Dr. G. Tacchini.

## References

1. American Psychiatric Association (1980) Diagnostic and statistical manual of mental disorders (3rd edn). American Psychiatric Association, Washington
2. Andersen R, Newman JF (1979) Social and individual determinants of medical care utilization in the United States. Milbank Mem Fund Q 51:95–124
3. American Psychiatric Association (1994) Diagnostic and statistical manual of mental disorders (4th edn). American Psychiatric Association, Washington
4. World Health Organization (1993) The composite international diagnosis interview, core version 1.1. American Psychiatric Press, Washington
5. Tacchini G, Janca A, Issac M (1993) Somatoform disorder schedule (SDS). WHO, Geneva

6. Kirmayer LK, Robbins JM, Paris J (1994) Somatoform disorders: personality and the social matrix of somatic distress. J Abnorm Psychol 103:125–136
7. Salkovskis PM, Clark DM (1993) Panic disorder and hypchondriasis. Adv Behav Ther 15:23–48
8. Janca A, Issac M, Costa e Silva JA (1995) World Health Organization international study of somatoform disorders—background and rationale. Eur J Psychiatry 9:100–110
9. Janca A, Issac M, Bennett LA, Tacchini G (1995) Somatoform disorders in different cultures—a mail questionnaire survey. Soc Psychiatry Psychiatr Epidemiol 30:44–48
10. Barsky AJ, Klerman GL (1983) Overview: hypochondriasis, body complaints and somatic styles. Am J Psychiatry 140:273–283

# The Influence of Depression and Anxiety on the Course of Somatization in Primary Case

Oye Gureje

*Summary.* Somatization often co-exists with depression or anxiety. The implications of such comorbidity on the course of somatization in primary care are unclear. In a large international study conducted in primary care settings of 14 countries, stability of somatization over a 12-month period was unrelated to the co-occurrence of depression or of generalised anxiety disorder (GAD). However, persistence of somatization was a risk factor for the emergence of new episodes of depression and of GAD after one year. Conversely, the incidence of somatization syndrome was increased among individuals who had either depression or GAD 12 months earlier. The data provide no evidence to suggest that the outcome of somatization is influenced by comorbidity with depression or GAD. However, somatization is more likely to develop among depressed or anxious primary care patients.

*Key words.* Somatization, Depression, Anxiety, Comorbidity, Course

## Introduction

Various published papers have shown an association between the occurrence of somatization on the one hand and depression or anxiety on the other [1–4]. In an earlier report, we showed that the risk of having a current depressive illness or generalized anxiety disorder (GAD) for patients with an abridged form of somatization was significantly elevated in 14 of 15 centres participating in an international collaborative study conducted in primary care settings: about 40% of patients with somatization also met the criteria for either ICD-10 depression or GAD.

The significance of the co-occurrence (or comorbidity) of somatization with depression and anxiety is unclear. First, the definition of what constitutes the syn-

Department of Psychiatry, University College Hospital, Ibadan, Nigeria
The data reported in this paper were collected as part of a World Health Organization's Psychological Problems in General Health Care project. The author acknowledges the work of all participating investigators and research workers at the 15 sites

drome of somatization is far from precise. There is evidence that a dimensional rather than a categorical description provides a better fit with clinical populations. Second, nosological descriptions of the syndromes of depression and anxiety include some somatic symptoms. Third, cross-sectional co-occurrence of syndromes is not unique to somatization but is a common observation in psychiatry [5]. In this regard, comorbidity as a phenomenon is probably only meaningful if it provides an understanding of the influence of one disorder on the course of the other.

Using an abridged definition of somatization that requires the presence of four current symptoms in men and six current symptoms in women [4, 6], this paper provides data on the longitudinal course of somatization in primary care in a large international study. It examines the impact of the co-occurrence of depression or GAD on somatization over a 12-month period. It also determines how the onset of somatization may be related to the presence of depression or GAD and vice versa.

## Method

This research formed part of the World Health Organization collaborative study on Psychological Problems in General Health Care (PPGHC). A full description of the methodology and rationale for the study is provided elsewhere [4, 7, 8]. Conducted among people contacting general health services in 15 centres in 14 countries: Ankara (Turkey), Athens (Greece), Berlin and Mainz (Germany), Bangalore (India), Ibadan (Nigeria), Groningen (Netherlands), Manchester (U.K.), Nagasaki (Japan), Paris (France), Rio de Janeiro (Brazil), Santiago (Chile), Seattle (U.S.A.), Shanghai (China), and Verona (Italy), it was designed to study the form, frequency and outcome of common psychiatric problems in primary care settings.

A two-stage epidemiological approach was used in which the screening stage involved the administration of the 12-item General Health Questionnaire (GHQ-12) [9] to a representative sample of persons aged 18 to 65 years making ambulatory visits to providers of health care services in primary care settings (total: 25,916; response rate: 96%). Respondents were selected for the second stage interview on the basis of site-specific GHQ thresholds: 100% of those with GHQ scores above the 80th percentile, 35% of those scoring between the 60th and 80th percentiles, and 10% of those scoring below the 60th percentile. A total of 8729 patients were eligible for interview out of which 5438 interviews were successfully completed (response rate was 62% but was not related to age, sex or screening GHQ score). The second-stage assessment included, among others, the primary care version of the Composite International Diagnostic Interview (CIDI) [10]. This version of the CIDI has a number of modifications, one of which was the inclusion in the somatization section of symptoms that clinicians from various cultural backgrounds had identified as being more typical of somatizing patients in their cultures. Data from this version allowed for the assignment of ICD-10 (and DSM-IV) diagnoses of somatization, anxiety, depression, neurasthenia, and alcohol use disorders.

Patients who exceeded a predetermined cut-off of a minimum number of symptoms in one or more of the CIDI sections, as well as a 20% random sample of "noncases", were asked to participate in 3- and 12-month follow-up assessments. This report is concerned with the 12-month follow-up. Assessment as this follow-up consisted of direct interviews with patients at their homes and involved identical instruments as used in the baseline interview. Thus, patients were interviewed with the CIDI and the other instruments used at the baseline assessment. The 12-month follow-up rate across the 15 sites was 68.5%. The rate was 65% or higher in 12 of the participating sites.

## Results

Of the 3201 patients who completed both the baseline and the 12-month assessments, 741 met the criteria for current abridged somatization (Table 1). When this is weighed back to reflect the probability of selection for the diagnostic interview, it represents a weighted prevalence of 16.7%. Out of the 1071 with the disorder at baseline, 522 continued to have it at 12 months follow-up, representing a weighted value of 46.2% for persistence of somatization. New episodes of somatization developed in 219 of 2130 individuals who did not have the syndrome at baseline, giving a weighted proportion of 7.1% for incidence.

Table 2 gives the weighted proportions of patients with somatization at baseline whose syndrome had either remained stable or remitted at 12-month follow-up in relation to whether generalized anxiety disorder (GAD) or depression was present at baseline or not. It can be seen that stability of somatization syndrome was unrelated to the presence or absence of GAD or depression at baseline. The proportions with stable syndrome were identical among patients with GAD at baseline as among those without GAD. The same lack of association was observed for depression at baseline.

The results in regard to the emergence of new syndromes were different (Table 3). While 15% of patients with GAD at baseline had developed somatization syndrome

TABLE 1. Abridged somatization at baseline and 12-month follow-up (unweighted number of cases)

|  | Follow-up No | Follow-up Yes | Total |
|---|---|---|---|
| Baseline No | 1911 | 219 | 2130 |
| Baseline Yes | 549 | 522 | 1071 |
| Total | 2460 | 741 | 3201 |

TABLE 2. Stability of abridged somatization at 12 months relative to presence or absence of depression and anxiety at baseline (weighted numbers and proportions)

|  | Baseline GAD No ($n = 575$) | Baseline GAD Yes ($n = 144$) | Baseline depression No ($n = 530$) | Baseline depression Yes ($n = 188$) |
|---|---|---|---|---|
| Somatization stable No, % | 54 | 53 | 56 | 48 |
| Somatization stable Yes, % | 46 | 47 | 44 | 52 |

GAD, generalised anxiety disorder.

TABLE 3. Onset of abridged somatization at 12 months relative to presence or absence of depression or GAD at baseline (weighted numbers and proportions)

| | Baseline GAD No ($n = 2088$) | Baseline GAD Yes ($n = 119$) | Baseline depression No ($n = 2055$) | Baseline depression Yes ($n = 152$) |
|---|---|---|---|---|
| Emergent somatization No, % | 93 | 85 | 94 | 83 |
| Emergent somatization Yes, % | 7 | 15 | 6 | 17 |

at follow-up, only 7% of those without GAD had emergent syndrome (chi square = 12.2, df = 1, $P < 0.001$). Among patients with depression at baseline, 17% had developed somatization while only 6% had done so among those without depression at baseline (chi square = 24.7, df = 1, $P < 0.001$).

Persistence of somatization increased the probability of the occurrence of GAD and depression at 12 months. At follow-up, 23.2% of individuals with persistent somatization had GAD compared with 8.2% of those with remittent somatization syndrome (chi square = 45.2, df = 1, $P < 0.001$). The relationship remained significant following a logistic regression analysis in which centre, age, sex, and anxiety at baseline were controlled for (odds ratio = 3.18, 95% confidence interval, 2.13–4.76, df = 1, $P < 0.0001$). The figures for depression were identical: among those with persistent somatization, 33.1% had depression at follow-up compared to 11.4% of those with remittent somatization. Also, the relationship remained significant following a logistic regression analysis controlling for centre, age, sex, and depression at baseline (odds ratio = 4.21, 95% confidence interval, 2.94–6.03, df = 1, $P < 0.0001$).

## Discussion

Over a period of 12 months, somatization as defined in this study showed a moderate degree of stability in this large primary care population: about one-half of patients with this syndrome at baseline continued to meet the operational definition 12 months later. It would appear that the traditional view of somatization as a chronic disorder is not always true for a large proportion of primary care patients. It is, however, possible that, rather than complete remission, the course of somatization, like that of some other psychiatric problems in primary care, is characterised by a pattern of waxing and waning [11, 12].

The stability of somatization was not related to the presence or absence of depression or generalized anxiety disorder at the baseline. If chronicity is a reflection of the severity of the illness, then clearly, neither the co-occurrence of depression nor of anxiety indicates severity of somatization. On the other hand, the presence of depression or GAD is a risk factor for the development of somatization. Contrary to earlier suggestions, this observation indicates that somatization is not a defence against the expression of depression (or anxiety) but may be a complicating feature of these disorders. This relationship is not, however, a simple one as the persistence of somatization was an independent risk factor for the emergence of new episodes of depression or anxiety. Individuals with persistent syndrome of somatization were at elevated risk of developing new episodes of GAD and of depression at 12 months. This observation would suggest that a clear distinction between the syndromes of depression and anxiety on the one hand and of somatization on the other is a tenuous one in primary care. It is no wonder that approaches in the management of depression and anxiety are also effective in the treatment of somatization.

## References

1. Escobar JI, Burnan A, Karno M, Forsythe A, Golding JM (1987) Somatization in the community. Arch Gen Psychiatry 44:713–718
2. Simon GE, VonKorff M (1991) Somatization and psychiatric disorder in the NIMH Epidemiologic Catchment Area Study. Am J Psychiatry 148:1494–1500
3. Gureje O, Obikoya B (1992) Somatization in primary care: patterns and correlates in a Nigerian clinic. Acta Psychiatr Scand 86:223–227
4. Gureje O, Simon GE, Ustun TB, Goldberg DP (1997) Somatization in cross-cultural perspective: a World Health Organization study in primary care. Am J Psychiatry 154:989–995
5. Sartorius N, Ustun TB, Lecrubier Y, Wittchen H-U (1996) Depression comorbid with anxiety: results of the WHO Study on Psychological Disorders in Primary Health Care. Br J Psychiatry Suppl. 30:38–43
6. Escobar JL, Ribio-Stipec M, Canino G, Karno M (1989) Somatic Symptom Index (SSI): a new abridged somatization construct. J Nerv Ment Dis 177:140–146
7. Ustun TB, Sartorius N (eds) (1995) Mental illness in general health care: an international study. Wiley, New York
8. Ormel J, VonKorff M, Ustun TB, Pini S, Korten A, Oldehinkel T (1994) Common mental disorders and disability across cultures. JAMA 272:1741–1748
9. Goldberg DP, Williams P (1998) The user's guide to the General Health Questionnaire. National Foundation for Educational Research, Nelson, Slough, UK
10. Wittchen H-U, Robins LN, Cottler L, Sartorius N, Burke JD, Regier D (1991) Cross-cultural feasibility, reliability and sources of variance of the Composite International Diagnostic Interview (CIDI): The Multicentre WHO/ADAMHA Field Trials. Br J Psychiatry 159:645–653; correction (1992) 1160:1136
11. Kessler LG, Cleary PD, Burke JD (1985) Psychiatric disorders in primary care: results of a follow-up study. Arch Gen Psychiatry 42:583–587
12. Katon W, Lin E, VonKorff M, Bush T, Walker E, Simon G, Robinson P (1994) The predictors of persistence of depression in primary care. J Affect Disord 31:81–90

# Somatization in Different Cultures (I). *Taijin Kyofusho* as One Aspect of Somatoform Disorders in Japan

Fumiko Maeda, Joichiro Shirahase, and Masahiro Asai

*Summary.* Although the ICD-10 and DSM-IV may seem to be adequate for most psychiatric diagnoses, they are far from ideal. The diagnostic process is clinical and relies on psychiatric symptoms that are often subjective and subtle. The classification resorts to a variety of information sources with little biological evidence. When making a diagnosis, other information sources are also necessary. The most important of all may be cultural factors. For example, when examining somatoform disorder in Japan, *taijin kyofusho* (*anthropophobia*, morbid fear of interpersonal situations) must be taken into consideration. In this chapter, somatoform disorders in Japan will be discussed. *Taijin kyofusho* will be taken as an example, although *taijin kyofusho* is usually categorized as social phobia. Specifically, this paper will discuss: (a) the prevalence of somatoform disorder in a general hospital outpatient clinic in Japan; (b) *taijin kyofusho* as a "primary" or "secondary" somatoform syndrome; (c) past studies on *taijin kyofusho*; and (d) Morita theory of *taijin kyofusho*.

*Key words.* Anthropophobia, Morita therapy, Psychotherapy, Somatoform disorder, *Taijin kyofusho*

## Introduction

Notions of somatoform disorder in ICD-10 and DSM-IV seem to be generally accepted and have been used internationally. However, there are a number of culture-specific disorders that are generally recognized as somatoform disorders but are significantly related to somatoform disorders.

In this chapter, somatoform disorders in Japan will be discussed. *Taijin kyofusho* (*anthropophobia*, morbid fear of interpersonal situations) will be discussed as an instance for rethinking the nosology of somatoform disorder. (It should be noted that *taijin kyofusho* is not usually categorized as a somatoform disorder.) More specifically, this paper will discuss: (a) the prevalence of somatoform disorder

Department of Neuropsychiatry, Keio University School of Medicine, 35 Shinanomachi, Shinjuku-ku, Tokyo 160–8582, Japan

in a general hospital outpatient clinic in Japan and its relation to *taijin kyofusho*; (b) *taijin kyofusho* as a "primary" or "secondary" somatoform syndrome (these terms "primary" and "secondary" somatoform syndromes were proposed by Escobar et al. in the late 1980s [1]); (c) the literature on *taijin kyofusho* in relation to somatoform disorder; and (d) Morita therapy's theory of *taijin kyofusho* and its place in nosology.

# Prevalence of Somatoform Disorder in a General Hospital Outpatient Clinic in Japan and Its Relation to *Taijin Kyofusho*

A study on somatoform disorder was carried out in Japan as a part of the WHO International Study of Somatoform Disorder. One of the main objectives in this study was to assess rates and culture-specific characteristics of somatoform disorder [2].

Data was obtained from 372 patients who visited a general hospital internist from October 1994 to July 1995. A total of 372 patients were screened with the WHO Screener for Somatoform Disorder (SSD) and 91 patients were found to have somatoform disorder. Those 91 patients were then interviewed with the Composite International Diagnostic Interview (CIDI) and the Somatoform Disorder Schedule (SDS) by Masters'-level psychologists. The overall prevalence rate of somatoform disorder in this setting was approximately 18%. In addition to these data, a study carried out in Yamanashi, Japan, (Ono et al., unpublished data) showed that there are a substantial number of patients having somatic symptoms in Japan. More interestingly, when their symptoms were reviewed in detail, there were a number of patients in this group that may have been given a dual diagnosis of *taijin kyofusho*. For this group, it was difficult to decide which feature was predominant.

According to DSM-IV, *taijin kyofusho* "refers to an individual's intense fear that his or her body, its parts or its functions, displease, embarrass, or are offensive to other people in appearance, odor, facial expressions, or movements. This syndrome is included in the official Japanese diagnostic system for mental disorders" [3] and somewhat resembles social phobia in DSM-IV. In ICD-10 [4], *taijin kyofusho* is included in social phobia. However, many studies have revealed that *taijin kyofusho* extends over several disorders including somatoform disorder, obsessive-compulsive disorder, social phobia, delusional disorder, and avoidant personality disorder in the ICD-10 and the DSM-IV (Figure 1).

In previous studies, the clinical prevalence of *taijin kyofusho* varies from 7.8% of patients with neurosis in a general university psychiatric outpatient clinic to 45.5% of patients with neurosis at a clinic offering Morita therapy [5]. One can see that *taijin kyofusho* is a commonly diagnosed disorder in Japan. As shown in the present WHO Japan study, a number of *taijin kyofusho* patients in these studies may overlap with somatoform disorder.

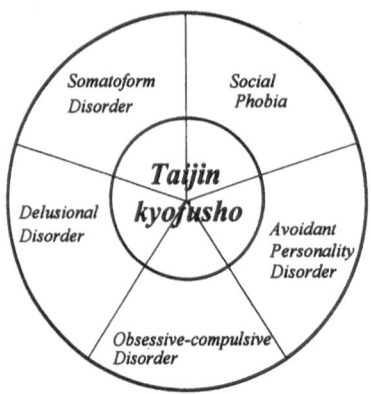

FIG. 1. *Taijin kyofusho* and its relation to disorders of other classifications

TABLE 1. Primary and secondary somatoform syndromes

| |
|---|
| "Primary" somatoform syndromes |
|     The syndromes in which the cluster of medically ill unexplained symptoms either come from or dominate the clinical picture |
|     *Example of symptoms*: fainting, paralysis, lump in the throat, deafness, blindness, and paresthesias |
| "Secondary" somatoform syndromes |
|     The syndromes that follow or are associated with another major psychiatric illness |
|     *Example of symptoms*: fatigue, headache, facial pain, generalized pain or aches, cardiorespiratory symptoms, gastrointestinal symptoms, and musculoskeletal symptoms |

## *Taijin Kyofusho* as a "Primary" or "Secondary" Somatoform Syndrome

In clinical practice, the central theme in the somatizing syndromes is the presentation of multiple symptoms, mainly physical but also psychological, and the overreporting of life events, frustrations, and misfortunes. Individuals affected with these traits generally display a tendency to amplify physical symptoms and sensations. They also are apt to endorse multiple physical symptoms involving various body areas. The tendency for these patients to amplify not only physical symptoms, but also psychiatric ones, has been documented as "high levels of psychiatric comorbidity." Also, somatizing syndromes are linked to high levels of psychopathology and psychological distress.

Patients enter a clinic not only with medically unexplained physical symptoms, but often with an accompanying anxiety and depressive mood. Escobar et al. [6] have proposed that these somatoform syndromes that follow or are associated with another major psychiatric illness should be distinguished from "primary" somatoform syndromes, and should be called "secondary" somatoform syndromes (Table 1) [1].

As mentioned earlier, especially (but not only) in Japanese culture, there is a group of *taijin kyofusho* patients with high levels of unexplained physical symptoms. If the basic pathology of *taijin kyofusho* lies in the fear of interpersonal relationships, then the somatic symptoms such as cardiorespiratory and gastrointestinal symptoms are the accompanying symptoms. In this case, the somatoform syndrome is a "secondary" somatoform syndrome. On the other hand, there may be cases in which the somatic symptoms are the primary symptoms and the fear of interpersonal relationships (*taijin kyofusho*) is the accompanying syndrome. Hence, *taijin kyofusho* would be a "primary" somatoform syndrome. This view of *taijin kyofushou* (as a "primary" somatoform syndrome) is the view supported by Morita theory.

## Past Studies on *Taijin Kyofusho*, Which Discuss Its Relation to Somatoform Disorder

There have been several studies and papers which have related *taijin kyofusho* and somatoform disorder. For example, Yamashita [7] discussed the common psychologi cal structure of *taijin kyofusho* and hypochondriasis. Other studies have stated that certain types of *taijin kyofusho* patients may fit an ICD diagnosis of *dysmorphophobia* (non-delusional) in hypochondriacal disorder or a DSM diagnosis of body dysmorphic disorder [5, 8, 9]. Similarly, Narita [10] and Nakamura [11] stated that the severe type of *taijin kyofusho* may be diagnosed as a somatoform disorder.

In our opinion, Yamashita [7] has made a provocative point in his discussion of *taijin kyofusho*. He discusses the similarity of *taijin kyofusho* and hypochondriasis in pathogenesis and not just in the superficial symptoms. He states that *taijin kyofusho* is the fear of self as social existence at its base, and somatoform disorder is the fear of self as physical existence at its base. Both disorders have a tendency to develop from a rather circumspect fear to strongly held convictions about the phenomenological world.

## Morita Theory of *Taijin Kyofusho* and Its Place in Nosology

As has been mentioned earlier, *taijin kyofusho* is generally classified as social phobia and is not considered to be a somatoform disorder. However, *taijin kyofusho* is closely related to Japanese culture and mentality, and is a type of Morita's *shinkeishitsu* (neurosis).

The psychopathology of *taijin kyofusho* was first explained by Masatake Morita (also known as Shoma Morita) utilizing the terms "hypochondriacal basic tone" and "psychic interaction" [12] (Table 2). "Hypochondriacal basic tone" is a personality characteristic or a temperament, relating to the *taijin kyofusho* condition. Morita's basic notion is that "hypochondriacal basic tone" needs to be given the highest priority in understanding the process of the onset of *taijin kyofusho*. The balance of introversion and extroversion in "hypochondriacal basic tone" is inclined towards introversion. Those with an introverted attitude have a fixation on their weak point and become anxious and depressive [13] (Table 2).

TABLE 2. Morita's theory of *taijin kyofusho*

| |
|---|
| [OCCURENCE OF *taijin kyofusho*] = [TEMPERAMENT] × [CHANCE EVENT] × [PATHOGENIC FACTOR] |
| Temperament: hypochondriacal basic tone<br>    A personality characteristic relating to the *taijin kyofusho* condition<br>    Introversion: introspective, self-punitive, vigilant, prudent, shy, wavering<br>    Extroversion: positive, self-centered, aggressive, stubborn, ambitious |
| Pathogenic factor: Psychic interaction<br>    "A mental process in which attention is concentrated on a certain sensation; this sensation becomes hyper-sensitized; this condition of hyper-sensitivity fixates attention; the hyper-sensitized sensation and the fixation of attention mutually interact to increasingly intensify the sensitivity of the sensation" (Morita) |

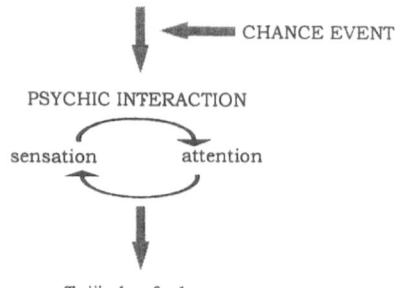

HYPOCHONDRIACAL BASIC TONE

CHANCE EVENT

PSYCHIC INTERACTION

sensation    attention

*Taijin kyofusho*

FIG. 2. Schema of development of symptoms

Morita expressed the mental mechanisms that trigger the onset of the *taijin kyofusho* condition with an equation (Table 2). An individual may start with a "hypochondriacal basic tone," and as a result of an accidental experience, which is called a "chance," the individual's receptiveness becomes highly sensitized. The tendency to impose a hypochondriacal interpretation of the events in the individual's life is reinforced. This tendency acts to further intensify sensations, and attention becomes more and more focused on these sensations. This process is what Morita called "psychic interaction" and ultimately sets up a "vicious circle of attention and sensation" [14] (Figure 2).

As an example, consider *erythrophobia* (morbid fear of blushing). One day, a person with a "hypochondriacal basic tone" experiences blushing all of a sudden after a chance event. He is embarrassed and his face becomes red and hot, and he becomes aware of his shyness. At the same time, the individual tries hard to overcome this condition. This process makes the person even more concerned about blushing and hence he becomes redder.

Morita therapy tries to restore the individual's psychology to its original *aruga-mama* (things as they are) condition. In Morita therapy, (a) the patient's specific symptoms, in this case, somatic symptoms, are ignored, to bring him/her into essential

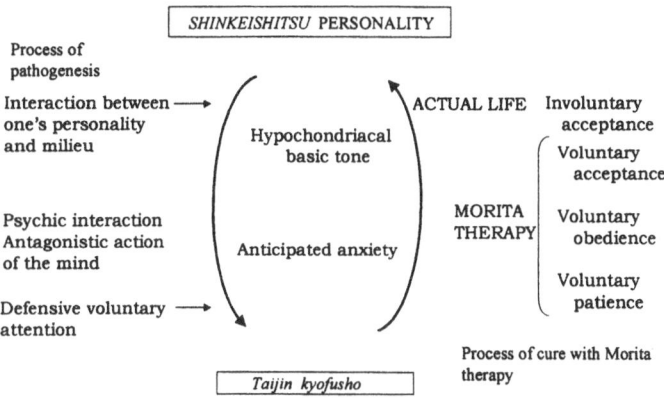

FIG. 3. Diagram of process of pathogenesis and cure

confrontation with reality; (b) the patient is induced to return to and accept his/her authentic human nature as *arugamama*; and (c) the patient begins the process of self-realization within the context of actual living conditions. Morita therapy seeks to direct the individual's energy from their previous concerns, such as somatic symptoms, to the "here and now" [12] (see Figure 3).

# Discussion

*Taijin kyofusho* is well understood by adopting Morita theory. In ICD-10 and DSM-V., it is usually translated as *anthropophobia*, and is included in social phobia of anxiety disorder. However, the various types of the single disorder *taijin kyofusho* may correspond to ICD-10 and DSM-IV categories of social phobia, somatoform disorder, obsessive-compulsive disorder, delusional disorder, and avoidant personality disorder (see Figure 1). The ICD-10 and DSM-IV categorical approach to psychiatric diagnosis differentiates among these groups, while the traditional Japanese conceptualization includes the various types of *taijin kyofusho* as a single disorder with a common psychological continuum of social anxiety [15]. Hence, when one tries to fit *taijin kyofusho* into these classifications, original conceptualization and related theory of treatment is lost. As Kirmayer [5] has stated, "different social contexts and clinical goals demand alternative diagnostic schemes."

We have been looking at typical somatoform disorders as well as more difficult ones, i.e., somatic representations primary to *taijin kyofusho*. This is just one example, but still, it makes us think of the need for further clinical oriented cross-cultural research to include cultural variation in psychiatric diagnosis, and hence make the ICD and DSM support international concerns.

*Acknowledgement.* The authors thank Dr. Jeffrey H. Nathan for his helpful comments.

# References

1. Escobar JI (1995) Transcultural aspects of dissociative and somatoform disorder. Psychiatr Clin North Am 18:555–569
2. Janca A, Isaac M, Bennett LA et al (1995) Somatoform disorders in different cultures— a mail questionnaire survey. Soc Psychiatry Psychiatr Epidemiol 30:44–48
3. American Psychiatric Association (1994) Diagnostic and Statistical Manual of Mental Disorders, edn. 4 (DSM-IV.). American Psychiatric Press, Washington
4. World Health Organization (1992) ICD-10 Classification of Mental and Behavioral Disorders, Clinical Descriptions and Diagnostic Guidelines. World Health Organization, Geneva
5. Kirmayer LJ (1991) The place of culture in psychiatric nosology: *taijin kyofusho* and DSM-III-R. J Nerv Ment Dis 179:19–28
6. Escobar JI, Burnman A, Karno M et al (1987) Somatization in the community. Arch Gen Psychiatry 44:713–718
7. Yamashita I (1982) Japanese diagnosis of neurosis and DSM-III (in Japanese). Rinshoseishinigaku (Clin Psychiatry) 11:205–212
8. Kirmayer LJ (1995) The cultural context of anxiety disorders. Psychiatr Clin North Am 18:503–521
9. Tseng WS, Asai M, Kitanishi K, et al (1992) Diagnostic patterns of social phobia: comparison in Tokyo and Hawaii. J Nerv Ment Dis 180:380–385
10. Narita Y (1988) *Taijin kyofusho*—recent perspectives (in Japanese). In: Kaketa K (ed) Gendaiseishinigakutaikei ('88A). Nakayamashoten, Tokyo, pp 171–185
11. Nakamura K (1994) Social phobia and *taijin kyofusho*—preliminary reports (in Japanese). Psychiatry (Seishinigaku) 36:131–139
12. Fujita C (1986) Morita therapy: a psychotherapeutic system for neurosis. Igaku-shoin, Tokyo
13. Maeda F, Nasen JH (1998) A view of multi-faceted, multi-layered object: Morita therapy treatment of *taijin kyofusho*. J Psychosom Res (in press)
14. Morita S (1974) Nature and treatment of nervosity, vol. 2 (in Japanese). Hakuyosha, Tokyo, 183 pp (original work published in 1928)
15. Kleinknecht RA, Dinnel DL, Tanouye-Wilson S et al (1994) Cultural variation in social anxiety and phobia: A study of *taijin kyofusho*. Behav Therapist 17:175–178

# Culture and Illness—Clinical Presentation and Management of Somatoform Disorders in Cambodia

Maurice Eisenbruch

*Key words*. Ethnographic techniques, Somatoform disorders, Traditional medicine, Clinical management

## Introduction

Western views of somatoform disorders are based on Western cultural assumptions about mind and body; linear time; cause-and-effect; and personal responsibility. Psychiatric research and clinical practice is embedded in these assumptions, but patients from non-Western backgrounds may hold radically different views.

Ethnographic techniques can help to uncover these cultural "organising principles." The method is illustrated with examples from research with traditional healers and their patients in Cambodia. The indigenous explanatory models for illness were explored. Attention was paid, through the use of narrative and drawing of homunculi, to local views of body structure and function; interpretations given to moral, super-natural and physical causes of the illness; rationale for diagnostic techniques and the traditional healing rituals employed. The metaphorical meaning of symptoms and the ritual treatments used to ameliorate them suggested the local logic by which illnesses were categorised.

The Cambodian example illustrates a non-Cartesian view of mind-soul-body, in which somatic symptoms are a product of moral and supernatural events. Work with traditional healers can help to refine nosologies of somatoform disorders and can guide the clinical management of patients from different cultural backgrounds suffering from somatoform complaints.

## Embodiment and Culture

In the early 18th century, the French surgeon Francois Gigot de Le Peyronie carried out autopsies in search of the soul; he failed [1]. He was early example of the quest to understand embodiment, i.e., how the society embodies its

Centre d' Anthropologie de la Chine du Sud et de la Péninsule Indochinoise (UPR413), Centre National de la Recherche Scientifique, 2 Carrefour de l'Odéon, Paris 75006, France

moral and social values in the way people see, use—and misuse—their bodies [2, 3].

How does culture influence the expression of the emotions through the body? Shweder [4] has framed the comparative study of emotions by six questions: (1) the *taxonomic* question, what types of feelings do people experience—lexical studies can be misleading as shown by Levy [5] for Tahitians who talk about feelings they don't feel and feel emotions for which they have no term; (2) the *ecological* question, what are the emotion-laden situations?—some situations are likely universal; (3) the *semantic* question, what do the feelings imply?—to study the meaning of emotions is not the same as identifying the lexical labels, and culture determines whether people believe that emotions, if unexpressed, are dangerous and do not go away or, alternatively, if expressed, are dangerous and do not go away [6]; (4) the *communication* question, what are the vehicles for communication of an emotion, which of these have universal readings and which are learned within the culture?; (5) the *social regulation* question, what feelings are appropriate for a person of this or that status to feel and to display?; (6) the *management* question, how emotions that are not expressed are handled—the techniques vary from denial to displacement to projection to somatisation (7, 8), and whether there is a generic human mind [9] or, against that, that the notions like somatisation or repression are in themselves products of Western thinking [10].

Kleinman and Kleinman [11] define somatisations as "the expression of personal and social distress in an idiom of bodily complaints and medical help-seeking." High rates of somatisation in depressive disorder are found in clinic-based studies in Saudi Arabia, Iraq, West Africa, India, Sudan, the Philippines, Taiwan and Hong Kong; it is also common in the West, and may not always represent pathology.

Kirmayer et al. [12], in pointing out that the explanatory model perspective of medical anthropology, directed by Kleinman, parallels the illness cognition models of Leventhal [13], has thrown a new perspective on symptom attribution in cultural perspective. Attributions are cognitive or conceptual links between experiences and knowledge structures that function as labels, categorisations and interpretations of events. Kirmayer also points out a difference between *diagnostic* interpretation, concerned with classification and legitimation through the production of authoritative truth, and *therapeutic* interpretation, which is concerned with "how to continue" and with the improvisation of meaning [14].

Many transcultural studies are limited by Western assumptions about mind and body, health and illness, nature and culture [15, 16]; and a nosology that ignores the religious and spiritual dimensions [17, 18]. The World Health Organisation international multi-centre study of culture and somatoform disorders [19] found a number of culturally shaped somatoform symptoms which do not fit the available nosologies [20]. Thousands complain of aches and pains which, to the Western eye, seem exotic, even imaginary, The laws of Western nosology can be adapted in the face of data about the cultural categorisation of mind and body—and soul. Not only could this advance knowledge concerning the body-mind, but it could improve health care.

Several of the somatoform disorders bear resemblance to many of the disorders described as affecting Cambodians [21]. Does this mean that Cambodians suffer from somatoform disorders? In this chapter, the traditional terminologies, taxonomies, explanatory models and ritual treatments for the common somatic symptoms are reported.

## Somatoform Disorders in Cambodia

The work reported in this chapter forms a part of a study on traditional healing in Cambodia, carried out by the author between 1990 and 1998. There were seven groups of healers: male Buddhist monks, their ritual assistants, who worked in the pagoda; male and female traditional healers or *kruu*; female or occasionally male mediums; Buddhist devotees; lay healers; and female traditional birth attendants.

The healers were found in the course of participant observation and by snowball sampling. The healers were observed, along with the families who sought treatment. The techniques they used for ritual diagnosis and treatment were documented. Attention was paid to the narrative and the interaction with the patient and how they and their families were reintegrated into their villages. After the treatment, we clarifi ed the healer's rationale and choice in examining, diagnosing and treating the person; his nosology of the illness; and the attention paid to eliciting physical symptoms and treating them.

### *"Thinking Too Much", Somatic Symptoms and Bad Humour*

The healers have a well-elaborated theory of neuroanatomy and physiology, including the nerve-tubules known as the *sAA say* which connect the vital organs to centres in the brain, and the embryological development of the person.

It was believed that thinking too much forces the blood into the gallbladder, known as *kAmraol*, "*KAmraol* that enters" means that it is as if something black descended on the face, until the person fell to the ground. The expression of anger was not always possible verbally, either because the society forbade it or because the patient suppressed it. Anger was said to emerge in the breathing, as befitted a culture in which breathing is closely identified with the state of mind. In *ñoa truuE*, the person felt terror and palpitations. The second sensation, known as "filled up chest" (*naen truuE*), or "tight chest" (*tBE truuE*), means that there was a sense of difficulty in breathing. It developed when the angry person had "tight chest, speech doesn't come out." Bottled-up stress can make the person shut down and appear dead for some days. This state, known as *plik*, signified that the soul had left the body. Doctors advised the families to wait and hope. After a few days, the patient came back to normal life, and some recalled a dialogue with Yama, the god of death.

### *"Wrecked Nerve-Tubule Illness," A Chronic Somatoform Condition*

Most lay Cambodians hold, at least, a consistent notion of the blood vessels, nerves and tendons known generally as the *sAA say*. Like people from Thailand, the Cambodians explained many serious somatic symptoms as caused by the wind or water elements blocked, or flowing in the wrong way through them. Headache, tightness in the chest, and abdominal pain are attributed to some local abnormality in the tubules interfering with the normal circulation.

When the nerve tubules become severely affected, the patient developed "nerve tubules" (*sAA say prA saat*). There were persistent headaches. The variant of "spinning head madness" was associated with excruciating stabbing pain in the head. There is a fear among Cambodians of abnormal sensations around the temples; the temple is literally "wearing a flower in the ear." People are also terrified of problems around the back of the neck, as it is believed that this is the junction of the nerve tubules ascending to the brain and, if injured, the brain will be damaged too. There were other somatic sensations, such as tightness in the chest, a sense of "weak" respiratory movements, heat in the chest and racing heartbeat. The sweat seemed sticky, not like the normal consistency, and it was noticeable even at rest. The patient felt nauseous as if the food swallowed had not been digested.

Damaged or disrupted nerve tubules needed direct treatment; the most direct was to apply a burning wick to the skin in the method of moxibusion. Occasionally the healers used medicinal ingredients to treat this illness. Since the disease is believed to stem from overheated nerves, some healers prescribe "cooling medicine" followed by ritual pouring of lustral water.

## *"Magical Action Illness," An Acute Somatoform Condition*

Individuals and groups inevitably come into conflict, and this is reflected in Cambodia by this category of illness, called "magical action" or "magical human intervention." For the most part the "object" was introduced through food or water, or through inhaling it in a cigarette—seemingly innocuous domestic routes. The patients complain of sharp severe abdominal pain. The pain may spread to the backbone and the chest, and it feels as if the bones are being pulverised by a hammer.

A Cham practitioner lay in wait to see what the intended victim liked to eat. If the person liked rice, for example, the practitioner placed a grain of normal rice into a bottle. If, later on, he saw that the intended victim liked a bowl of sour soup, the practitioner added sour soup to the contents. The sorcerer case the bottle into the river and, after a while, the water which had filled the bottle was absorbed by the food which inflated. At that moment, the food in the victim's stomach expanded and inflated his belly. Once the soggy rice in the bottle rotted, the victim's intestines rotted too. At midday, this Cham practitioner used a second ritual, "magic done by water buffalo hide." He placed seven grains of rice into a segment of bamboo. He added a grilled small fish, a cord made of cowhide, and a fragment of bone from a corpse, and placed the bamboo tube into a well, or he planted it in front of the intended victim's house. Whenever the intended victim happened to eat cow or buffalo the cowhide entered his stomach, or when he ate grilled fish, the grilled fish expanded, and the patient developed pain.

Such popular accounts help to frame the somatic sensation within the tension existing in the local community. No-one needs to know *who* was responsible; the fact that the blame has been laid upon the social network of the patient is enough.

## The Magical Removal of Spirits, Agents of Acute Somatic Pain

When a wandering spirit, dispossessed of its own body, attacked a victim, the Khmer term for this interference was "touched their place." The patient felt hot and stabbing sensations in the body, sometimes pressure, often starting in the abdomen and migrating to the chest and the limbs, including the elbows and knees. A classic description was that during the night the spirit was sitting on the chest, compressing and suffocating.

Before attacking the spirits, the healer had first to "put the patient's mind back together." After that, using a sequence of Pali stanzas, he tied the spirits, and vitiated their power, and them untied the effete spirit. A spirit cornered is most dangerous, and the healer had to calm it. In the pre-operative sedation, healers recited a stanza with which to charm the spirit to become infatuated with them. To exorcise a *priey* spirit, the sequence was (1) untie the spirit → (2) induce the sedating love charm → (3) force the *priey* spirit out of the patient's body. The healers demand that the spirit leave through the patient's anus. Spirits, hating this route, pleaded to be allowed to leave through the legs. When the spirit left, the patient declared "I'm going!" and promptly defecated the spirit's last word through the patient's body. In this neat symmetry, the patient got sick because bad words came out of his mouth and, as a result, the bad spirit entered his body orifice. The healer had put something good—the medicine and the Pali stanzas—into the patient's mouth and ears, and the spirit had to leave through an inauspicious orifice—the anus; the spirit's last words from the patient's mouth completed the circuit.

## "Incompatibility Illness," A Postpartum Somatoform Disorder

The Khmer term *toah* means "in conflict, and incompatible." It is the name given to the illness affecting a woman after childbirth because of overwork, violation of a dietary taboo, or premature sexual behaviour with her husband, any of which was "incompatible" with her delicate post-partum physical state. One form, known as "incompatibility of the way of sleeping," was caused when the husband forced his wife to have sex within the months after she had given birth.

A woman came, three months after her confinement, to see a medium. She told him that, since her husband had forced sex on her, she had had tightness in the chest, and a hot and agitated feeling in the head. The healer motioned her to turn with her back facing him again. He placed his fingers between her shoulder blades. Then he moved his left hand to press into her left waist. Holding his hands in this position, he told her she had a problem with the nerves of her heart and her tubules that suspended her uterus from her backbone. He said she had a fallen uterus. This drawing by the medium showed the uterus as a small circle just above the top of the legs (Fig. 1).

The healer has constructed a detailed map of the somatic symptoms that makes sense to the woman. The husband had put his sexual products into his wife's lower orifice. Now the healer got the wife to put an extract of them into her upper orifice, her mouth; in this way, the medicine cancelled out the effects of the violation. Or they got the husband to wash his penis to extract its secretions. In the traditional family, the couple sleeps on the woven mat placed on top of the bamboo. Several male healers took the frayed bits of that heavily used old mat, where the couple had intercourse, added pubic hair, and burned them, and the woman drank the mixture.

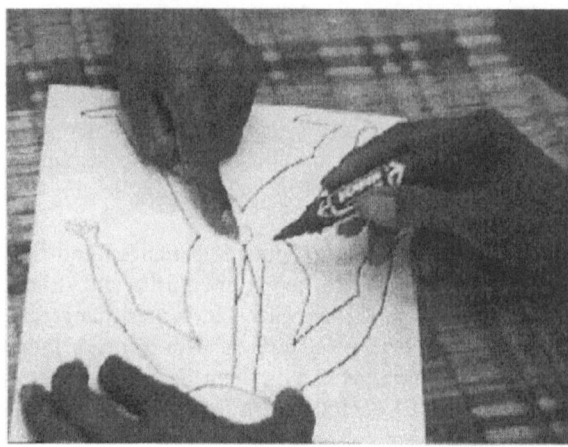

FIG. 1. Drawing of tubules flowing from uterus to kidney and brain. The healer points out uterus location where husband's forced sex with wife after childbirth started disorder, symptoms spreading to brain

## The Fatal Kiss of the Preceding Mother (skAn), or Childhood Epilepsy

Childhood epilepsy is a major problem faced in developing countries and, in Cambodia, the condition is commonly known as *skAn* [22]. The *kruu* in drawing his homunculus—the long tresses of the preceding mother flowing into the child's brain—shows the shared beliefs of patient and healer about how the preceding mother enters her child's body and induces somatic symptoms, recounted more often by the healer, or the parents, than the child (Fig. 2).

It was believed that the child dreamt of its preceding mother coming to embrace him. In "dog or wolf *skAn*," (s)he dreamt of a dog or wolf with bared fangs about to pounce, and he awakened in a rage. In "cartwheel *skAn*," (s)he saw the mythical form of Indra's rainbow or bow, waxing and waning, and was said to experience "dizziness" as the chest spun around. In "crocodile *skAn*," (s)he saw the approach of the crocodile to bite his/her legs and, in a reflex to escape, (s)he violently contracted them. The somatic symptoms were assumed from the diagnosis, rather than the other way around. There was no need to ask the patient.

## Discussion

The body is not simple something on which cultural values are passively inscribed, but as an existential ground for culture and self [2]. The Cambodian traditional healers chart "culture" and "self" through the body. They classify somatic disorders according to the indigenous anatomy which, in itself, is morally based. As diagnosticians, they "see" the workings of the body by physical examination which, in itself, is inspired by folk and Buddhist beliefs. As healers, they act as metaphoric

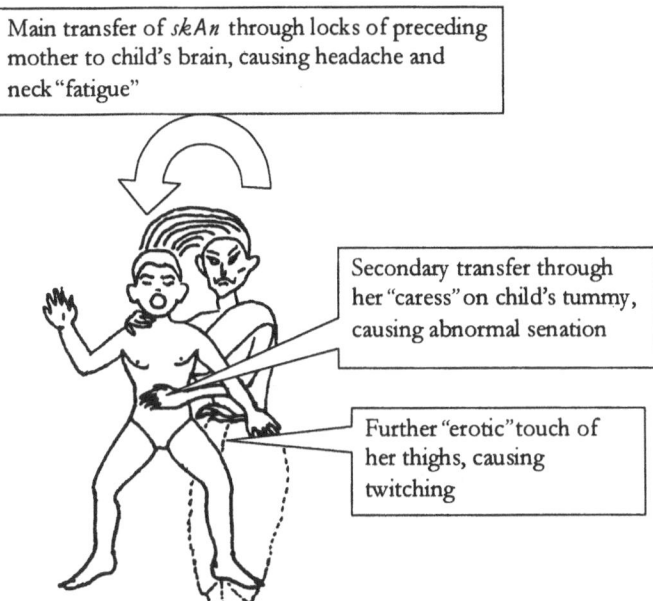

Main transfer of *skAn* through locks of preceding mother to child's brain, causing headache and neck "fatigue"

Secondary transfer through her "caress" on child's tummy, causing abnormal senation

Further "erotic" touch of her thighs, causing twitching

FIG. 2. *SkAn* of preceding mother showing transfer of illness to child, with development of somatic symptoms at metaphorical points of contact

surgeons, for example, treating the organs in the body by supernatural and natural means.

Magical action madness is a remarkable example of an embodied illness in which the patient, an embodiment of the community, shows symptoms of "breaking up", almost as a mirror of the break-down of the patient's community relations.

We can see a line running through the treatment of "incompatibility illness"—the goal being to reverse the disruption. Fed up with a sexually demanding husband? Eat a symbolic part of his sexual products. None of the treatments materially changed the woman's social circumstances. But she joined a group of women in the village with a socially acceptable label—she was not "mad"—and they gathered strength as a group, despite and perhaps because of the license afforded by their somatic symptoms.

In attributing pain and somatic symptoms, the healer worked out the causal path, which spanned "natural" and supernatural" (mystical, animistic and magical) events. Then he located the illness in a Euclidean vertical axis (deities and ancestors above; the patient and community in the middle; and spirits beneath), and a unipolar horizontal axis (patient in the middle; protective spirits around the house; and illness-causing spirits in the forest).

The indigenous view of *neuroanatomy* is one of structures which are nerves and tubules; that the contents and the "walls" are not easily differentiated; that substances flow up the body into the brain and then down again; that critical centres occur outside the brain, for example, in the eyes. It is worth recalling Descartes' assertion that the body moved with the assistance of small organisms called "animal spirits" that were produced and stored in the brain, and which travelled through nerves supposed to resemble hollow tubes [23]. His legacy, the Doctrine of the Hollow Nerve [24], which transmitted animal spirits [25], was the forerunner of modern neurology "which strips away the fabric of cultural experience that once enfolded pain" [26].

Studies of anatomy in Japan, China, and India show the importance of meridians which do not necessarily follow the Western division into organ-tissues. The vertical gradient of the body, identifi ed in Cambodia, seems to bear a resemblance to the systems of yoga found in India and Tibet.

In decoding somatoform disorders, it is essential to elicit the indigenous views of the body's structure and function. The Cambodian view of somatic symptoms shows that the *topology* and *axes of the body* are not well represented in three-dimensional Euclidean co-ordinates. A better way to depict the body is by a combination of a vertical axis with a radial horizontal polar axis. The vertical axis includes a moral gradient up to the head as the most sacred part. Disturbance to the body may ascend from the morally inferior territory of demons and evil spirits or, less commonly, it may descend, as in the example of attack by the preced-ing mother. The metaphoric treatment must reverse the gradient of this interference. The horizontal polar axis suggests the core of the body, surrounded by a sort of sausage-shaped integument. Illness has to be categorised, then, depending on whether it *penetrates* or *emerges* from this tubular structure. These directions are metaphorical, as shown by the healer's use of substitution rituals to "reverse" or "focus" the progression of physical symptoms to the surface and away from the body core. The ritual ensemble of Cambodian healing, such as reciting mantra, spraying saliva and blowing on the apex of the patient's head to drive the spirit down the patient's body, may be keyed by the idea that illness goes up the body, across tissues and organs—one principle of illness and the body, in vertical space [27–29].

The Cambodian taxonomy and ritual management of somatic symptoms shows well how many "somatic" symptoms are almost impossible to translate into English terms. As shown in this chapter, however, it is not simply an issue of translation–back-translation of somatic terminology. Like all taxonomies, diagnostic systems of medicine are based on Linnaean classification; on the law of parsimony; and on the General Systems Theory Law, defi ned by A.N. Whitehead, that "no class shall be a member of itself" (so, an illness can be subdivided, but cannot recur in the hierarchy). This law works in the world of linear thinking and Euclidean space. In Cambodia, where logic is based on what Condominas [30] called the system of *embôitement* and on non-Euclidean space, the taxonomy breaks the law—and somatic symptoms are clear cultural "ciphers" of the body and illness and, beyond that, of the system of classification itself.

The indigenous views of the body are constantly changing—witness the precipi-tous Westernisation of anatomical drawing in eighteenth century Japan [31] and, more recently, the partial "medicalisation" in local views of the anatomical pathology of AIDS [32]. further research is needed to consider how, under the influence of Western health education, the somatoform disorders might change.

# References

1. Kaitaro T (1996) La Peyronie and the experimental search for the seat of the soul: neuropsychological methodology in the eighteenth century. Cortex 32:557–564
2. Csordas TJ (1994) Words from the Holy People: a case study in cultural phenomenology. In: Thomas JC (ed) Embodiment and experience: the existential ground of culture and self. pp 269–290. Cambridge University Press, New York, pp 269–290
3. Desjarlais R (1994) The Bridge People: daily life in a camp of the homeless (see IRPS No. 71/94c01853). Am Anthropol 96:765
4. Shweder RA (1985) Menstrual pollution, soul loss, and the comparative study of emotions. In: Anonymous (ed) Culture and depression, University of California Press, Berkeley, pp 182–215
5. Levy RI (1973) Tahitians: mind and experience in the Society Islands. University of Chicago Press, Chicago
6. Rosaldo M (1980) Knowledge and passion. Cambridge University Press, Cambridge
7. LeVine R (1973) Patterns of personality in Africa. Ethos 1:123–152
8. Kleinman A, Gale JL (1982) Patients treated by physicians and folk healers: a comparative outcome study in Taiwan. Cult Med Psychiatry 6:405–423
9. Spiro M (1984) Karma: an anthropological inquiry. Am Anthropol 86:1002–1004
10. Rosaldo R (1984) Towards and anthropology of self and feeling. In: Shweder R, LeVive RA (eds) Culture theory: essays on mind, self and emotion. New York: Cambridge University Press, New York, pp 137–157
11. Kleinman A, Kleinman J (1985) Somatization: the interconnection in Chinese society among culture, depressive experiences, and the meanings of pain. In: Anonymous (ed) Culture and depression, University of California Press, Berkeley, pp 429–490
12. Kirmayer, LJ, Young A, Robbins JM (1994) Symptom attribution in cultural perspective. Can J Psychiatry 39:584–595
13. Leventhal H (1986) Symptom reporting: a focus on process. In: McHugh S, Vallis TM (eds) Illness behavior: a multidisciplinary perspective. Plenum Press, New York, pp 111–133
14. Kirmayer LJ (1994) Improvisation and authority in illness meaning. Cult Med Psychiatry 18:183–214
15. Escobar JI (1995) Transcultural aspects of dissociative and somatoform disorders. Psychiatr Clin North Am 18:555–569
16. Lee AM, Lee S (1996) Disordered eating and its psychosocial correlates among Chinese adolescent females in Hong Kone. Int J Eat Disord 20:177–183
17. Manson SM (1995) Culture and major depression. Current challenges in the diagnosis of mood disordes. Psychiatr Clin North Am 18:487–501
18. Fabrega H (1992) Culture and the psychosomatic tradition. Psychosom Med 54:561–566
19. Jablensky A, Sartorius N, Ernberg G, Anker M, Korten A, Cooper JE, Day R, Bertelsen A (1992) Schizophrenia: manifestations, incidence and course in different cultures. A World Health Organization ten-country study [published erratum appears in Psychol Med Monogr Suppl 1992 Nov; 22(4): following 1092]. Psychol Med Monogr Suppl 20:1–97
20. Janca A, Prilipko L, Costa (1997) The World Health Organization's global initiative on neurology and public health. J Neurol Sci 145:1–2
21. Task Force on DSM-IV (1994) Diagnostic and statistical manual of mental disorders, 4th end. American Psychiatric Association, Washington, DC
22. Eisenbruch M (1991) From post-traumatic stress disorder to cultural bereavement: diagnosis of Southeast Asian refugees. Soc Scie Med 33:673–680
23. Descartes R (1664) De l' homme, translated by Thomas Steele Hall. Harvard University Press, Cambridge, MA, 1972

24. Clarke E (1968) The doctrine of the hollow nerve in the seventeenth and eighteenth Centuries. In: Stevenson LG, Multhauf RP (eds) Medicine, science and culture: historical essays in honor of Oswei Temkin. Johns Hopkins University Press, Baltimore, pp 123–141
25. Riese W (1959) A history of neurology, MD Publications, New York
26. Morris DB (1991) The culture of pain. University of California Press, Berkeley
27. Ang C (1986) Les êtres surnaturels dans la religion populaire khmère. Cedoreck, Paris
28. Eisenbruch M (1992) Toward a culturally sensitive DSM: cultural bereavement in Cambodian refugees and the traditional healer as taxonomist. J Nerv Ment Dis 180: 8–10
29. Lemoine J, Eisenbruch M (1997) L'exercise du pouvoir de guérison chez les chamanes hmongs et les maîtres-guérisseurs khmers d'Indochine. l'Homme 144:69–103
30. Condominas G (1968) Notes sur le bouddhisme populaire en milieu rueal lao. Archives de Sociologie des Religion 13:81–110
31. Kuriyama S (1992) Between mind and eye: Japanese anatomy in the eighteenth century. In: Leslie C, Young A (eds) University of California Press, Berkeley, pp 21–43
32. Eisenbruch M (1997) Why I hate condoms: traditional healers and their patients in Cambodia (abstract). Fouth International Congress on AIDS in the Asia and Pacific, 5–5

# Post-Traumatic Somatic and Psychological Problems

Naotaka Shinfuku

*Summary.* The writer had a rare experience as medical doctor to become victim and observer of a major disaster. His office at the Kobe University Medical School was located at the center of the Hanshin-Awaji earthquake. The writer experienced the Great Hanshin-Awaji earthquake on January 17, 1995, in Kobe. He analyzed the physical and psychological consequence of the earthquake based on his experience. Stress-related physical symptoms and psychological symptoms have greatly changed at many phases after the earthquake. The Great Hanshin-Awaji Earthquake has been tragic. However, it has provided an invaluable opportunity to study physical and psychological problems of the population under severe stress. The importance of a long-term and wide-ranging program for the victims including housing, employment, and financial support is stressed.

*Key words.* Hanshin-Awaji earthquake, Somatic symptoms, Psychological symptoms, Post-traumatic stress disorder

## Introduction

The earthquake took place at 5:46 AM on January 17, 1995. The Richter-scale measurement was 7.2.

The earthquake hit just below the major city areas of Hanshin, which includes Kobe City, of approximately 1.5 million population. One year after the earthquake, Kobe City had lost almost 100,000 population due to migration to nondamaged areas.

The number of the population affected by the earthquake was estimated as 2.4 million. City gas supply was cut to 857,400 households. Every household would have three family members on average. This enabled a very rough estimation of the population affected by the earthquake. The number of the people who lost their housing and had to stay at shelters was over 320,000. In April 1995, the number of the dead was reported as 5502. But it was revised in July to 6048 as some of the victims who died at

International Center for Medical Research, Kobe University School of Medicine, Kusunoki-cho, 7-chome, Chuo-ku, Kobe 650-0017, Japan private hospitals were not included in the initial counts. The official number of the dead due to the earthquake was once again revised to more than 6500 in August 1995 as some of the delayed death cases, such as pneumonia and suicide, were certified as resulting from the earthquake.

Three quarters of the immediate death was due to asphyxia by house furniture and roof materials. Other major causes were due to burn, multiple fractures including cervical area, and traumatic shock.

Many people were unable to understand what had happened soon after the earthquake. This period is sometimes known as "6-hour vacuum." When the earthquake struck, the writer was unable to realize that it was an earthquake. He thought that it was some kind of an explosion under his house. Also, it took a long time for many people in Kobe to realize that the epicenter of the earthquake was near Kobe. Nobody expected an earthquake in the Kobe area. Kobe University was the center of the hard-hit area. Many victims in the Kobe area could realize the magnitude of the earthquake only after watching the burning scene of Nagata district on television. It is important to know that the population affected by the disaster is sometimes the least informed on the magnitude and nature of the disaster [1].

# Health Problems at Acute and Subacute Phases

## Immediately After the Earthquake

Immediate medical needs were emergency medicine. At Kobe University Medical School a considerable number of victims brought to emergency services were found to be DOA, dead on arrival. For medical services, many were for orthopedic surgery. Several cases of crash syndrome were also reported. The forensic department of our medical school was extremely busy for administrative autopsy and certification of death [2].

Soon after the earthquake, most of victims experienced emotional numbness. A writer's friend who lost his parents said that he felt out of touch with reality. He said that he could not feel sadness. A shaking feeling continued due to frequent aftershocks. The writer experienced a kind of depersonalization (feeling that everything is unreal). Depersonalization could be a psychological protection from the disaster.

Two or three days after the earthquake, the majority of the victims became talkative and joyful. Some people even became hypomaniac and showed signs of psychomotor excitement. These symptoms might be caused by the joy of survival.

Major psychiatric problems at the early stage were recurrence of mental disease and epileptic seizure due to the suspension of habitual medication. Loss of memory and disorientation were reported, particularly among the elderly. In general, manic depressive patients turned manic.

## By Week

For the first week, everybody was anxious to secure food, water, and information. A kind of a battlefield friendship existed for a certain period. This resulted in the sustainment of mental excitement and friendship among victims. However, fear of aftershock and general anxiety were experienced at the same time. Survivor's guilt was strong for those who lost family members.

The writer had an abnormal sense of time. One day was felt as eternal. But he could not remember the events of the previous day.

After 1 week, the focus of health care was shifted from emergency medical care to care for chronic patients. Treatment of the chronic patients including those with hypertension, diabetes mellitus, and mental diseases was resumed [3]. Care for senile demented and mentally handicapped in shelters posed difficult problems for managers of shelters. Insomnia was common at crowded shelters. Acute stress responses such as nightmare were reported. Psychiatric emergency care was established at some shelters.

The Hyogo Prefectural Mental Health Center played a key role in coordinating mental health care to victims. Volunteers including medical professionals such as psychologists and psychiatrists flooded Kobe and damaged areas. It is reported that almost 1.5 million volunteers from all over Japan, and some from abroad, came to the Hanshin area to assist after the Earthquake [4].

After 10 days, the life in shelters became very stressful for many victims. Increase of acute stress response, including serious stress ulcer, was reported. The department of Internal Medicine of Kobe University Medical School was busy with the treatment of many cases of extremely serious bleeding ulcers. Anxiety reaction and sleep disorder were common [5].

Increase of pneumonia and bronchitis was reported among the elderly. The earthquake took place in January, which was winter-time in Japan.

After 2 weeks, victims started facing the reality and the loss including family members, housing, and job. Depression became manifest among victims.

A few suicide cases were reported. Acute symptoms of post-traumatic stress (ASD) such as flashback continued among victims.

## By Month

After 1 month, a considerable number of the aged people became unable to cope with the continued stressful events of their lives. Among elderly victims, dementia, disorientation, and incontinence were often reported. The consumption of alcohol was increased among victims, which led to an epidemic of alcohol-related problems in some shelters. Alcohol-related violence was sometimes reported. Children showed regression. Burnout syndrome of volunteers became commonplace.

After 2 months, most victims had been transferred from shelters to temporary housing by lot. Later, this arrangement was criticized. In shelters, neighborhoods stayed together.

At one time, more than 320,000 people lived in shelters such as schools and public buildings. The government started the building of temporary housing which was similar to military barracks. In total, 47,000 temporary houses were constructed by public fund and almost 80,000 people lived in temporary housing.

Many victims lost their jobs and faced economic difficulties. Unlucky victims had to repay their loans for houses destroyed by the earthquake. In the process of rehabilitation and relocation, many victims faced degradation in social status and economic difficulty which, in turn, caused depression.

Among the victims, the most disadvantaged population groups included the following:

- the elderly who lost kin
- a family of mother and children
- physically and mentally disadvantaged
- foreigners from developing countries

After 2 years, victims moved gradually from temporary housing to condominiums built by the local government. In February 1998, only 23,700 households (43%) of 47,000 temporary housing units were occupied.

# Long-Term Health Consequences

A wide range of physical and psychological problems have been observed among victims even 3 years after the earthquake.

These long-term effects include both physical and psychological problems. These problems are mainly related to stressful experiences and conditions of the victims. However, other environmental factors and direct physical damage also play an important role. It should be noted that many factors contribute to one specific problem. For example, hypertension among victims could be caused by several causes such as salty instant food, stressful living conditions, and nightmares. There are many unknown health effects among victims. It will take a long time to obtain concrete data on the effects of the earthquake on such issues as long-term effects on psychosocial development of children, lowering of immunity and its effects on the incidence of allergy, cancer, etc.

## Long-Term Physical Effects

The risk factors of physical impacts of the disaster are not the only effects of the disaster. There are many factors. The biggest one is housing and the nutritional condition of victims. The isolated lifestyle has increased alcohol use and cigarette smoking, thus increasing the risk of hypertension and coronary heart diseases. In addition, the lack of intake of fresh vegetables and the increased intake of "fast food" would increase the risk of coronary heart disease among victims.

Cold temperature and insufficient air conditioning have caused common colds, bronchitis, and emphysema.

Some experts suggest the lowering of immunity among victims and predict a higher prevalence of cancer.

A small number of victims have been chronically disabled by the earthquake. They are suffering from head injuries and spinal cord injuries, and some have developed paraplegia. Continuous stress has affected the normal functioning of brain activities. Pseudodementia has been suspected among a sizable number of elderly victims. Heavy drinking caused alcoholic hepatitis in some victims. A high-risk group for chronic stress disorders is elderly males who lost their family members.

However, the scientific and large-scale epidemiologic studies have yet to be completed for the victims of the Great Hanshin-Awaji earthquake [6]. Table 1 summarizes a list of earthquake-related physical problems at each stage after the earthquake.

TABLE 1. Earthquake-related physical problems

|  | Direct | Stress-related |
|---|---|---|
| Acute | Immediate Death (5502) | Bleeding ulcer |
|  | Crash syndrome | Hypertension |
|  | Pneumonia | Coronary heart attack |
| Subacute | Earthquake-related death (900) | Atopic dermatitis |
|  | Influenza | Endogenous uveitis |
| Chronic | Head injury | Pseudodementia |
|  | Spinal cord injury | Alcoholic hepatitis |
|  | Paraplegia |  |

Number of deaths is shown in parentheses.

## Long-Term Psychological Effects

Among the major problems affecting the victims are psychological difficulties resulting from isolated life in temporary housing. This isolation and the loss of community sometimes have led to many tragedies such as suicides and so-called solitary death (unattended death in temporary housing). Upto February 1998, more than 200 cases of solitary death have been reported among victims of the earthquake. This has become a major social concern among the population in Kobe and a reason to blame the local government. Lack of local health personnel was cited as one of the contributing factors for this tragedy. It is well known that strong life-threatening experiences cause long-term psychological effects. Those who experienced disastrous life events suffer from post-traumatic stress syndromes (PTSD) characterized by nightmare, insomnia, flashback of the event, and various neurotic and depressive symptoms. Victims of the Hanshin earthquake have been no exception [7].

According to our study on school children, psychological effects have been marked among girls of a younger age who lost families and friends. Neurotic symptoms decreased after 6 months but depressive symptoms and physical complaints continued even after 12 months [8]. A few articles from the Kobe area report a relatively low prevalence of PTSD among victims compared with data in other countries [9].

Table 2 summarizes the earthquake-related major psychological symptoms among the victims of the Great Hanshin-Awaji earthquake.

## Discussion

### Time Factors and Bio-Psycho-Social Layers

A series of bio-psycho-social symptoms appeared after the Great Hanshin-Awaji earthquake. Table 3 shows the relationship between the phases after the Great Hanshin-Awaji earthquake and bio-psycho-social symptoms observed after the earthquake. Stress-related physical symptoms were the first group which appeared soon

TABLE 2. Earthquake-related psychological symptoms

| | |
|---|---|
| Acute phase (day) | Joy to be alive |
| | Depersonalization |
| | Disorientation |
| | Survivor's guilt |
| Subacute phase (week) | Anxiety |
| | Sleep problems |
| | Depression |
| Chronic phase (month to year) | Alcohol-related problems |
| | Interpersonal difficulties |
| | Apathy |
| | Post-traumatic stress disorder |

TABLE 3. Time factor and bio-psycho-social layers

| Layer | Symptoms | Course |
|---|---|---|
| Bio | Bleeding ulcer | Peak: 2–3 weeks |
| | Hypertension | Decrease by 6 months |
| Psycho | Anxiety symptoms | High at the beginning, decreasing with time |
| | Depression symptoms | High among those who lost home and family |
| | | Not decreasing with time |
| | | Increasing up to 6 months |
| Social | Alcohol problems | Increasing gradually with time |
| | Interpersonal difficulties | |

after the earthquake. Hemorrhagic ulcer and hypertension increased soon after the disaster, peaked at 2–3 weeks, and gradually decreased by 6 months. They were rather short-lived. Among psychological symptoms, anxiety symptoms were prevalent from the beginning and decreased with time. Sympathy and guilt symptoms appeared together with anxiety and decreased by 6 months.

However, depressive symptoms did not decrease with time. Depressive symptoms increased up to 6 months. Also, depressive symptoms were high among those who lost their home and family.

Social problems became dominant after 1 year. Alcohol problems and interpersonal difficulties increased gradually with time, and they continue to exist as major problems among victims.

This change of symptoms shows the stress caused a series of bio-psycho-social symptoms among victims after the disaster. Also, it was observed that biological, psychological, and social problems appeared consequently in the above order as time went on.

Figure 1 illustrates in a schematic way the relationship between bio-psycho-social layers, major symptoms, and their courses after the Hanshin-Awaji earthquake.

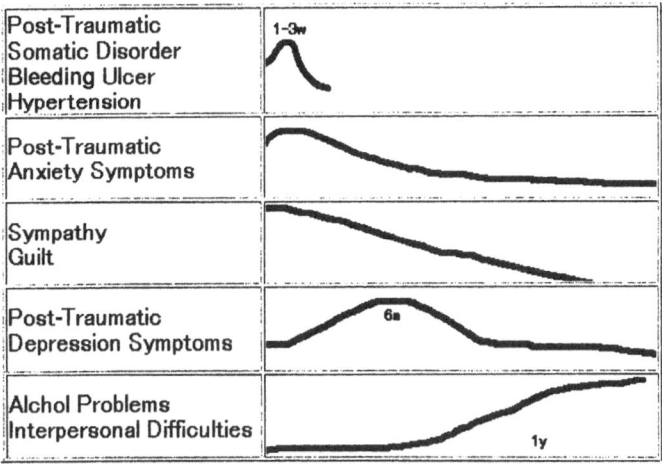

Fig. 1. Time factor and symptoms. *w*, week; *m*, month; *y*, year

## PTSD

ASD (acute stress disorder) and PTSD (post-traumatic stress disorders) are not adequate to cover the full range of trauma-related psychological problems. Studies at the Psychological Care Center of Hyogo Prefecture have demonstrated that among 1,956 cases consulted at the Center after the earthquake, PTSD complex positive (Symptoms A, B, C, D according to DSM-4R) cases were 2.5% of all cases and 4.5% among cases who lost their homes, and 13.1% among cases who lost their family members. This figure could be interpreted in many ways. PTSD was clearly related to the severity of damage such as loss of home and loss of family. However, a complete form of PTSD so far has been rather rare among the victims in Kobe.

There may be many reasons and possible interpretations for the low rate of PTSD among the victims in Kobe. One explanation was the low reporting of PTSD symptoms. Victims might have had some reservations in reporting such symptoms as dissociation to medical professionals due to the stigma attached to mental symptoms. A second explanation would be the low recognition of PTSD by medical professionals. There was no particular motivation among medical professionals to ask about the existence of PTSD among victims. No compensation was involved in its diagnosis in Japan. However, the above two explanations may not be sufficient to explain a rather low prevalence of PTSD after the Hanshin-Awaji earthquake. The PTSD concept became so popular soon after the earthquake that the widespread use of the concept PTSD contributed to reducing even the stigma attached to psychological problems in general. The media reported almost every day about PTSD. Almost all Japanese psychiatrists have become familiar with DSM-IV and its criteria for PTSD. A third explanation would be the commonly stipulated hypothesis that Asians including Japanese tend to somatize more rather than to develop psychological symptoms such as dissociation under a stressful situation. We have no accountable data to prove this explanation.

This explanation would instead invite discussion on the relationship between PTSD and somatoform disorder, and even the clinical accountability of PTSD among Asian victims [10].

A fourth explanation would be that many victims in Kobe did not feel abandoned or neglected after the earthquake. The communal-oriented Japanese society might have contributed to lowering the incidence of PTSD in Kobe. Also, no political and financial incentives have been involved, for patients or doctors, in the diagnosis of PTSD in the Kobe area. This explanation seems more plausible. However, we have not yet completed any epidemiological study with scientific vigor on PTSD among the victims of the Great Hanshin-Awaji earthquake. PTSD might increase with time. PTSD could be a cry for "Don't forget me" or "Don't forget Kobe." We have to continue careful observation regarding psychological status of the victims in the Kobe area.

# Conclusion

For health professionals living in Kobe, the most important concern at present is how to promote health among victims of the disaster and especially how to prevent so-called solitary death (unattended death) among victims. Immediately after the earthquake, there was a flood of volunteers to the Kobe area to take care of victims. It has been reported that almost 1.5 million volunteers came to Kobe and vicinity after the earthquake. Three years later, all volunteers have gone. Local governments mobilized public health nurses to visit temporary housing. However, the number of public health nurses is extremely limited. In each temporary housing community, autonomous committees have been set up to foster self-help among residents. These mechanisms have been working to prevent solitary death and long-term health problems.

It is very difficult for those who lost their homes, money, friends, and partners in old age to hold on to the meaning of life and hope.

Victims need a human network to find meaning in life and to hope for the future. A minimum amount of compensation to rebuild homes and to start small-scale businesses will be indispensable for victims to find meaning in life. Personal compensation to the victims is a hot political issue at present. We have to continue to promote the awareness of the public on long-term health consequences from the disaster and to find effective measures to reduce these problems.

# References

1. Baba S, Taniguchi H, Nambu S et al (1996) Essay, the great Hanshin earthquake. Lancet 347:307–309
2. Ueno Y, Nishimura A, Tatsuno Y et al (1998) Analysis of the result of inquests in the Great Hanshin earthquake. In: Comprehensive medical studies on the earthquake victims, Kobe University School of Medicine, Kobe, Japan, pp 27–34
3. Saito K, Kim JL, Maekawa K et al (1997) The Great Hanshin Awaji earthquake—aggravated blood pressure control in treated hypertensive patients. Am J Hypertens 10(2):217–221
4. Shinfuku N (1996) Psychological care and international cooperation (In Japanese). Kokorono-Kagaku 65:68–77

5. Aoyama N, Kinoshita Y, Kasuga M et al (1998) Peptic ulcer after the Hanshin-Awaji earthquake—increased incidence of bleeding gastric ulcers. In: Comprehensive medical Studies on the earthquake victims. Kobe University School of Medicine, Kobe, Japan, pp 45–52
6. Shinfuku N, Future task (In Japanese). Hanshin Awaji Dai-shinnsai-shi, Asahi Shinnbunn Syuppann-sha, pp 528–532
7. Shinfuku N (1998) Psychological consequences of the Great Hanshin-Awaji earthquake. In: Comprehensive medical studies on the earthquake victims. Kobe University School of Medicine, Kobe, Japan, pp 189–193
8. Shinfuku N, Honda M, Uemoto M et al (1998) Epidemiological Study of the Great Hanshin-Awaji earthquake's psychological consequences on affected school children. In: Comprehensive medical studies on the earthquake victims. Kobe University School of Medicine, Kobe, Japan, pp 194–197
9. Kokai M, Takeuchi S, Ohara K et al (1998) PTSD among victims of the Great Hanshin Awaji earthquake (in Japanese). Sheishin-Igaku 478:1061–1068
10. Kokai M, Shinfuku N (1998) Post-traumatic stress disorder and somatoform disorder (in Japanese). Psychosom Med 2(3):193–197

# Somatoform Disorders in China

Shu Liang

*Summary.* Since somatoform disorders were first included in DSM-III, Chinese psychiatrists have been concerned about these disorders. Some reviews and lectures were published in Chinese journals. During 1987–1992, the definition and diagnostic criteria were introduced in ICD-10 and DSM-III-R, and some Chinese doctors took an interest in these disorders and began to carry out clinical studies. However, the classification was not included in the Chinese Classification of Mental Disorder (CCMD) and its second revision (CCMD-II-R). The probable reasons are: (1) Until now the medical administration departments in China only authorize all hospitals to adopt the ICD-9 which does not include somatoform disorder. (2) CCMD-II-R still classifies hysteria as a disease (3) Chinese specialists are in dispute regarding somatoform disorder. Some claim that the definition of this disorder is unclear, its etiology and pathogenesis are unclear, and its symptoms are difficult to differentiate from those of depression, anxiety, hypochondriasis, neurasthenia, and medical problems. The proponents claim that patients with this disorder are commonly seen in general and mental hospitals. Keeping this disorder in the classification system of mental disorders is helpful in clinical treatment. The CCMD-III protocol is now being edited and tested. The disagreements will be discussed.

*Key words.* Somatoform, Somatization, Depression, Classification, Neurosis, Hysteria

## Studies on Somatoform Disorders Published in China

### Hospital Epidemiological Studies

(1) Data from the WHO/China Mental Health Information System showed the diagnosis of 896 hospitalized neurosis patients at ten mental hospitals in China during 1994–1996. The neurosis-involved somatoform symptoms are: 300.1, 300.7, 300.8 and 300.9 (according to ICD-9). See Table 1.

Institute of Mental Health, Beijing Medical University, Beijing, Republic of China
References were not provided by the author.

TABLE 1. Diagnoses of 896 hospitalized neurosis cases in ten hospitals in China between 1994 and 1996

| Diagnoses | No. 1 | No. 2 | No. 3 | No. 4 | No. 5 | No. 6 | No. 7 | No. 8 | No. 9 | No. 10 | Total n | Total % |
|---|---|---|---|---|---|---|---|---|---|---|---|---|
| 300.0 Anxiety | 28 | 12 | 11 | 1 | 9 | 59 | 4 | 3 | 9 | 0 | 136 | 15.2 |
| 300.1 Hysteria | 8 | 70 | 38 | 5 | 12 | 49 | 28 | 1 | 112 | 15 | 338 | 47.4 |
| 300.2 Phobia | 10 | 0 | 1 | 0 | 0 | 3 | 0 | 0 | 0 | 0 | 14 | 1.6 |
| 300.3 OCD | 51 | 0 | 1 | 3 | 2 | 12 | 8 | 4 | 7 | 2 | 91 | 10.2 |
| 300.4 Dysthymia | 39 | 2 | 3 | 0 | 9 | 38 | 0 | 2 | 22 | 0 | 115 | 12.8 |
| 300.5 Neurasthenia | 4 | 0 | 0 | 0 | 1 | 2 | 0 | 2 | 1 | 0 | 10 | 1.1 |
| 300.6 Depersonalization | 0 | 0 | 0 | 0 | 0 | 2 | 0 | 0 | 0 | 0 | 2 | 0.2 |
| 300.7 Hypochondriasis | 12 | 0 | 1 | 0 | 0 | 4 | 0 | 0 | 4 | 0 | 21 | 7.27 |
| 300.8 Other | 10 | 8 | 0 | 0 | 0 | 5 | 1 | 0 | 2 | 1 | 27 | 7.54 |
| 300.9 NOS | 0 | 0 | 0 | 0 | 0 | 0 | 0 | 0 | 0 | 142 | 142 | 15.8 |

Data from WHO/China Mental Health Information System.
No.1, Beiyi; No.2, Ankang; No.3, Shengh, No.4, Xicheng; No.5, Tianjin; No.6, 261; No.7, Jihn; No.8, Huilongguan; No.9, Xi'an; No.10, Shanghai.

TABLE 2. Mental disorders in patients of the General Hospital International Collaborative Study

| Diagnosis | Prevalence | |
| --- | --- | --- |
| | Shanghai | Mean of 15 centers |
| Alcohol dependence (F10.2) | 1.1 | 2.7 |
| Alcohol abuse (F10.1) | 1.6 | 3.3 |
| Depression (F32/33) | 4.0 | 10.4 |
| Dysthymia (F34) | 0.6 | 2.1 |
| Social phobia (F40.0) | 0.1 | 1.5 |
| Panic disorder (F41.0) | 0.2 | 1.1 |
| General anxiety (F41.1) | 1.9 | 7.9 |
| Somatization disorder (F45.0) | 1.5 | 2.7 |
| Hypochondriasis (F45.2) | 0.4 | 0.8 |
| Neurasthenia (F48.0) | 2.0 | 5.4 |
| More than one diagnosis | 9.7 | 24.0 |

1673 subjects were sampled in 20 municipal or district hospitals. In subjects who completed the General Health Questionnaire (GHQ), 583 had mental disorder and were diagnosed with CIDI/ICD10.

(2) Mental disorders of outpatients in general hospital—an international collaborative study. The results showed that the prevalence of somatoform disorder is lower than the mean of 15 international centers. See Table 2.

## Clinical Studies

(1) Zou YiZhuang has used the CIDI-c/ICD-10 Category 5 to test 100 neurosis patients (according to CCMD-II-R). He found that 9 cases were diagnosed somatoform disorders: 2 cases F45.2 (hypochondriasis); 7 cases F45.4 (pain disorder). The percentage of somatoform disorder in neurosis is 9%.

(2) In 1989, Wang reported on the relationship between somatoform symptoms and hysteria in the inpatients of Nanjing Brain Hospital during 1977–1987, whose original diagnoses included 18 cases of hysterical paralysis and 82 of hysteria; these were reevaluated with the DSM-III criteria of somatic disorder in 1987. Twenty-two were diagnosed as somatoform disorder. The clinical diagnoses of hysteria were retained for these 22 patients after 1–6 years of follow-up (according to CCMD-II). The mental symptoms appearing in these 22 patients included depression, suicide, excitement, impulsiveness, hallucination, refusing food, and mannerism. All 36 symptoms of somatization disorder occurred in these 22 patients. The occurrence frequencies were: repeated headache (19/22), dizziness (15/22), fatigue (14/22), seizure-like attack (14/22), palpitation (13/22), abdominal pain (12/22), fainting (10/22), walking difficulty (10/22), nausea (10/22), other pain (10/22), amnesia (9/22), back pain (9/22), hypermenorrhea (8/22), unconsciousness (8/22), dysphasia (7/22), vomiting (7/22), irregular menses (7/22), extremity pain (7/22), thoracic pain (7/22).

(3) The relationship between masked depression or depression and somatic (physical) symptoms was also investigated. Shengli Oil Field Hospital (San Dong) and Longquan Shan Hospital (Guangxi) reported on the relationship between depression and somatic symptoms (see Table 3). In our clinical practice, the depression patients

TABLE 3. "Depression" and physical symptoms—1997

| Research center | Department | No. | Mental symptom | Physical symptom | Treatment |
|---|---|---|---|---|---|
| Shengli Oil Field Hospital, Shangdong | Medicine, traditional medicine, pain treatment-department | 37 M·F = 1225 | Mild depression | Headache, leg pain, fatigue, anorexia, chest stiffness, short breath, back pain, abdominal discomfort, palpitation, dizziness, nausea, vomiting | TCAs 8 weeks Recovered 67.6% (25/37) improved 21.6% (8/37) ineffective 10.8% (4/37) |
| Longquan Shan Hospital, Guangxi | Whole hospital | 80 M·F = 4535 | Depression, lowered interest, sleep disoarder etc. | Chronic pain, headache, back pain, extremity pain, etc. Dizziness, chest stiffness, palpitation, burning sensation, etc. GL anorexia, nausea, vomiting, abdominal discomfort, etc. 80 patients mainly complained of physical symptoms | TCAs 6 weeks 100% significantly improved |
| Beijing Medical University | Institute of Mental Health | 32 8 | Depression neuroses | CIDI-C Section C Items 2–14 CIDI-C Section C Items 1–14 | |

mainly complain of somatic symptoms and always overlook the feeling of depression. Using CIDI-C to interview the depression patients revealed that all 32 cases experienced somatic symptoms (see Table 3).

## Comment

The data from the above studies suggested:

1. Somatic symptoms are commonly seen in our clinical practice. Patients present often with multiple symptoms referring to any body part or function or organ system, and unexplained by physical illness. These symptoms often persisted for more than several months.
2. The somatoform symptoms occurred in some mental disorders, such as major depression, "masked depression", neurosis, hysteria, etc. This shows that is difficult to diagnose the somatoform disorder as a disease.

3. Using the Composite International Diagnostic Interview, CIDI/ICD-10 Category 5 to test the neurosis patients (according to CCMD-II-R), about 9% of them may be diagnosed as somatoform disorder (according to ICD-10).

4. In China, the published literature on somatoform and somatization disorders is rare. The limited studies were clinical surveys. It is difficult to establish the classification of pure somatization and somatoform disorder. Many more studies need to be done.

# Preliminary Research on the Clinical Features of Somatoform Disorders in Three General Hospitals*

Fanqiang Meng[1], Yuhua Cui[1], Yucun Shen[1], Kai Lin[1], Dongfen Hou[2], Yuanli Qi[3], and Aleksandar Janca[4]

*Summary.* We investigated the clinical features and incidence of ICD-10 Somatoform Disorders (SD) in an outpatient population from general hospitals. Outpatients were first screened with the Screener for Somatoform Disorder (SSD). Those SSD-positive were further examined with the Somatoform Disorder Schedule (SDS). A total of 3346 outpatients were screened. The estimated incidence of SD in outpatients was 18.2%. SD outpatients went to see doctors 13.1 times on average in the past 12 months, and 60% of them reported being unchanged or even worse after treatments. Overlaps among the subtypes of SD were observed. Thirty-six outpatients with SD also met the criteria for neurasthenia. The frequency of the symptom groups of somatization disorder, from the most to the least, appeared in the following order: (1) dissatisfied with the doctors' diagnosis and treatments; (2) weakness; (3) biological symptoms such as sexual symptoms; (4) pain symptoms; (5) gastrointestinal symptoms, vegetative, and conversion symptoms. The incidence of SD is rather high in the outpatient population of general hospitals. Outpatients with SD go to see doctors very frequently, but most of them are dissatisfied with the diagnoses and treatments.

*Key words.* Somatoform, Somatization, Neurasthenia, Incidence, Outpatient, Diagnosis

## Introduction

Somatoform Disorders (SD) is a new diagnostic entity in The ICD-10 Classification of Mental and Behavioral Disorders [1]. It was estimated that 30%–40% of patients who went to their GP have medically unexplained symptoms [2]. Most patients with

---

[1] Institute of Mental Health, Beijing Medical University, Beijing 100083 P. R. China
[2] Department of Acupuncture and Moxibustion, Second Affiliated Hospital of Tianjin Traditional Chinese Medicine College, Tianjin 300193, P. R. China
[3] Department of Psychiatry, The First Affiliated Hospital of Haerbin Medical University, Haerbin 150001, P. R. China
[4] Division of Mental Health, World Health Organization, 1211 Geneva 27, Switzerland
* The research was part of a WHO International Study of Somatoform Disorders, organized by Dr. A. Janca.

SD were misdiagnosed or underdiagnosed, and many negative investigations or fruitless operations may be carried out [3]. The situation could be even worse in China, since SD was not included in the Chinese Classification and Diagnostic Criteria for Mental Disorders—2nd edition–Revised (CCMD-2-R) [4]. The diagnoses are quite unfamiliar to Chinese physicians. Although some of the patients with SD could be diagnosed as hysteria, hypochondriasis, and neurasthenia, that remain in CCMD-2-R, it was hard to find a proper place for many ICD-10 SD patients in CCMD-2-R in clinical practice. The clinical features of SD have never been studied in China. As a part of the WHO International Study on Somatoform Disorders, the present article investigated outpatients in three general hospitals affiliated to medical universities. The purpose of our study was to examine the clinical features and the incidence of SD in the outpatient population of general hospitals.

# Patients and Methods

## Subjects

Outpatients from departments of neurology and internal medicine were investigated. Those who were unable (even with the help of others) to participate in a 1- to 2-hour interview of Somatoform Disorder Schedule (SDS) [5] were excluded.

## Instruments

Two instruments were used: The Screener for Somatoform Disorder (SSD) [6] and SDS. SSD is a 12-item self-rating scale. Patients were regarded as SSD-positive if they presented three or more symptoms persisting for more then 1 month without physical basis. SDS was a structured clinical interview and consisted of two parts. Part one was designed to assess various somatoform symptoms. Part two was taken from the Composite International Diagnostic Interview-core version (CIDI-C) to assess panic attack, depression, and alcoholic disorders. SDS consisted of 80 medical symptoms. Each symptom was asked after, according to the "Probing chart flow for SDS" and was coded. Code 1 meant the symptom does not exist; code 2 indicated the symptom was not clinically significant; code 4 indicated the symptom was caused by medication, drugs, alcohol, injuries, or physical illness; and code 5 indicated the symptom was of clinical significance.

## Clinical Assessment

All the investigators were psychiatrists and received standard training for the use of SSD and SDS. They were directed by an experienced rater to interview at least 5 patients before they worked independently.

## Research Procedure

Every outpatient who went to departments of internal medicine and neurology was screened with SSD. Those who were disabled or unable to read and write were helped by trained nurses to complete the SSD. SSD-Positive patients could be interviewed by a psychiatrist with SDS on a voluntary basis.

## Statistical Analysis

Data were analyzed with SPSS 6.0⁺. Subtype diagnosis was based on ICD-10 research criteria. Two or more clinical diagnoses were accepted for each case should they were applicable. Frequency analysis was used for symptom analysis.

# Results

## General Data

Of the 3346 outpatients, 632 patients (18.9%) were SSD-positive; 140/632 patients completed SDS; 135/140 patients met ICD-10 criteria for at least one type of SD. The estimated incidence of SD in our 3346 outpatients was 18.2%.

Of the 135 patients with SD, 59 were male (43.7%)and 76 were female (56.3%). The age of the 135 patients ranged from 14 to 67 years, 36.2 ± 10.2 (mean ± SD) years on average. The age group distribution of SD was: 7 patients in the 14–20 age group, 36 patients in the 21–30 age group, 52 patients in the 31–40 age group, 30 patients in the 41–50 age group, 8 patients in the 51–60 age group, and 2 patients in the 61–67 age group. Of the SD patients 87.4% were aged between 21 and 50 years.

The average education of the 135 SD patients was 11.1 ± 3.5 years, equal to high school education in China. Their marital status was 27 single (20.0%), 99 married (73.3%), 9 widowed or divorced or separated (6.7%).

SD patients came to see doctors 13 times on average in 12-month period. Only 46/135 (34%) patients felt a little better; 81/135 (60%) patients complained they were unchanged or even worse after medical treatment, 8/135 (6%) patients did not give therapeutic assessment since some symptoms emerged while the old symptoms disappeared after treatment..

## Subtypes of SD

The 135 SD patients could be classified into various subtypes of SD as well as neurasthenia (see Table 1). There were no statistical differences of age, sex, and work influence due to somatoform symptoms among the subtypes.

The subtypes of SD overlapped with each other (see Table 2). Thirty-six patients with SD also met the ICD-10 criteria for neurasthenia.

## Clinical Features of Somatization Disorder

All the 80 symptoms were presented in 55 patients with Somatization Disorder. Analyzing symptoms occurred in 10 persons or more; 52 symptoms were included (Table 3). These symptoms could be grouped into five syndromes. From the highest frequency to the lowest, they were: (1) Dissatisfaction with doctors' diagnosis and treatments; (2) Physical or mental weakness; (3) Physiological symptoms (such as sleep or sexual disorder); (4) Pains; and (5) Gastrointestinal, autonomic, conversion, and dissociation symptoms (see Table 3).

## Comorbidity with Other Disorders

Of 135 patients with SD, no patients were found to be associated with ICD-10 depression, panic disorder, or alcoholism.

TABLE 1. Subtypes of 135 patients with somatoform disorders

| Subtypes | n (%) | Percentage of outpatients (%) | Age (mean ± SD) | Sex (%) | | Work time |
|---|---|---|---|---|---|---|
| | | | | Male | Female | |
| Somatization[a] | 55 (40.7) | 7.4 | 38.2 ± 10.8 | 21 (38.2) | 34 (61.8) | 7.6 ± 5.1 |
| Undifferentiated[b] | 23 (17.0) | 3.1 | 38.2 ± 9.0 | 10 (43.5) | 13 (56.5) | 7.5 ± 5.5 |
| Hypochondriac[c] | 11 (8.1) | 1.5 | 30.4 ± 9.4 | 7 (63.6) | 4 (36.4) | 7.4 ± 5.8 |
| Autonomic[d] | 9 (6.7) | 1.2 | 36.7 ± 11.6 | 6 (66.7) | 3 (33.3) | 7.5 ± 5.2 |
| Pain Disorder[e] | 3 (2.2) | 0.4 | 28.0 ± 4.6 | 1 (33.3) | 2 (66.7) | 5.7 ± 6.0 |
| Others[f] | 40 (29.6) | 5.4 | 35.1 ± 9.2 | 18 (45.0) | 22 (55.0) | 8.5 ± 4.9 |
| Neurasthenia | 36 (26.7) | 4.9 | 34.3 ± 8.7 | 16 (44.4) | 20 (55.6) | 7.3 ± 5.0 |

Work time, months worked in the past 12 months.
[a] Somatization disorder.
[b] Undifferentiated somatoform disorder.
[c] Hypochondriacal disorder.
[d] Somatoform autonomic dysfunction.
[e] Persistent somatoform pain disorder.
[f] Other somatoform disorders.

TABLE 2. Subtypes overlap among somatoform disorders

| Subtypes | | | | | | |
|---|---|---|---|---|---|---|
| A | 55 | | | | | |
| B | 21 | 36 | | | | |
| C | 7 | 4 | 11 | | | |
| D | 0 | 4 | 1 | 9 | | |
| E | 0 | 5 | 1 | 4 | 23 | |
| F | 0 | 1 | 1 | 0 | 0 | 3 |
| G | 0 | 0 | 0 | 0 | 0 | 0 | 40 |
| | A | B | C | D | E | F | G |

A, somatization disorder; B, neurasthenia; C, hypochondriacal disorder; D, somatoform autonomic dysfunction; E, undifferentiated somatoform disorder; F, persistent somatoform pain disorder; G, other somatoform disorders.

# Discussion

Our results showed that 18.2% outpatients from general hospitals suffered from SD. This incidence was quite close to that of Gureje and Obikoya [7], who found 16.7% of Nigerian patients in primary care setting meeting the criteria for at least one somatoform disorder. However, our incidence was much lower than that of Portegijs et al. [8], who found the prevalence of somatization to be 45%. The difference of incidence in these studies might be related to the different diagnostic criteria and research instruments used across studies, as well as the different patient population investigated. Our subjects were outpatients from university hospitals and many of them were referred from primary care settings. Perhaps this was why our population had a much higher

TABLE 3. Symptom frequency of the patients with somatization disorders

| Clinical symptoms | No. of patients | Frequency (%) | Clinical symptoms | No. of patients | Frequency (%) |
|---|---|---|---|---|---|
| Dissatisfied with treatment | 48 | 82.3 | Trouble with a dry mouth | 21 | 38.2 |
| Dissatisfied with diagnosis | 48 | 82.3 | Hot or cold sweats | 21 | 38.2 |
| Tiredness | 39 | 70.9 | Menstrual-period irregularity | 21 | 38.2 |
| Being tired all the time | 38 | 69.1 | Trouble in keeping balance | 20 | 36.4 |
| Easily tired | 37 | 67.3 | Frequent body shock | 20 | 36.4 |
| Pounding heart | 36 | 65.5 | Worrying about health | 20 | 36.4 |
| Unrecoverable fatigue | 36 | 65.5 | Abdominal pain | 18 | 32.7 |
| Unable to relax | 36 | 65.5 | Dissatisfied with management | 18 | 32.7 |
| Sleep disorder | 34 | 61.8 | Blurred vision | 16 | 29.1 |
| Irritability | 34 | 61.8 | Ear ringing or buzzing | 16 | 29.1 |
| Digestive problem | 33 | 60.0 | Numbness or tingling | 16 | 29.1 |
| Sexual problem | 33 | 60.0 | Lump in throat | 15 | 27.3 |
| Headaches | 29 | 52.7 | Clumsiness | 15 | 27.3 |
| Back pain | 28 | 50.9 | Pain in arms or legs | 14 | 25.5 |
| Chest pains | 27 | 49.1 | Worrying physical deformity | 14 | 25.5 |
| Being sickly most of time | 25 | 45.5 | Cause or diagnosis was incorrect | 14 | 25.5 |
| Worry about illness | 25 | 45.5 | Amnesia | 12 | 21.8 |
| Bodily weakness | 25 | 45.5 | Urinating too frequently | 12 | 21.8 |
| Excessive gas or bloating | 24 | 43.6 | Unusual feeling in/on the body | 12 | 21.8 |
| Burping or hiccups | 24 | 43.6 | Heavy or fast breathing | 12 | 21.8 |
| Discomfort in stomach | 24 | 43.6 | Excessive menstrual bleeding | 11 | 20.0 |
| Weakness | 24 | 43.6 | Diarrhea | 10 | 18.2 |
| Heaviness or lightness | 24 | 43.6 | Blushing | 10 | 18.2 |
| Requesting tests | 24 | 43.6 | | | |
| Dizziness | 24 | 43.6 | | | |
| Shortness of breath | 23 | 41.8 | | | |
| Nausea or sickness | 22 | 40.0 | | | |
| Worrying about having illness | 22 | 40.0 | | | |
| Bad taste or coated tongue | 21 | 38.2 | | | |

percentage of patients with somatization disorder (7.4%) than the patient population in primary care (1.1%) and the general population (0.2%–0.3%) [7,9]. Our results showed that the incidence of somatization disorder was the highest among all the subtypes of SD (see Table 1), perhaps due to the long-term nature of somatization disorder.

Our results suggested that the treatment outcome of SD was usually very poor. As high as 60% of patients complained there was no change or were even worse after medical treatment. That could explain why patients went to hospitals so often: seeing doctors 13 times in the past 12 months. The high frequency of "hospital-shopping" and poor treatment outcome might worsen patients' dissatisfaction with doctors' diagnosis and treatments.

Approximately similar to those of other investigations [10, 11], our results showed that the average age of SD patients was 36 years. Moreover, 87.4% of our patients with SD were aged between 21 and 50, a crucial age for both the individual and the family.

It was reported that women were suffering more frequently from somatization disorder [12]. Our results showed that female patients comprised two-thirds of patients with somatization disorder. However, there were no sex differences among the other subtypes of SD.

Little research had been done on the differential diagnosis of SD subtypes. The present results showed that the subtypes of SD overlapped with each other. Except for somatization disorder, all the other four subtypes (undifferentiated somatoform disorder, hypochondriacal disorder, somatoform autonomic dysfunction, persistent somatoform pain disorder) interlaced with each other (see Table 2). It was hard to make a differential diagnosis of the subtypes according to ICD-10 diagnostic criteria alone. We suggest that the ICD-10 diagnostic criteria for SD subtypes needs to be further specified.

A prominent and impressive result of this study was patients' distrusting attitude toward doctors. A total of 82% patients with somatization disorder were dissatisfied with doctors' diagnosis and treatments. This was in accordance with the finding that somatizing patients obtained higher scores on bodily preoccupation and hypochondriacal beliefs [13]. Physical and mental weakness presented in 70% of SD patients. Unlike the findings of Gureje and Obikoya [7], headache and palpitation were not the first rank symptoms of our somatization disorder. However, 52% and 65% of patients, respectively, with somatization disorder presented these two symptoms. It seemed SD patients with different cultural backgrounds manifested similar clinical symptoms. Therefore, somatic expression of psychological distress could be a universal phenomenon, and somatization was unlikely to be a culture-bound syndrome [14].

It has been reported that somatoform disorders often coexist with anxiety disorders or depressive disorders [3, 10]. In our present study, we did not find such comorbidity. The result corresponded with a community survey in Florence [15].

Neurasthenia was and still is a controversial diagnostic entity. It has been removed from DSM-IV [16] but remains in ICD-10 and CCMD-2-R [1, 4]. Our results suggested that ICD-10 criteria for neurasthenia lacked specificity because in 36 patients diagnosed with neurasthenia, 21 patients could be diagnosed as having somatization disorder, 4 hypochondriacal disorder, 4 somatoform autonomic dysfunction, 5 undifferentiated somatoform disorder, and 1 persistent somatoform pain disorder. We believe further study on the clinical applicability of the ICD-10 criteria for neurasthenia is needed.

## References

1. World Health Organization (1992) The ICD-10 Classification of mental and behavioral disorders: clinical descriptions and diagnostic guidelines. World Health Organization, Geneva, pp 132–173
2. Fava A (1992) The concept of psychosomatic disorder. Psychother Psychosom 58:1–12

3. Lipowsky Zl (1988) Somatization: the concept and its clinical application. Am J Psychiatry 145:1358–1368
4. Society of Psychiatry, Chinese Medical Association (1995) Chinese Classification and Diagnostic Criteria for Mental Disorders—2nd edition-revised (CCMD-2-R) (in Chinese). Southeast University Press, pp 1–43
5. Janca A, Burker JD, Isaac M et al (1995) The World Health Organization somatoform disorders schedule—a preliminary report on design and reliability. Eur Psychiatry 10:373–378
6. Issac M, Tacchini G, Janca A (1993) Screener for somatoform disorders. World Health Organization, Geneva
7. Gureje O, Obikoya B (1992) Somatization in primary care: pattern and correlates in a clinic in Nigeria. Acta Psychiatr Scand 86:223–227
8. Portegijs PJM, Van-der-Horst FG, Proot IM et al (1996) Somatization in frequent attenders of general practice. Soc Psychiatry Psychiatr Epidemiol 31:29–37
9. Robins LN, Helzer JE, Weissman MM et al (1984) Lifetime prevalence of specific psychiatric disorders in three sites. Arch Gen Psychiatry 41:949-958
10. Katon K, Lin E, Korff MV et al (1991) Somatization: a spectrum of severity. Am J Psychiatry 148:34–40
11. Yutzy Sh, Cloninger R, Guze SB et al (1995) DSM-4 field trail: testing a new proposal for somatization disorder. Am J Psychiatry 152:97-101
12. Chadda RK, Bhatia MS, Shome S et al (1993) Psychosocial dysfunction in somatising patients. Br J Psychiatry 163:510-513
13. Labott SM, Preisman RC, Torosian T et al (1996) Screening for somatizing patients in the pulmonary subspecialty clinic. Psychosomatics 37:327–338.
14. Isaac M, Janca A, Orley J (1996) Somatization—a culture-bound or universal syndrome? J Ment Health 5:219–222
15. Faravelli C, Salvatori S, Galassi F et al (1997) Epidemiology of somatoform disorders: a community survey in Florence. Soc Psychiatry Psychiatr Epidemiol 32:24–29
16. American Psychiatric Association. (1994) Diagnostic and statistical manual of mental disorders (4th edn.) (DSM-IV). APA, Washington, pp 13–24

# Neurasthenia: Transpacific Comparisons

Keh-Ming Lin

*Summary.* This paper reports key findings from two large-scale studies examining the clinical features, epidemiological characteristics, and cultural meaning of neurasthenia as defined by ICD-10. These studies are: (1) the Chinese American Psychiatric Epidemiologic Study, an ECA type community-wide survey ($n = 1747$) using stratified sampling methods and standardized structured instruments including the CIDI; and (2) a multinational comparative study ($n = 448$) utilizing standardized clinical and anthropological instruments to systematically study neurasthenia patients recruited from sites (China, Hong Kong, Taiwan, and Los Angeles) divergent in socioeconomic development and political structures. Issues explored include the clinical features, pattern of distress, perceived cause, help-seeking patterns, stigma, and other sociocultural factors related to the phenomenon of neurasthenia. The results showed that ICD-10 neurasthenia is highly prevalent both in the clinical and community settings and can be distinctively differentiated from other psychiatric conditions. The symptom profiles of neurasthenia are strikingly similar among patients studied at divergent sites, as well as between Chinese neurasthenic and non-Chinese CFS patients. However, sociocultural correlates of neurasthenia diverge remarkably across sites and study groups. These results have important implications regarding the validity of ICD-10 definition of the condition, as well as the care of a large number of patients with clinical features compatible with such a diagnosis.

*Key words.* Neurasthenia, Chronic fatigue syndrome, Somatoform, Epidemiology, Ethnography

## Introduction

Originally coined and popularized by the American neurologist George Beard in the 1860s [1, 2], the concept of neurasthenia went through a series of fascinating transformations and permutations, and at present represents one of the most controver-

Research Center on the Psychobiology of Ethnicity and the Department of Psychiatry, Harbor-UCLA Medical Center, 1124 West Carson Street, B-4 South, Torrance, CA 90502, USA
Supported in part by NIMH Research Center on the Psychobiology of Ethnicity MH47193 and MH47460, and the UC Regent Pacific Rim Research Center #A92-1224A-00

sial issues in psychiatric nosology and cultural psychiatry [3–10]. The rapid ascendency of such a concept in the West, as well as its subsequent decline in the beginning of the 20th century, both as a diagnostic category for the professionals and an illness label for the lay public, most likely reflected changes in social attitudes and medical ideologies rather than scientific progress [6]. Interestingly, exactly around the time when neurasthenia was beginning to lose its foothold in the West, its introduction to the East, especially among the Chinese, was quickly followed by its "indigenization," such that within the time span of several decades, it became one of the most commonly used idioms of distress in these communities. In the last several decades, whereas the term neurasthenia has become practically obsolete in the United States and in most Western European countries, its currency in Asian communities has remained strong [7, 9, 10]. In Mainland China, where neurasthenia has remained as an official diagnostic category in the medical classification system, its prevalence has been reported to be extremely high, with some studies showing that up to 10% of community samples suffering from such a condition [11, 12]. In other Asian communities, where clinicians have been more profoundly influenced by contemporary "Western" medical practices, neurasthenia typically has not been recognized as an official diagnostic entity, and thus little information is available regarding its prevalence in the clinical or community settings. However, despite its neglect by professionals, neurasthenia remains an extremely common idiom of distress for patients and their families. The currency and tenacity of such an illness label in these societies indicate that, irrespective of its nosological status, there may be powerful cultural and sociopolitical forces that continue to render the concept of neurasthenia meaningful and useful for the general public [3, 13].

Further complicating the picture, in the West where neurasthenia has faded from professional and public consciousness, numerous "epidemics" of severe chronic fatigue, often in association with symptoms and signs that may be interpreted as subtle manifestations of infection and/or immunological dysfunctions (mild fever, muscle and joint pain, swelling of lymph nodes, etc.), have emerged [6, 8, 14–16]. The clinical features of these patients, now commonly labeled with the term "chronic fatigue syndrome" (CFS), have been noted by a number of authors to be similar to those suffering from neurasthenia in the past in Western countries, raising the question of whether CFS represents "old wine in a new bottle" [8].

To start to address these fascinating issues, we have initiated a series of cross-cultural research projects in recent years. Key results of two of these studies will be reported in the following.

# The Epidemiology of Neurasthenia Among Chinese Americans in Los Angeles

This was conducted in the context of a large-scale, community-wide psychiatric epidemiological study [17] aiming at determining the prevalence and incidence of major psychiatric conditions and their associated risk factors. Using a stratified cluster sampling method, the study included 1747 adult Chinese American subjects randomly selected from the Los Angeles County area. A modified version of the Composite

International Diagnostic Interview (CIDI) was used for the identification of DSM-III-R psychiatric diagnoses including major depression, dysthymia, and anxiety disorders. In addition, a supplemental neurasthenia module was constructed for the diagnosis of International Classification of Diseases, Version 10 (ICD-10) defined neurasthenia. Dimensions of social stress and social support were measured by the use of established instruments.

Unlike DSM-III-R and DSM-IV, neurasthenia is included as an official diagnostic category in the ICD-10 system. The diagnosis is operationally defined by the existence of persistent and distressing mental fatigue or bodily weakness that are not explainable by other specific disorders, as well as at least two of the following seven symptoms believed to be commonly seen among these patients: muscular aches and pains, dizziness, tension headaches, sleep disturbance, inability to relax, irritability, and dyspepsia. The CIDI neurasthenia supplemental module was constructed to capture cases fulfilling these definitions. In addition, to reach a diagnosis of neurasthenia, they should also have suffered from these symptoms for a duration greater than 6 months, experienced significant impairment in functioning, and/or severe distress that were disabling. Using this module, the study first identified all cases with symptom patterns compatible with ICD-10 criteria listed above, irrespective of whether they also fulfilled other psychiatric diagnoses ("all neurasthenia"). They were then further divided into those "comorbid," with one or more lifetime DSM-III-R diagnoses ("mixed," neurasthenia), and those without such comorbidity ("pure" neurasthenia).

The results showed that a remarkably high proportion of the Chinese Americans interviewed in this study experienced significant distress and functioning impairment secondary to symptoms compatible with a diagnosis of ICD-10-defined neurasthenia. As shown in Figure 1, this diagnosis represented the most prevalent condition as compared to all the other psychiatric syndromes. This is true not only when all cases with neurasthenic symptom profiles ("all neurasthenia") were included (6.4%; 112/1747),

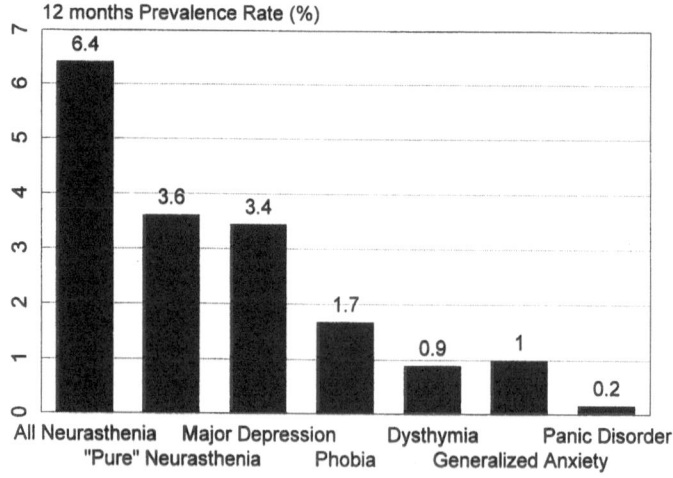

FIG. 1. Prevalence of mental disorders in Chinese-Americans

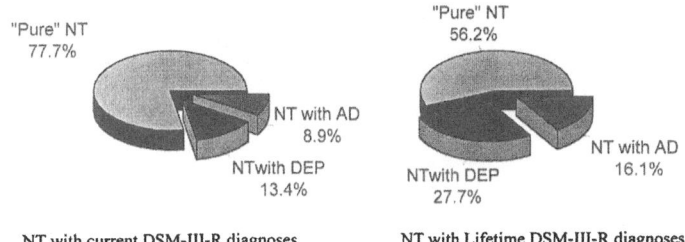

FIG. 2. Overlaps of neurasthenia (*NT*) with other psychiatric conditions. *AD*, anxiety disorder; *DEP*, major depressive disorder

but also when the comparison was limited only to those without comorbid DSM-III-R diagnosis ("pure" neurasthenia).

As shown in Figure 2, the overlap between neurasthenia and DSM-III-R diagnoses appeared to be quite limited. Approximately 78% (87/112) of these neurasthenic cases did not have any current DSM-III-R diagnosis, and approximately 56% (63/112) of them did not have any lifetime DSM-III-R diagnosis. Of the "mixed" or comorbid cases, approximately two thirds (31 cases) were identified with a current diagnosis or past history with major depression (22 cases) or dysthymia (9 cases). Of the 18 cases who were comorbid with anxiety disorders, 12 had a lifetime diagnosis of generalized anxiety disorder, and 6 had a lifetime diagnosis of phobia.

## A Cross-Cultural Comparison on Neurasthenia: Chronic Fatigue Syndromes in East Asia and North America

Conducted from 1992 to 1995, this multisite collaborative study utilized an identical research protocol to examine the phenomenology and culture meaning of neurasthenia and CFS in divergent populations on both shores of the Pacific Ocean. Together, the study included a total of 348 subjects with chronic fatigue, recruited from the following sites: Los Angeles (76 Chinese Americans and 93 Caucasians), Hong Kong (100 Chinese), and Changsha, China (79 Chinese) (Data from Taiwan with 100 cases are not complete and are not included in this report). All subjects were assessed with the use of structured interview instruments and standard rating scales, and were evaluated for DSM-III-R diagnoses, as well as as the existence of CFS and neurasthenia according to established operationalized criteria (ICD-10 for neurasthenia and the CDC criteria for CFS). Explanatory Model Interview Catalogue (EMIC), a semi-structured interview instrument designed to systematically collect information on patients' illness experiences, was also used at all participating sites to assess cultural influences on the patterning of distress, beliefs on the nature and meaning of their afflictions, help-seeking preferences, and stigma [18].

Figure 3 shows that, irrespective of research sites and cultural affiliations, the majority of the patients suffering from chronic fatigue could be classified as neurasthenic patients with the use of the ICD-10 criteria. In contrast, the applicability of the CDC-defined CFS appeared to be extremely limited, capturing only 4%–20% of all

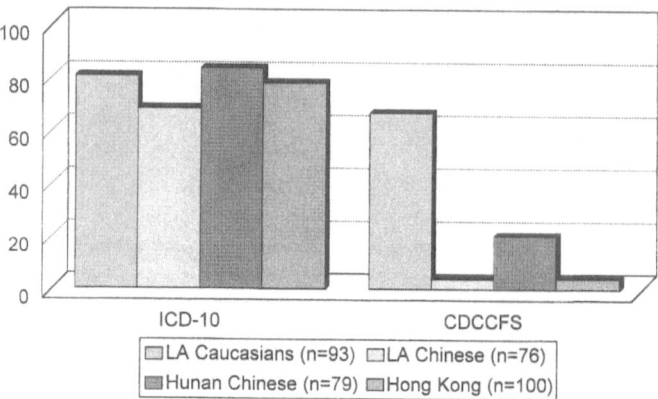

FIG. 3. Diagnostic characteristics of chronic fatigue patients. *LA*, Los Angeles; *HK*, Hong Kong

subjects with persistent fatigue in these populations. Even among the Caucasians, substantially more chronic fatigue patients were identifiable with the ICD-10-defined neurasthenia than with CFS as originally defined by CDC [19]. These data suggest that, relative to CFS, the concept of neurasthenia, particularly as defined by ICD-10, may be more clinically useful and cross-culturally applicable for patients suffering from chronic fatigue and related symptoms. This is congruent with the development in CFS research in recent years, suggesting that the earlier emphasis on signs of infection might not have been useful. Responding to such observations, attempts have been made to minimize the emphasis on infection and immunological deficiency in the definition of CFS. Reflecting such a trend, the revised CDC criteria for CFS, as formulated in 1994 [20], became remarkably similar to the ICD-10 definition of neurasthenia.

Similar to findings derived from the epidemiological study described above, ICD-10 defined neurasthenia overlaps only to a limited extent with DSM-III-R syndromes. Irrespective of study location and cultural grouping, less than one third of the patients studied suffered from concurrent DSM-III-R conditions, and less than half had a lifetime diagnosis of any of these psychiatric problems. In contrast to the prevailing beliefs by many clinicians and researchers that neurasthenia and CFS might represent depressive conditions masked with somatizing presentations, our data thus indicate that neurasthenia/CFS is to a large extent separable from depression and other psychiatric syndromes as defined by the DSM system. At present, there is no place for these significantly distressed patients in the DSM-IV schema except the extremely ambiguous category of "undifferentiated somatoform disorder" or "somatoform disorder NOS," neither of which adequately or accurately depict these patients' clinical features, nor do they point to treatment strategies or facilitate research activities.

Overall, the clinical features of these fatigue patients were remarkably similar across sites and ethnicity. As an example, the SCL-90 profiles of all four study groups closely resemble one another (Figure 4), despite the fact that these patients came from drastically divergent cultural backgrounds and lived in societies crucially different in many ways. Such similarity suggests that the clinical condition captured by the

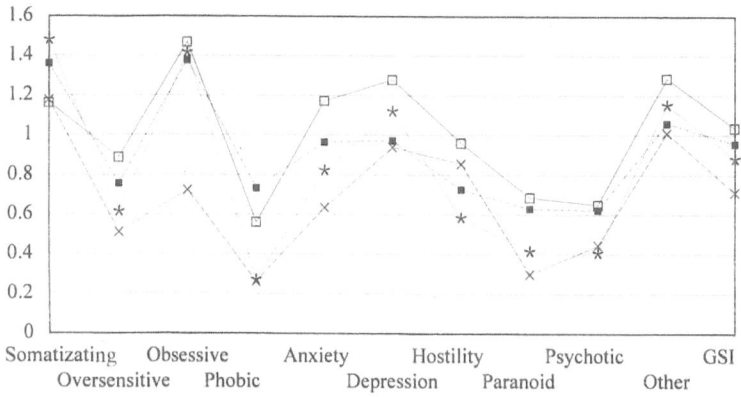

Fig. 4. ICD-10 neurasthenia patients without major current DSM-III-R diagnosis: Caucasians (*asterisks*) Chinese Americans (*open squares*), Hunan Chinese (*crosses*), and Hong Kong Chinese (*closed squares*)

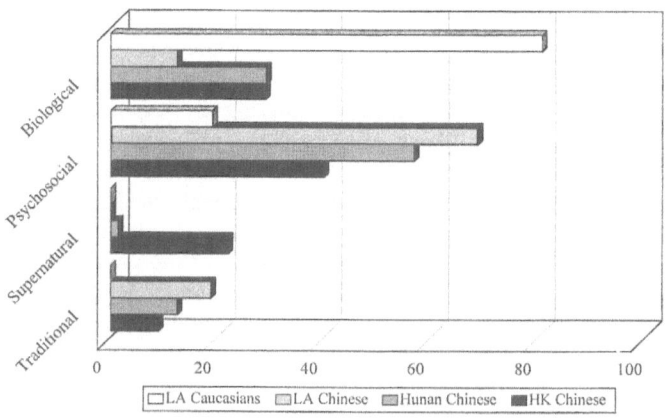

Fig. 5. Perceived cause of patients' neurasthenia

concept of neurasthenia/CFS may be a worldwide phenomenon that transcends cultural, socioeconomic, and political boundaries. These data also support the thesis that neurasthenia and CFS are related concepts that may be regarded as variants of one another.

Such a strikingly high degree of homogeneity in the clinical domain notwithstanding, patients interpret the meaning of their affliction in divergent ways, subscribe to unique explanations regarding the etiology, pathogenesis, and potential outcome of their problems, and seek help from varied sources. Data covering these issues, both quantitative and qualitative, are still in the process of being analyzed. Figures 5 and 6 present some of the initial results in a highly summarized format, which does not adequately reflect the rich nuances patients cope with and attempt to make sense of

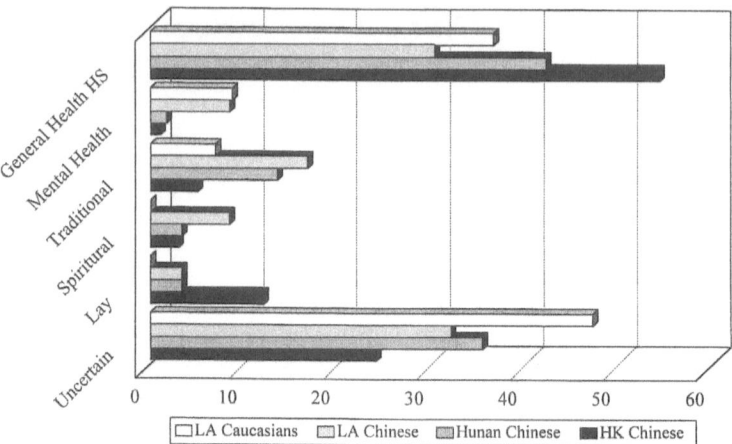

Fig. 6. Most important help-seeking preference of neurasthenia/chronic fatigue syndrome patients

their puzzling and debilitating problems. However, they are presented here to show that (1) culture does play a significant role in shaping patients' beliefs, outlooks, and reactions vis-a-vis their afflictions; (2) considering the magnitude of differences in many aspects of their lives (lifestyles, social structure, economic development, etc.) among the three Chinese groups, the similarity in the way they conceptualize and attempt to manage their ailment is quite remarkable, which possibly reflects the tenacity of cultural influences; (3) and for all groups, mental health services rarely appear to be an important part of their treatment options. At the same time, a remarkably high proportion of the patients, irrespective of site and ethnicity, could not identify any system of care that is regarded as substantially helpful.

## Conclusions

This paper briefly describes two recently completed studies on neurasthenia and CFS. The results showed that patients suffering from symptoms compatible with the formulation of the ICD-10 for neurasthenia is commonly seen in the clinical settings as well as in the communities. In fact, for Chinese Americans, the prevalence of such a syndrome exceeds all other psychiatric conditions as currently defined. Contrary to prevailing beliefs that neurasthenia represents a somatic equivalent of depression, most of these patients did not manifest sufficient symptoms that allow for the diagnosis of any psychiatric disorders as currently defined. The cross-cultural similarity in the clinical features of such patients argues for the universality of such a clinical phenomenon. At the same time, similarities as well as variations in the way the afflictions are perceived and interpreted, as well as the patterns and pathways of help-seeking, attest to the importance of culture in shaping patients' responses to their afflictions, which are likely to play a significant role in determining the course and outcome of their conditions.

# References

1. Beard G (1869) Neurasthenia or nervous exhaustion. Boston Med Surg J 3:217–220
2. Beard G (1881) American Nervousness. edition. G.P.Putnam, New York
3. Kleinman A (1982) Neurasthenia and depression: a study of somatization and culture in China. Cult Med Psychiatry 6:117–190
4. Lee S, Wong KC (1995) Rethinking neurasthenia: the illness concepts of shenjing shuairuo among Chinese undergraduates in Hong Kong. Cult Med Psychiatry 19: 91–111
5. Zheng YP, Lin KM, Zhao J, Zhang MY, Yong D (1994) Comparative study of diagnostic systems: Chinese classification of mental disorders—second edition (CCMD-2) versus DSM-III-R. Comp Psychiatry 35:441–449
6. Abbey SE, Garfinkel PE (1991) Neurasthenia and chronic fatigue syndrome: the role of culture in the making of a diagnosis. Am J Psychiatry 148(12):1638–1646
7. Zhang MY (1989) The diagnosis and phenomenology of neurasthenia: a Shanghai study. Special issue: neurasthenia in Asian cultures. Cult Med Psychiatry 13:147–161
8. Wessely S (1990) Old wine in new bottles: neurasthenia and "ME". Psychol Med 20: 35–53
9. Cheung FM (1989) The indigenization of neurasthenia in Hong Kong. Cult Med Psychiatry 13:227–241
10. Rin H, Huang MG (1989) Neurasthenia as nosological dilemma. Cult Med Psychiatry 13:215–226
11. Liu X, Song W (1986) An epidemiological study of neuroses in Chengdu city. Chin J Neuropsychiatry 19:318–321
12. Epidemiological Study Group of Mental Disorders in 12 Areas in China (1986) 12 Areas epidemiological survey of neuroses. Chin J Neuropsychiatry 19:87–91
13. Kleinman A, Kleinman J (1985) Somatization: the interconnections in Chinese society among culture, depressive experiences, and the meanings of pain. In: Kleinman A, Good BJ (eds) Culture and depression: studies in the anthropology and cross-cultural psychiatry of affect and disorder. University of California Press, Berkeley
14. Demitrack MA, Abbey SE (1996) Chronic fatigue syndrome. Guilford, New York
15. Greenberg DB (1990) Neurasthenia in the 1980s: chronic mononucleosis, chronic fatigue syndrome, and anxiety and depressive disorders. Psychosomatics 31:129–137
16. Manu P, Lane TJ, Matthews DA (1993) Chronic fatigue and chronic fatigue syndrome: clinical epidemiology and aetiological classification. Ciba Found Symp 173:23–31
17. Zheng YP, Lin KM, Takeuchi DT, Kurasaki KS, Wang Y, Cheung F (1997) An epidemiological study of neurasthenia in Chinese Americans in Los Angeles. Compr Psychiatry 38:249–259
18. Weiss MG (1997) Explanatory Model Interview Catalogue (EMIC): framework for comparative study of illness. Transcult Psychiatry 34:235–263
19. Holmes G, Kaplan JE, Gantz NM, Kamaroff AL, Schonberger LB, Straus SE, Joneo JF, Dubois RE, Chunninsham-Rundles C, Pahwa S (1988) Chronic fatigue syndrome: a working case definition. Ann Intern Med 108:387–389
20. Bates DW, Buchwald D, Lee J, Kith P, Doolittle TH, Umali P, Komaroff AL (1994) A comparison of case definitions of chronic fatigue syndrome. Clin Infect Dis 18 Suppl 1:S11–S15

# Somatization in Papua New Guinea

U. AMBIHAIPAHAR

*Summary.* Somatoform disorders occur in Papua New Guinea. A total of 50 patients were interviewed randomly from April 1996 to April 1997 at Port Moresby General Hospital. Ninety percent of the patients were within the age-range of 25 to 40 years. Eighty percent of the patients visited the primary care personnel; of those, 60% were females. A majority of patients had body aches/pains, insomnia, and headache. In this group, 60% of patients had some form of improvement with the use of anti-depressants, anxioletics, and small doses of chlorpromazine with individual psychotherapy.

*Key words.* Somatoform disorders, Papua New Guinea, Somatization in Papua New Gulnea, Bougainville crisis

## Introduction

Papua New Guinea is an independent nation in the South Pacific. It has many health problems, among which mental illness has low priority.

Public health programmes have important roles in controlling some infectious diseases such as malaria, tuberculosis, and other parasitic infections. With increasing psychiatric problems in Papua New Guinea, it has become clear that not only the frequency of mental disorders but also their presentation to some extent is culturally determined.

In Papua New Guinea, the mainland population is 4.7 million and has 800 languages, which is a unique situation. Papua New Guinea has 19 provinces. It is a beautiful tropical forest in the mainland and wide swamps along the coastal boarder, in addition to a complex cultural background [1] with 99% Christianity and 1% Muslim influence.

With regard to somatization in Papua New Guinea, a morbidity study (1980–1989) showed 12.1% was depression, 1.9% psychoneurosis, and 1.7% anxiety state [2]. However, there has been no formal epidemiological study conducted to date. Most of

Department of Health, P.O. Box 195, Port Moresby, Papua New Guinea the patients are not aware that somatic symptoms can be secondary to a psychiatric disorder.

## Method and Materials

A questionnaire was designed specifically to study the various clinical presentations of somatoform disorders. A total of 50 patients were interviewed randomly by the author.

From April 1996 to April 1997, the subject matter originated from random outpatient individuals at Port Moresby General Hospital with an array of clinical symptoms consistent with the ICD-10 criteria for somatoform disorder.

## Results/Discussions

Ninety percent of the patients were within the age range of 25 and 40 years. Sex distribution accounted for 60% female, with 20 male patients making up the remainder. Literacy level among the patients was less than 25% which comprised tertiary and higher education.

As many as 80% of patients visited primary care personnel such as nurses, health extension officers, and traditional healers; depending on attributing factors, even before actually visiting the major referral centres such as hospitals.

Table 1 shows that the majority of the patients had body aches/pains, insomnia, and headache, with a reduced percentage having dizziness.

With the complexity of a multilingual and multicultural scenario, the somatoform disorders seem to increase in incidence clinically. The morbidity study by Bradley [3] did not show any case of depression or post-traumatic stress syndrome but had one case of anxiety state. However, Johnson [2] later reported that 12.1% had depression, which was the third most common cause of admission to hospital.

Since independence, the education system in Papua New Guinea, urbanisation, intercultural marriage, teenage marriage with increased marital breakdown, domestic violence, increased psychosocial pressure in the community, and the Bougainville crisis are some of the contributing factors in developing somatoform disorder.

It is clear that some of the somatic symptoms were secondary to depression, anxiety, and post-traumatic stress disorder.

TABLE 1. Clinical presentation

| No. | Clinical features | Number | Percentage (%) |
|-----|-------------------|--------|----------------|
| 1 | Aches/pains | 44 | 90 |
| 2 | Insomnia | 41 | 80 |
| 3 | Headache | 39 | 80 |
| 4 | Dizziness | 32 | 65 |
| 5 | Skin disorder | 11 | 20 |
| 6 | Peptic ulcer | 6 | 10 |
| 7 | Breast pain | 2 | 5 |

Regarding management, 60% of the patients had some form of improvement with the usage of anti-depressant, anxiolytic, small dosage of chlorpromazine, and individual psychotherapy. Those who were treated had somatic symptoms secondary to depression, anxiety state, and post-traumatic stress disorder. The remaining patients showed not much satisfactory improvement with the above treatments.

## Conclusion

It is clearly evident that in Papua New Guinea, somatoform disorder exists as it does in many developed societies. The management of this disorder is currently ranked as unsatisfactory. There is a need to seriously put in place epidemiological research to gauge the impact of this disorder.

The International Symposium on Rethinking Somatoform Disorder has taught us that somatization does exist in different cultures and that it varies with age groups. Our perception of management has been broadened, particularly when the socioeconomic aspects of the disorder are diverse and not unique.

## References

1. Burton Bradley BG (1993) Culture and psychiatry. PNG Med J 36:33–40
2. Johnson FYA (1990) Historical review and admission statistics from 1980–1989
3. Burton Bradley BG (1969) Papua and New Guinea transcultural psychiatry (Ib). The first one thousand referrals. Aust NZ J Psychiatry 3:130

# Somatization in Thailand

KASEM TANTIPHLACHIVA

*Summary.* Somatization, the somatic expression of psychological distress, is a universal clinical syndrome found in every country. Some aspects of somatization and somatoform disorders in Thailand are discussed with regard to clinical manifestation, cultural influences, psychodynamics, and future trends affected by changing social attitudes toward psychiatry.

*Key words.* Culture, Somatization, Somatoform disorder, Social attitude

The ICD-10 classification of mental and behavioural disorders has proposed the terms Somatoform Disorders and Somatization Disorders for international usage since 1992. Although these disorders have been found by psychiatrists and general health care professions for a long time, they used to be diagnosed as other disorders, and have often been unrecognized.

In clinical practice, it is not always possible to clearly differentiate somatoform, somatization, psychosomatic, and somatic symptoms. Medically unexplained symptoms are common in the general population and in all medical settings [1].

Somatization has been proposed to be the somatic expression of psychological distress [2]. Those patients who communicate their psychosocial distress in the form of physical symptoms are called somatizers [3].

Most studies reinforce the view that culture exerts a powerful influence in shaping symptom presentation and determining health-related attitudes [4].

In Thailand, it is common that patients with psychosocial distress would come to see general care physicians with some forms of somatic complaints. They are more likely to be diagnosed as anxiety disorder and given some kinds of antianxiety drugs. In recent years, more patients in general practice are diagnosed as depressive disorder and given antidepressant agents. Rarely are the diagnoses of somatoform disorder and somatization disorder given by nonpsychiatric practitioners, since they are not quite accustomed to the diagnoses. On the contrary, there can also be some occasions when a physical disorder is misdiagnosed as a psychiatric disorder and the patients are sent for psychiatric consultation [5]. Some psychiatric symptoms like

---

The Psychiatric Association of Thailand, Somdet Chaopraya Hospital, Bangkok 10600, Thailand

globus hystericus can also be demonstrated to have underlying pathology in the majority of cases when studied by videofluorography and manometry [6].

Most of the patients who seek psychiatric care come by themselves or at their relatives' advice. Only a small proportion are referred by medical practitioners. Those who come to see psychiatrists at their own will have the advantage of having some insight into their illness. In any case, they will present with some somatic complaints at the beginning. Headache is the most common symptom among the group of formerly-called "neurotic" patients.

Dejatiwongse [7] proposed the psychodynamic of somatization in Thai people as the influence of traditional child-rearing technique that teaches overinhibition of emotions, feelings, and inexpressiveness of sex and aggression, with stronger pressure on females, who have the predominance of somatization. Physical symptoms are a more acceptable way of attention-seeking for the suffering. The patients subsequently find an outlet for their repressed emotions by rechanneling through a physiological mechanism. Another factor that plays a part in patients who present with somatization disorder or somatoform disorder is the avoidance of the stigma of being a psychiatric patient, by manifestation of more socially acceptable "physical" symptoms.

During the last 2 years, the role of psychiatrists in Thailand has been quite successfully promoted by both the governmental and nongovernmental sectors. Thai people have increasingly become familiar with the role of psychiatrists and are utilizing more psychiatric services than they used to. With this change of attitudes toward psychiatry, presenting clinical symptoms are also changing. More patients are complaining that they are worried, depressed, or in distress, rather than complaining of somatic symptoms. My personal clinical experience suggests that fewer cases are presenting with multiple somatic complaints or somatization and somatoform disorders. But whether these changes in clinical manifestations will significantly alter the epidemiologic findings of somatoform disorders necessitates further study.

## References

1. Mayou R (1993) Somatization. Psychother Psychosom 59(2):69–83
2. Noyes R Jr, Holt CS, Kathol RG (1995) Somatization. Diagnosis and management. Arch Family Med 4(9):790–795
3. Ford CV (1995) Dimensions of somatization and hypochondriasis. Neurol Clin 13(2): 241–253
4. Esocobar JI (1995) Transcultural aspects of dissociative and somatoform disorders. Psychiatr Clin North Am 18(3):555–569
5. Witoonchart C, Boonyaprakob V (1995) Primary torsion dystonia misdiagnosed as conversion disorder: a case report. Siriraj Hosp Gazette 47 (suppl):175–182
6. Leelamanit V, Geater A, Sinkitjaroenchai W (1996) A study of 111 cases of globus hystericus. J Med Assoc Thailand 79(7):460–467
7. Dejatiwongse S (1986) Classification and diagnosis in relation to service provision and training. J Psychiatr Assoc Thailand 31:99–110

# Somatization in Field Studies

BENJAMÍN VICENTE, MARIO URIBE, MABEL VIELMA, PEDRO RIOSECO, and SANDRA SALDIVIA

*Summary.* The prevalence of DSM-III-R somatization disorder in a general population sample is analyzed. Risk factors, psychiatric co-morbidity, symptom profile, disability, and pattern of utilization of services are identified and described. The information was collected in a general population psychiatric disorder survey undertaken in Concepción, Chile. The sample size was 800 adults interviewed with the CIDI, which was previously adapted and validated. The results show a relatively low prevalence of somatoform disorders but a high frequency of gastrointestinal symptoms. The disorder is clearly more prevalent in women, young adults between 15 and 39 years old, single, unemployed, and with very low education. The presence of somatoform symptoms is related to the diagnosis of depressive and anxiety disorders. The strongest association is found with somatoform pain and dysthymia. The utilization of services by these patients is not as high as expected. Results are compared with other available data in the literature.

## Introduction

General medical practice usually handles polysymptomatic patients who show different somatic symptoms, and a clinical condition of difficult evolution and unexplained origin. Such patients very frequently resist for a long time a psychogenic explanation of their symptoms and look for an organic explanation of their problems without results. The economic impact of this type of iterative consultation to the health care services makes these patients an administrative focus of interest [1].

The first precise descriptions of hypochondria are found in the works of Gallen who defines it as "a form of melancholy where abdominal and psychic symptoms coexist" [2]. During the seventeenth century this classic etiopathogenic conception changes and puts the initial perturbation in the nervous system. Boissier de Sauvages, in 1770, defined this disorder as an "hallucination of man for his own health," and J.P. Falret introduced the distinction between a deliriant hypochondria and a simple one. The latter will be classified within the domain of "neurasthenia" by Beard, being supported

Department of Psychiatry and Mental Health, University of Concepción, Casilla 60-C, Concepción, Chile

later by several authors [2, 3]. It was Freud who first classified it within the category of current neurosis.

Parallel to the adjectival use of the hypochondria concept in the clinical area, the Diagnostic and Statistical Manual (DSM) of the American Psychiatric Association places it within the category of somatoform disorders with operationalizing purposes [4, 5].

The somatizer prototype is a female of low socieconomic status from a developing country [1, 6]. The current tendency related to somatization is to make the concept operational using as a baseline the list of somatic symptoms proposed by the DSM. Along this line several authors have proposed to define the somatizer not only from counting the somatic symptoms, but considering also its degree of disability [1]. To do this, complex statistical methods have been used which include discriminant function analysis and logistic regression.

## Epidemiology of Somatoform Disorders

Two classic community studies have estimated the prevalence of DSM-III disorders including the Somatization Syndrome: ECA (Epidemiologic Catchment Area) [7] in the United States and the Psychiatric Epidemioliogy Study of Puerto Rico [8]. Both studies used DIS (Diagnostic Interview Schedule) [9] and identical methodology. According to ECA, Somatization Disorder ranged from 0.06% to 0.6% [10]. In Puerto Rico the lifetime prevalence of the Somatization Disorder was 0.7%. As in the United States, the somatization disorder in Puerto Rico was significantly more prevalent in people of low educational level (2%) compared to those of high level of education (0.0%). Different from what was found in ECA, the Puerto Rican study revealed a similar prevalence of the Somatization Disorder in both genders (0.7%, respectively). The five most frequent somatic symptoms in Puerto Rico were: excessive gas, abdominal pain, thoracic pain, heart pounding, and limb pain. It is a remarkable fact that four of those symptoms were among the five somatization symptoms most prevalent in two ECA sites (Durham and Los Angeles), and that these symptoms are all included in the list of 11 key symptoms required by DSM-III for Somatization Disorder [10].

In Chile a community study of similar methodology used the CIDI CORE Version 1.0, translated, adapted and validated [11] in order to obtain lifetime prevalence of some psychiatric disorders including Somatoform Disorders in the province of Concepción (Chile) [12]. The prevalence of Somatoform Disorders in our sample was also low, reaching 0.25% for Somatization and 1.75% for Somatoform Pain. This paper presents the most relevant sociodemographic risk factors, DSM-III-R associated diagnosis, most prevalent somatic symptoms, disability, and utilization of services associated with Somatization.

## Method

The analysis uses part of the information collected in the Lifetime Prevalence Study of some mental disorders in the province of Concepción, Chile [12]. The target population was people of 15 years of age and older living in Concepción, excluding institutionalized individuals and those with no residence. The original study considered a representative randomized and probabilistic sample of 800 subjects distributed in 4 subsamples (Concepción, Talcahuano, Tomé, and Hualqui counties). Stratification by gender and age was obtained from the Population Census of 1982. The data for diagnostic purposes of Somatoform Disorders have been analyzed through the CIDI Program of WHO and the Statistical Package SAS.

# Results

The most relevant demographic characteristics of the sample used in this study are gender predominantly female (52.5%); the largest age group is 25 to 39 years old (35.5%); followed by the age group of 15 to 24 (28.2%). Nearly half of the sample were married (48%) while 40.7% were single. In relation to education a quarter of the sample reached some degree of tertiary education (more than 12 years of schooling), 30% had elementary education, either complete or incomplete, and 2.3% were illiterate. Only 38% of the sample had a paid job at the time of the study.

## Characterization of the Somatizer

According to our study the subjects that present somatoform symptoms are mainly women (58%), young adults from 15 to 39 years of age (60%) having low schooling level (under 11 years) (61%), unmarried (52%), and had no occupation (65%).

Escobar et al. [1] and Kirmayer [6] find similar sociodemographic characteristics to ours for their somatizers.

The most frequent somatoform symptoms found in our study are stomachache (22.5%), food intolerance (22.5%), headache (20.9%), lump in the throat (19.1%), and fainting (15.3%).

Only stomachache is shared as most frequent symptoms when comparing our results with what was found in two sites of ECA (Durham and Los Angles) [13] and in Puerto Rico [10].

It is remarkable that only one out of the five most frequent somatoform symptoms in our protocol is found within the seven key symptoms for the diagnosis of Somatization Disorder according to the DSM-III-R (lump in the throat). Among these key symptoms, those with greater representation in our somatizers are: lump in the throat, 96 cases; painful menstruation, 53 cases; limb pain, 52 cases; shortage of breath, 48 cases; and burning in genitals and rectum, 27 cases.

If we are to accept that the somatoform phenomenon derives from a culturally determined mechanism [6], our "target organs" seem to be different from those studied by the Americans and Puerto Ricans.

## Measurable Aspects of the Somatoform Phenomenon

When measuring the frequency of the somatoform symptoms, we conclude that their presence is a very frequent factor in a randomized field study. In fact, 68% of our respondents showed one or more significant somatic symptoms. Most have had one to three (46.4%), followed by the 14% who presented four to six symptoms. There is only 32% that has never showed them.

Undoubtedly the presence of only one symptom is a frequent fact which does not make a diagnosis per se. Such consideration may depend on the instrument used, as well on the fact that "in one week only 80% of healthy subjects experience body symptoms" [13]. The reference to this analysis based on "symptom counting" opens the discussion on cutoff points on which a person complaining of somatoform symptoms may be categorized as a sick person. This must necessarily consider the study of the variables that modify the mean of the symptoms to be presented. In our sample this mean was 2.66, with a standard deviation of 3.57. The variables gender, age, schooling, marital status, and occupation modify these means significantly; that is, the mean of symptoms in women is higher than in men; those with no occupation have more symptoms than those with an occupation; married people have more symptoms than the unmarried; and those with less schooling have more symptoms than the more educated ones. These results confirm the findings of other studies such as those mentioned from Puerto Rico and ECA.

These low prevalences of somatoform disorders demand a significant effort since the naive impression of clinicians is that the disorder could be more frequent and/or the DSM-III-R criteria too strict. Furthermore, our patients request care and demand a solution to their problems even if they do not meet such cutoff points. In our study only six respondents met more than the 13 points required for the diagnosis of Somatization Disorder and out of the six, only two met the required age criteria (over 30 years of age).

In our study 14.4% of men and 16% of women were placed over the cut-off points of four and six defined by Escobar et al. [1]. In Puerto Rico these percentages were 18% and 20%, respectively.

When analyzing the 16 cases in which the DSM-III-R diagnosis was confirmed we observe that the studied risk factors become more conspicuous: 56% of women, mean age 44 years, 81% married, and 62% with low educational levels (complete or incomplete elementary education).

Finally, if we consider our population as from a young country from a sociodemographic point of view in relation to United States, we could ask and then reflect upon the true validity of the criteria of age required by the DSM-III-R in order to qualify as somatizer (30 years of age).

## Somatoform Symptoms, Somatoform Disorders, and DSM-III-R Diagnosis

The respondents that presented with somatoform symptoms clearly had greater concentration of DSM-III-R diagnosis, Anxiety and Depressive Disorders being the ones with the highest prevalence.

In relation to total DSM-III-R Somatoform Disorders, the low prevalence of somatization disorder does not allow for an adequate analysis of its comorbidity. Regarding Somatoform Pain, Dysthymia (19.4%), Severe Organic Brain Syndrome (16%), Major Depression (12.9%), Generalized Anxiety Disorder (12.9%), and Agoraphobia without Anxiety (6.5%) represent the most relevant comorbidity.

## Disability and Use of Services in Somatoform Symptoms and Disorders

Our overall sample showed 11.9% of disability due to pain and 2.1% due to social disability. If we consider only the respondents of the group that presented one or more somatoform symptoms, 63% of those that presented with disability due to pain show more than four somatoform symptoms.

The mean of symptoms of those with disability due to pain is significantly higher, replicating the findings of the Puerto Rico and the ECA studies. Nearly 7% of the respondents that presented more than four symptoms and 0.8% of those who presented less than four symptoms revealed some degree of social disability. In Puerto Rico these percentages were 15.5% and 4%, respectively. The mean of the symptoms of the socially disabled people was also significantly higher.

In relation to the utilization of services, it was not possible to establish in a significant way that those with higher numbers of somatoform symptoms consulted more frequently without referral. Such a lack of association remains unexplained in the light of the methodology used. In the Los Angeles ECA sample, the association is strong and categorical. As a possible explanation we could speculate that the CIDI section of Services is not applied immediately after the Somatoform Disorders section, but practically at the end of the interview which, due to its duration, could introduce a bias that might have influenced the results.

However, when comparing the mean of consultations of the general sample (0.05) with the mean consultation of the subjects that presented with DSM-III-R Somatoform Disorders (1.5 consultations), the differences are significant.

Considering the level of satisfaction with the medical care received by the subjects that showed somatoform symptoms, the association is slightly significant in the sense that "the higher number of symptoms, the lower the level of satisfaction," confirming what has for long been known by clinicians. In the group with Somatoform Disorders, dissatisfaction (22%) is higher compared to that of the general sample (9.6%).

## Conclusions

This first descriptive phase has allowed to corroborate that associated risk factors of the somatoform phenomenon in Concepción, Chile, are not that much different from those described in the specialized literature. The prevalence of DSM-III-R somatoform disorders is low; however, the presence of somatoform symptoms is a very frequent phenomenon. In our sample the presence of a high number of digestive symptoms is marked in relation to the studies of Puerto Rico and ECA. This different body location of the somatoform phenomenon must be considered when designing local instruments to measure these disorders.

In a second phase we believe it is necessary to design an instrument which should be the result of a treated prevalence study of somatoform disorders. The new instrument should improve the sensitivity and specificity found for CIDI [11]. The nosological discussion is an open topic where the conclusions are not definitive, and can be focused from the point of view of reliability and validity of the instrument used, as well as from a clinico-ethiopathogenic perspective based on the analysis of comorbidity. The need to have adequate instruments relevant to our own situations to measure the phenomenon under study is a clear and imperious goal. This would facilitate the early detection of unexplained somatic disorders, making it possible to treat them at the right time, improving outcome and the use of the always scarce resources.

## References

1. Escobar J, Rubio-Stipec M, Canino G, Karno M (1989) Somatic symptom index (S.S.I.). A new and abridged somatization construct. J Nerv Ment Dis 177:140–146
2. Mai FM, Merskey H (1980) Briquet's treatise on hysteria. Arch Gen Psychiatry 37:1401–1405
3. De Souza C, Othmer E (1984) Somatization disorder and Briquet's syndrome. Arch Gen Psychiatry 41:334–336
4. Asociación Psiquiátrica Americana (A.P.A.) (1980) DSM-III: manual diagnóstico y estadístico de los trastornos mentales. Massons
5. Asociación Psiquiátrica Americana (A.P.A.) (1990) DSM-III-R: manual diagnóstico y estadístico de los trastornos mentales. Massons
6. Kirmayer LJ (1984) Culture, affect and somatization. Transcult Psychiatry Res Rev 21:159–188
7. Regier DA, Myers J, Kramer M, Robins L, Blazer D, Houg R (1984) The MINH epidemiologic catchment area program. Arch Gen Psychiatry 41:934–941
8. Canino GJ, Bird H, Shrout P, Rubio-Stipec M, Bravo M, Martínez R, Sesman M, Guevara L (1987) The prevalence of specific psychiatric disorders in Puerto Rico. Arch Gen Psychiatry 44:727–735
9. Robins LN, Helzer J, Croughan J, Ratcliff K (1981) National Institute of Mental Health diagnostic interview schedule. Arch Gen Psychiatry 38:381–389
10. Robins LN, Helzer J, Weissman M, Orvaschel H, Gruenberg F, Burke J, Recier D (1984) Lifetime prevalence of Specific psychiatric disorders in three cities. Arch Gen Psychiatry 41:949–958
11. Vielma M, Vicente B, Rioseco P, Castro N, Torres S (1992) Validación en Chile de la entrevista diagnóstica estandarizada para estudios epidemiológicos CIDI. Rev de Psiquiatría 9:1039–1049
12. Vicente B, Rioseco P, Vielma M, Uribe M, Boggiano G, Torres S (1992) Prevalencia de vida de algunos trastornos psiquiátricos en la provincia de Concepción. Rev de Psiquiatría 9:1050–1060
13. Lolas F, Retamal P (1992) La depresión en la práctica médica. Servicio de Cooperación Científica Saval

# Part 3
# Management and Economic
# Aspects of Somatoform Disorders

# Psychotherapy of Somatoform Disorders

Wolfgang Hiller and Winfried Rief

*Summary.* Strategies for the psychotherapy of somatoform disorders have been developed during the past years mainly from cognitive-behavioral models. This article summarizes some recent findings and describes a controlled inpatient study with 251 patients from the Roseneck Center in Germany. We found significant improvements in patients with somatoform disorders concerning the severity of somatic symptoms, hypochondriacal fears, depression, dysfunctional cognitions, and psychosocial disabilities. The rationale of cognitive-behavioral treatment is outlined and some principal techniques are described. It seems essential in the future to provide effective training programs for medical and mental health specialists in order to enhance the efficacy of psychotherapeutic approaches.

*Key words.* Psychotherapy, Cognitive-behavioral treatment, Somatization disorder, Hypochondriasis

## Introduction

The history of psychotherapy for somatoform disorders is still young. The first controlled studies were reported by Smith and colleagues, who sent information letters to general practitioners in rural areas of Arkansas (USA) and conducted short group therapies based on cognitive-behavioral principles [1]. They showed that this intervention reduced the annual medical costs for this patient group. The decrease was more than 50% for patients with somatization disorders and around 33% for patients with a less strictly defined somatization syndrome. The group intervention improved the patients' general physical and mental health status as well as their level of physical functioning. It is known from many studies that patients with somatoform disorders suffer from various psychological complaints such as depression and anxiety, and their low psychosocial functioning is frequently linked to some forms of "doctor-shopping" behavior [2]. Recent studies from other research groups have confirmed that psychotherapy is effective in a large number

Roseneck Center for Behavioral Medicine, Am Roseneck 6, D-83209 Prien, Germany of patients with multiple somatoform symptoms [3, 4] and hypochondriacal disorder [5].

One important prerequisite for conducting psychotherapy is an explanatory model for the disorder and its components. Specific interventions may be derived from the model shown in Fig. 1. It is assumed that the bodily symptoms are not due to a medical disease but to psychophysiological mechanisms (e.g., somatosensory amplification, correlates of emotional states, benign dysfunctions). These bodily changes are perceived by the person and misinterpreted as signs of a serious disease or as untolerable. Two vicious circles explain why the symptoms are further amplified and how the disorder is maintained over a long period of time. Symptom amplification may be due to an increased selective attention on bodily functioning and increased levels of autonomic arousal. Maintenance mechanisms include all kinds of avoidance and "illness behaviors" such as repeated checking of the body, increased worry about one's health, overuse of the medical system, inadequate drug consumption like longstanding use of analgesics, and withdrawal from familial, social, and occupational obligations.

Psychotherapeutic strategies should not be uniform for all mental disorders. They should be derived systematically from the specific symptoms and functional clinical characteristics which characterize a specific disorder. In the case of hypochondriasis, Warwick et al. [5] and Barsky et al. [6] were the first to develop such treatment programs taking into account the needs and expectations of this particular patient group. We expanded on these approaches to include also specific interventions for patients with multiple unexplained somatic symptoms.

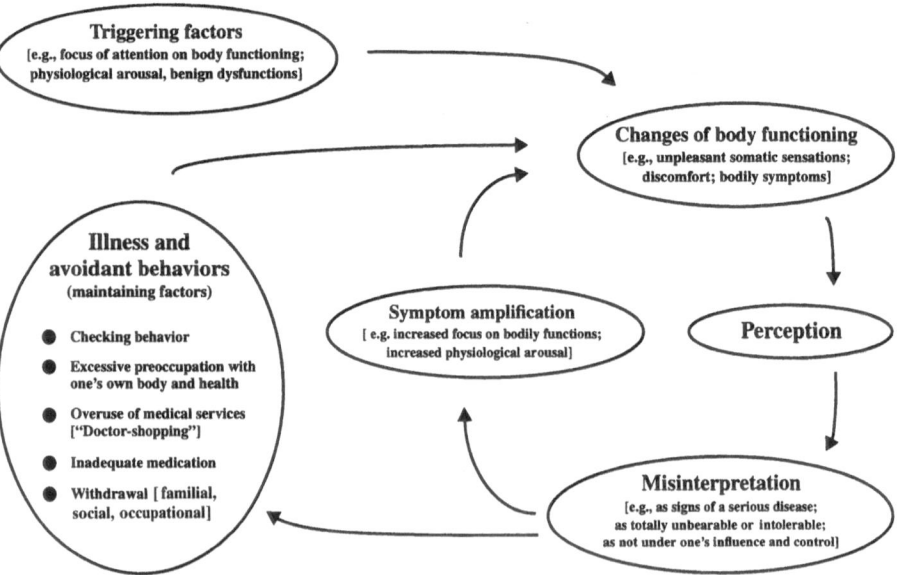

Fig. 1. A cognitive-behavioral model of somatoform disorders

In short, the following main suggestions for the psychotherapy of patients with any of the somatoform disorders (including hypochondriasis) can be regarded as a logical consequence of the model outlined above:

an explanation of the individual patient's somatoform symptoms considering both biological and psychosocial aspects should be introduced as a more adequate alternative to a purely medical perspective;

the patient may be encouraged to use symptom diaries in order to evaluate more closely the everyday interactions between psychological variables such as mood or stress and his physical complaints;

practical demonstrations can enhance the patient's understanding of psychological mechanisms affecting his physical state (e.g., biofeedback, stress experiments);

relaxation techniques can be employed to reduce high levels of autonomic arousal;

inadequate disease convictions (e.g., "my headaches are most certainly due to a brain tumor") or conclusions (e.g., "I can't do anything on my own and without my doctor to gain some relief from my complaints") should be identified and re-attributed;

the patient should be encouraged to give up withdrawal behavior and he should actively enhance his physical fitness;

dysfunctional avoidance and "illness behaviors" are to be reduced.

These strategies are applied in the Roseneck Center as part of the routine treatment program for all patients presenting with a somatoform disorder. In the next sections of this article we will briefly describe a preliminary evaluation of our treatment effects.

## Materials and Methods

We studied the data of 251 inpatients who had been consecutively admitted to the Roseneck Center in Prien, Germany. This is a regular tertiary care hospital as part of the general German health care system. Our treatment programs are accessible to patients of all levels of social and vocational status. The patients of this study reported to suffer from somatic or psychological problems when they were initially applying for admission. They were treated in our hospital for a mean number of 57.8 days (SD = 16.7). The treatment period was compared with a waiting period before admission lasting 123.7 days (SD = 87.9). The sample was divided up into two separate diagnostic subgroups:

(i) *Somatoform group.* 158 patients presented with a somatoform disorder according to the criteria of DSM-IV. Within this group, 53 patients were found to have the complete clinical picture of somatization disorder, while the remaining 105 fulfilled the symptom requirements of at least eight somatoform symptoms from the DSM-IV list of somatization disorder (similar to Escobar's definition of abridged somatization disorder; see also [7]). Therefore, we combined patients with full somatization disorder and the less strictly defined somatization syndrome. These 158 patients had a mean age of 46.0 years (SD = 10.9), and the female percentage was 67.7%.

(ii) *Control group.* The other 93 patients had mental disorders other than somatoform disorders. Most of them presented with the clinical picture of a depressive or anxiety disorder according to DSM-IV. The mean age of this group was 45.1 years (SD = 11.8), and the female proportion was 63.4%.

The diagnostic evaluation included a thorough examination of mental disorders according to DSM-IV using the Structured Clinical Interview (SCID) as well as diagnostic checklists. We also employed a number of different self-report measures. Among these were well evaluated psychometric instruments assessing somatoform symptoms (SOMS—a list of bodily complaints as listed in either DSM-IV or ICD-10), hypochondriacal fears and convictions (Whiteley-Index), the degree of depressive symptomatology (Beck Depression Inventory), psychosocial impairments (DAQ—Dysfunctional Analysis Questionnaire), and dysfunctional cognitions related to somatoform disorders (CABAH—Cognitions About Body and Health Questionnaire). Patients completed these instruments at three points of time: at registration, admission, and discharge.

## Results

A significant decrease of complaints and psychopathology was observed for all scales in the somatoform disorder group. As can be seen from Table 1, this change took place only during the phase of treatment, while the symptomatology remained practically unimproved during the waiting period. Therefore it can be concluded that the treatment had specific effects on the condition of somatoform patients and that these changes cannot be explained by the natural course of the disorder. All improvements not only reached statistical significance, but their magnitude was also in the range of clear clinical relevance. A significant change was found even for the key feature of somatoform symptom distress (SOMS). This scale was the only one not administered at the time of registration so that a comparison with the waiting period was not available.

For the control group of patients with non-somatoform disorders, the values of all measures were clearly and significantly lower than those for the somatoform patients. The differences were most evident for the somatoform symptom distress (SOMS), hypochondriasis as assessed by the Whiteley-Index, and for the CABAH scales indicating dysfunctional cognitions. For these three features it can be stated that both groups had qualitatively different levels with the somatoform patients in the pathological range and the control patients in the more or less "normal" range. In contrast, both groups had relatively high levels of depression and psychosocial impairments at registration and admission. However, patients with somatoform disorders were still significantly more pathological in these scales than control patients, indicating the enormous amount of subjective distress and psychosocial dysfunction in the particular diagnostic group of somatoform disorders.

In a second step we analyzed in more detail whether there were differences in the degree of respondence or non-respondence to our treatment program. We calculated correlation coefficients for a number of variables that were considered as potential predictors of treatment success. The change scores of psychosocial functioning (DAQ), i.e., the difference between admission and discharge, were to be predicted. We found that best predictors were (i) a catastrophizing style of thinking (e.g., self-statements like "bodily complaints are always a sign of disease"), (ii) high scores in

TABLE 1. Treatment effects in patients with somatoform disorders, and as compared with the control group

| | Registration[a] | Admission[a] | Discharge[a] | Significance | | |
| --- | --- | --- | --- | --- | --- | --- |
| | | | | Change in waiting period[b] | Change in treatment period[b] | Difference of both groups at admission[c] |
| *Somatoform disorders (n = 158)* | | | | | | |
| Somatoform symptom distress (SOMS) | – | 20.2 (9.6) | 16.5 (9.2) | – | $P < 0.01$ | |
| Hypochondriasis (Whiteley-Index) | 7.4 (3.3) | 7.2 (3.3) | 5.4 (3.6) | n.s. | $P < 0.01$ | |
| Depression (Beck Depression Inventory) | 22.7 (10.6) | 22.6 (10.4) | 13.2 (9.4) | n.s. | $P < 0.01$ | |
| Dysfunctional cognitions (CABAH) | 56.3 (21.1) | 57.6 (20.9) | 50.2 (21.3) | n.s. | $P < 0.01$ | |
| Psychosocial impairments (DAQ) | 65.7 (14.0) | 66.0 (14.9) | 54.6 (16.8) | n.s. | $P < 0.01$ | |
| *Other mental disorders (n = 93)* | | | | | | |
| Somatoform symptom distress (SOMS) | – | 12.5 (7.1) | 9.1 (7.3) | – | $P < 0.01$ | $P < 0.01$ |
| Hypochondriasis (Whiteley-Index) | 4.6 (3.0) | 4.4 (3.2) | 3.2 (3.0) | n.s. | $P < 0.01$ | $P < 0.01$ |
| Depression (Beck Depression Inventory) | 19.7 (10.4) | 18.1 (10.5) | 8.7 (8.6) | $P < 0.05$ | $P < 0.01$ | $P < 0.01$ |
| Dysfunctional cognitions (CABAH) | 44.9 (15.9) | 44.3 (15.7) | 38.6 (17.3) | n.s. | $P < 0.01$ | $P < 0.01$ |
| Psychosocial impairments (DAQ) | 50.4 (13.9) | 59.0 (14.3) | 47.5 (16.0) | n.s. | $P < 0.01$ | $P < 0.01$ |

[a] Mean (SD).
[b] t-test with repeated measures.
[c] pairwise t-test comparisons.
n.s., not significant.

the Beck Depression Inventory, and (iii) the presence of an additional major depression according to DSM-IV. The correlation coefficients for these three main predictors were 0.26, 0.23 and 0.22, respectively (all $P < 0.01$). In other words, the more patients showed a catastrophizing thinking (at admission), the more they were depressed, and in case of the presence of a major depression, the more likely they were to improve unusually well from our treatment program.

Less powerful predictors at the $P < 0.05$ level were the presence of an additional panic disorder ($r = 0.20$), agoraphobia (0.18), cognitions indicating a high intolerance of bodily discomfort (0.17), and a tendency towards the self-perception as being bodily weak and disabled (0.16). Other variables such as health behavior, hypochondriacal fears and convictions, specific and social phobia, age, and gender were not able to predict the magnitude of treatment success (all $P > 0.05$).

# Discussion

Different approaches have been suggested to treat patients with somatoform disorders. It will certainly be sufficient in many cases that the general pracitioner or familiy physician, if understanding the underlying mechanisms of this disorder, give support to their patients by explaining the (not life-threatening) nature of the somatic symptoms, and by refraining from unnecessary medical examinations and treatments. In more severe cases, however, such strategies of "clinical managment" within the frames of general medicine may fall short and intense psychotherapy is then needed. Although this field has been neglected for many years [8], the time has come that systematic and differentiated approaches be developed and evaluated through empirical trials.

The controlled study described in this article shows that somatic symptoms and associated psychopathology improved during an intense treatment program lasting several weeks. Since the Roseneck Center is a highly specialized facility of the German tertiary care system, these results cannot be generalized to other settings. However, the patients treated in our study are likely to belong to the most severely disturbed subgroup of somatoform disorders with high levels of comorbidity and chronicity. We feel encouraged that our patients improved despite this selection of severe cases. To our surprise, the presence of an additional depressive or anxiety disorder was even a positive predictor of therapy success. One interpretation of this finding could be that these patients with comorbidity were more pathological and thus more likely to improve (i.e., regression towards the mean). On the other hand, these results demonstrate that even the most severe patients with somatoform disorders are not "untreatable" if systematic cognitive-behavioral strategies are applied.

# References

1. Smith G (1995) Treatment of patients with multiple symptoms. In: Mayou R, Bass C, Sharpe M (eds) Treatment of functional somatic symptoms. Oxford University Press, Oxford, pp 175–187
2. Hiller W, Rief W, Fichter MM (1997) How disabled are patients with somatoform disorders? Gen Hosp Psychiatry 19:432–438

3. Rief W, Hiller W, Geissner E, Fichter MM (1995) A two-year follow-up study of patients with somatoform disorders. Psychosomatics 36:376–386
4. Speckens AEM, van Hemert AM, Spinhoven P, Hawton KE, Bolk JM, Rooijmans HGM (1995) Cognitive behavioural therapy for medically unexplained physical symptoms: a randomized controlled trial. Br Med J 311:1328–1332
5. Warwick HMC, Clark DM, Cobb AM, Salkovskis PM (1996) A controlled trial of cognitive-behavioural treatment of hypochondriasis. Br J Psychiatry 169:189–195
6. Barsky AJ, Geringer E, Wool CA (1988) A cognitive-educational treatment for hypochondriasis. Gen Hosp Psychiatry 10:322–327
7. Hiller W, Rief W, Fichter MM (1995) Further evidence for a broader concept of somatization disorder using the Somatic Symptom Index. Psychosomatics 36:285–294
8. Rief W, Hiller W (1998) Somatization—future perspectives on a common phenomenon (Editorial). J Psychosom Res 44:529–536

# The Psychological Treatment of Somatoform Disorders

WINFRIED RIEF and WOLFGANG HILLER

*Summary.* Psychological factors are assumed to be of major importance in the maintenance of somatoform disorders. Therefore psychological interventions can play a pivotal role in the treatment and management of somatoform disorders. These interventions, however, should be based on empirical findings concerning the origins of the symptomatology. We present a psychological treatment program which is based on studies about cognitive, behavioral, psychobiological, and further aspects of the disorder. This treatment package includes interventions such as relaxation training, cognitive restructuring, exposure, biofeedback, communication training, family interventions, and medical management.

*Key words.* Somatization, Somatoform disorder, Psychological treatment, Comorbidity, Evidence-based medicine

## Introduction

The general healthcare system can be categorized into three parts. Most patients with unclear somatic symptoms are treated in primary care. For some of these patients, primary care is not sufficient and the patients are referred to specialists who use psychopharmacology or brief psychological interventions. However, these specialist treatments fail to succeed for some patients with somatoform symptoms. These patients may be characterized by comorbidity with other mental and physical disorders, by high chronicity, or severe psychosocial problems. Therefore some countries propose a third step of treatment using multiprofessional and intensive approaches (Fig. 1).

In a previous paper we presented the results of a treatment approach of tertiary care in an inpatient treatment-setting [1]. We found that an integrative behavioral medicine approach can help to improve patients with somatization syndromes. Patients of this study were treated in 1991 and reassessed 2 years later. Meanwhile,

Klinik Roseneck, Center for Behavioral Medicine, Am Roseneck 6, D-83209 Prien am Chiemsee, Germany

FIG. 1. Cascade model for the management of somatization

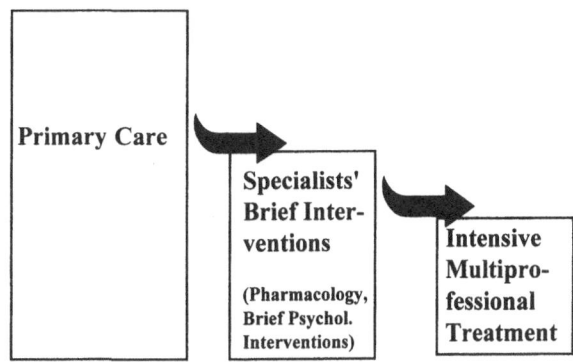

multiple studies investigating the properties of patients with somatization syndrome have been published. Therefore, we can now improve our treatment approach considering more specific results about the process of somatization.

# Components of a Psychological Treatment Programme

## Normalization of Psychobiological Processes

A series of studies has demonstrated that somatoform disorders are characterized by psychobiological and psychophysiological abnormalities. Somatization as well as associated disorders can covary with psychoendocrinological and psychoimmunological changes. While some authors found reduced scores for cortisol in disorders such as chronic fatigue syndrom or posttraumatic stress disorder, we could demonstrate that some patients with somatization are characterized by increased morning cortisol concentrations (see Fig. 2). Further findings for psychophysiological overarousal were also presented [2].

Many patients with somatization syndrome show further signs of psychophysiological dysfunction which may contribute to the maintenance of physical symptoms (such as dysfunctional breathing, elevated muscle tension, etc.). All of these psychobiological properties can be of major importance for the treatment of the patients. Psychobiology presents a bridge between the organic health belief of the patients and the more psychosomatic health beliefs of the therapists. The therapist can demonstrate that he doesn't believe that all symptoms are "just in the mind," but the physical symptoms also have organic, but nonthreatening correlates. This information may help to constitute a positive relationship between therapist and patient.

The psychobiological results point to the necessity of psychological treatment approaches including interventions which help to reduce psychophysiological dysfunctions. Such interventions may include relaxation training, biofeedback, or breathing retraining.

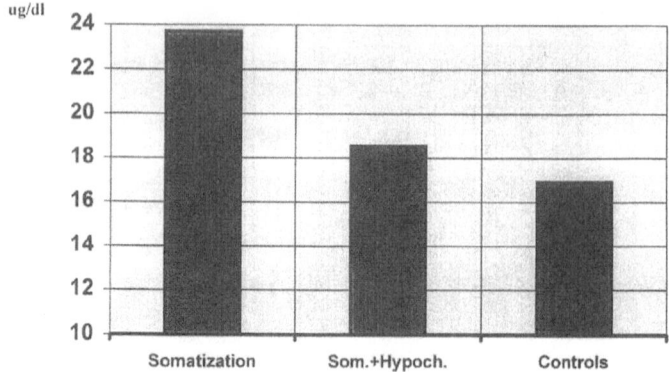

FIG. 2. Salivary morning cortisol. *Som. + Hypoch.*, somatization and hypochondriasis

## Normalization of Attributions and Cognitions

Somatization can be understood as abnormal perception and misinterpretation of physical symptoms. Physical symptoms are an everday phenomenon [3]. Nearly everyone experiences such sensations as slight dizziness after standing up, hot feet after a long walk, or breathlessness after going up some steps.

To investigate how people with somatization syndromes interpret such bodily signals, we developed a questionnaire (the CABAH, cognitions about body and health [4]). We could demonstrate that people with somatization syndrome as well as people with hypochondriasis have elevated scores for the factor "catastrophizing interpretation of bodily signals." These patients tend to misinterpret typically benign physical symptoms as potentially threatening (e.g., headache is often a sign of a brain tumor). The resulting health concerns lead the patient to observe even minor bodily sensations. This selective attention process may lead to an amplified style of perception, as Barsky [5] points out.

These results demonstrate that in psychological treatment approaches it is necessary to normalize the perception and interpretation of bodily symptoms. Sensky et al. [6] emphasize that the focus should not be on eliminating catastrophizing cognitions, but the psychological treatment should strengthen possible alternatives and neutral interpretations of physical symptoms.

How can this be reached in psychological treatments? One possibility is the provocation of benign physical symptoms. Patients should be encouraged not to avoid, but to be exposed to as many as possible physical sensations. This approach resembles to the exposure therapy for agoraphobic fears. Another possibility is the demonstration of psychophysiological changes after psychological tasks. Using biofeedback equipment, therapists can demonstrate to patients how heart rate, muscle tension and other variable change after tasks such as mental arithmetic, remembering difficult social situations, or relaxing. These interventions help to reduce a catastrophizing interpretation of physical symptoms and to look for possible psychological influences on bodily well-being.

## Reducing Abnormal Illness Behaviour

Patients with somatoform symptoms are characterized by abnormal illness behavior. Often they cannot sustain body misperceptions without visiting doctors. Many patients take unnecessary and sometimes even harmful medication. Others permanently ask reassurance that the physical symptoms are not threatening. In psychological terms, these behavioral aspects are reinforced as they lead to the consequence of reductions of health anxiety. Moreover, they prevent the patient from developing self-help strategies. Therefore the psychological interventions have to follow the aim of a reduction of abnormal illness behavior and to encourage the patient to develop coping strategies which reduce the dependency on other persons.

Some patients cannot manage to reduce or give up doctor visits due to the somatoform symptoms. The doctor visits, however, can reinforce abnormal illness behavior as described above. A solution to this dilemma may be to propose regular doctor visits which should be independent of subjective or physical well-being and which only depend on time (e.g., every 4–6 weeks). In this way, the doctor visits can lose the reinforcing function due to the reduction of health anxiety. Furthermore, in the time period between doctor visits, patients are encouraged to develop and to test self-help strategies.

The avoidance of physical exercise is a further behavioral aspect of somatization. This leads to a reduction of physical fitness. The physically weak person, however, experiences more bodily symptoms than the well-trained person. Thus the more the person avoids physical activity, the more he/she will experience body symptoms. Therefore it is necessary to encourage people with somatoform symptoms to do regular physical activities such as jogging, swimming, or gymnastics.

A further behavioural problem may arrive when patients with somatization syndrome reduce their social activities as consequence of the disorder. A reduction of external stimulation however leads to an amplified perception of physical symptoms [3]. Thus the more a patient with somatoform disorders lives in social isolation, the more he/she will experience the somatoform symptoms. Therefore, the psychological treatment has to encourage these patients to look for social contacts and to communicate with other persons.

The communication with other persons, however, can be disturbed when the patients tend to complain a lot. The chronically ill patient is in danger of using his/her complains to get his/her needs satisfied. To reduce the "secondary gain" of the symptomatology, the psychological interventions should enhance the person's possibilities to communicate in a self-fulfilling manner. Communication training and role playing may be means to stimulate a normal expression of needs, emotions, and assertiveness behavior [10].

Sometimes "significant others" take part in the maintenance of illness behaviour. Family members, the head of the employment, or colleagues can motivate the patient to search for further medical specialists or to visit new treatment centers offering nonevaluated therapies. In these cases, it can be helpful to contact these persons and to try to motivate them for a coordinated intervention. Moreover, family interventions can be helpful to reduce illness-oriented family communications.

# The Psychological Treatment of Comorbid Problems

Many patients presenting with somatoform symptoms have further psychiatric disorders. Major depression and other affective disorders are common, but also panic and other anxiety disorders are frequent [8]. Most of these problems can be treated effectively by psychological interventions [9]. Comorbidity should not only be viewed as a problem but can sometimes provide further possibilities in the treatment of somatoform disorders. In the case of anxiety disorders, psychological and physical interactions can be demonstrated very convincingly. In the case of depressive disorders, the interaction between affective well-being and physical well-being can be demonstrated using symptom diaries.

## Medical Management

In a subgroup of patients with somatoform symptoms an accompanying medical management is necessary. As decribed above, the doctor visits should be provided in an time-contingent manner and not well-being-contingent. Some authors suggest that the principal treatment goal is to prevent iatrogenic harm. Therefore unnecessary examinations should be avoided. Moreover, pseudodiagnosis and pseudotreatments can reinforce the organic health beliefs of the patients; therefore they are not helpful in the long-term course.

# The Evaluation of Psychological Treatments

As the tradition of research in somatoform disorders is short, there is a lack of controlled and randomized treatment trials. However, the first studies have demonstrated that psychological treatments can help to improve the subjective well-being, to reduce health anxieties, and to normalize the interpretation and attribution of physical symptoms (cf. [1, 10, 11]). As the knowledge about psychological processes in somatoform disorders is rapidly increasing, further improvements of the effectiveness of psychological interventions can be expected for the following years.

## References

1. Rief W, Hiller W, Fichter MM (1995) A two-year follow-up study of patients with somatoform disorders. Psychosomatics 36:376–386
2. Rief W, Shaw R, Fichter MM (1998) Elevated levels of psychophysiological arousal and cortisol in patients with somatization syndrome. Psychosom Med 60:198–203
3. Pennebaker JW (1982) The psychology of physical symptoms. Springer, Berlin Heidelberg New York
4. Rief W, Hiller W, Margraf J (1998) Cognitive aspects of hypochondriasis and the somatization syndrome. J Abnorm Psychol 107:587–595
5. Barsky AJ (1992) Amplification, somatization, and the somatoform disorders. Psychosomatics 33:28–34
6. Sensky T, MacLeod AK, Rigby MF (1996) Causal attributions about common somatic sensations among frequent general practice attenders. Psychol Med 26:641–646
7. Liberman RP, de Risi WJ, Mueser KT (1989) Social skills training for psychiatric patients. Pergamon, New York

8. Rief W, Heuser J, Mayrhuber E, Stelzer I, Hiller W, Fichter MM (1996) The classification of multiple somatoform symptoms. J Nerv Ment Dis 184:680–687
9. Barlow DH (1993) Clinical handbook of psychological disorders, 2nd edn. Guilford, New York
10. Warwick HMC, Clark DM, Cobb AM, Salkovkis PM (1996) A controlled trial of cognitive-behavioural treatment of hypochondriasis. Br J Psychiatry 169:189–195
11. Speckens AEM, van Hemert AM, Spinhoven P, Hawton KE, Bolk JH, Rooijmans GM (1995) Cognitive behavioural therapy for medically unexplained physical symptoms: a randomised controlled trial. Br Med J 311:1328–1332

# Schematic Understanding of the Worried Patient with Somatoform Disorder

Takaaki Koyazu

*Summary.* The problem of "doctor shopping behavior" of the somatizing patient resides in the big deviation between the patient's self-diagnosis and the doctor's medical diagnosis. The former is subjective, the latter objective. The doctor's reply "there is nothing wrong with you" does not work well. Rather it results in a feeling of distrust of the doctor in the patient's mind. The importance of making use of a collaborative therapeutic relationship in cognitive therapy is asserted.

*Key words.* Schema, Somatoform disorder, Therapeutic relationship, Collaboration, Cognitive therapy

## The Aim of the Study

The aim of this study is to obtain knowledge about appropriate treatment of somatizing patients from the psychological viewpoint. Why does the patient with somatoform disorder perform the so-called doctor shopping behavior? Now, conceptualization of the behavior of the patient is necesary.

## Conceptualization of "Doctor Shopping Behavior"

First, a macroscopic model of the patient's behavior is shown in Fig. 1. In the first stage the patient perceives physical symptom(s) (e.g., pain sensation in the abdomen, head, etc.) with an uncomfortable feeling. If it is weak in intensity, coarse in quality, generalized, not localized, and/or just temporary, then he will forget or sometimes neglect it (as in Fig. 2). But if it is painful enough, clearly confirmed, and/or frequently occurring, then he will take it aversively and will suspect some illness (e.g., stomach cancer).

Here the problem is whether the patient is vulnerable to such (a) symptom(s) or not. In general, the worried patient has a tendency to amplify it and sometimes to focus too much attention on it. He may complain that he feels it extremely unpleas-

Faculty of Letters, Keio University, Mita, Minato-ku Tokyo 108-0073, Japan

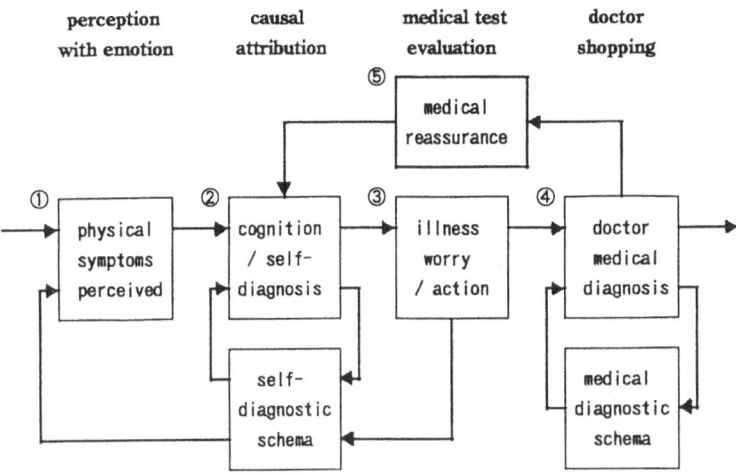

FIG. 1. A model of the patient's behavior

| The quality of the image of the physical symptom | |
|---|---|
| ⟨fine⟩ | ⟨coarse⟩ |

|  | ⟨fine⟩ | ⟨coarse⟩ |
|---|---|---|
| ⟨hard⟩ | aversive<br>want to remove<br>suspect specific illness<br>appropriate coping | extremely unpleasant<br>followed by anxiety<br>suspect serious illness<br>chaotic consultation |
| ⟨weak⟩ | slightly interested<br>half-hearted<br>cautiously watched<br>at one's convenience | forgotten<br>ignored or neglected<br>take it easy<br>unnoticed |

The intensity of the image of p.s.

FIG. 2. The perceptual image of the physical symptom (*p.s.*)

ant and aversive. What we could then do is just to accept him empathetically and to understand his feeling of unpleasantness as subjectively real, whether or not it be due to his diathetic condition.

In the next stage the patient tries "self-diagnosis," making use of his "self-diagnostic schema." The schema is so defined as a memorized set of knowledge and experiences concerning what the illness is, which one of the coping strategies may work well for it, and so on. A great deal of the patient's knowledge is pseudo-medical as the layman's used to be, but all certainly has been formed and accumulated through his long-term life history. So, some patients strongly believe it, and evaluate their bodily symptoms on the basis of it. It is hard even for the doctor to change the patient's self-evaluation and self-diagnosis without giving him any agreeable reasons and a feeling of trust for the doctor himself. Thus, the doctor-shopping behavior concerns both the rigidity of the patient's self-diagnostic schema and the trustworthiness of the doctor.

Note, by the way, that the patient's self-diagnosis is carried out in an attributive way. That is he attributes, with reasoning, his perceived physical symptoms to some external cause (e.g., attributing his stomachache to the mushroom he ate last night) or to some other internal cause (e.g., to the possible stomach cancer he fears). In the latter, problems tend to occur. False or faulty information about illness gleaned from his friends and various other media, if any, might drive these kinds of illness attributions.

In addition, the diathesis which dominates the self-diagnostic schema should not be set aside. Neuroticism allows the patient to be vulnerable to somatization and worry about illness. Irrational belief tends to work in a way that his attribution style would become so complicated that he might not get out of worrying about illness he has been afraid of. So he decides to visit a doctor at a clinic for consultation.

We now arrive at the fourth stage. The doctor assesses the patient's complaint, and gives him an explanation of the medical evaluation with medical test results, but in vain. The patient never wants to believe what the doctor explains, especially in the case when he is confident with his sensation and evaluation of his physical disorder according to his self-diagnostic schema.

Concerning this, Wise [1] asserted that "nothing wrong with you" would not work well for the somatizing patient, especially with hypochondriasis. In fact, the patient's complaints and illness worry seem to have matured so that he might have the basic feeling of distrust toward the doctor.

The reason is that the physical symptom of his illness still exists, and never disappears despite the repeated medical reassurance by the doctor. It might be said that the feeling of distrust would direct the patient to go to another doctor, and also strengthen his automatic thought which would thwart the ongoing reassurance, leading to more distrust toward the doctor. It is really a vicious cycle. This will tentatively be a plausible explanation for "doctor-shopping behavior." So, the problem concerns not only the patient's illness anxiety but also his feeling of distrust toward the doctor. It is quite a delicate balance.

## Therapeutic Relationship in Cognitive Therapy

Now we return to the problems in five stages stated before. They are primarily: (1) perceptual amplification of physical symptoms, (2) causal attribution with poor self-diagnostic schema, (3) too much worry about illness, (4) the resort to clinical consultation, and (5) medical assurance and the feeling of distrust. They are all related to the cognitive or cognitive-behavioral function of the mind. To settle each of those problems, cognitive therapy (e.g., Beck [2]) as well as cognitive-behavioral therapy seem most attractive. Strategies of cognitive and cognitive-behavioral therapy work on perception, cognition, emotion, and behavior of the patient to change his irrational belief, negative automatic thought, etc., which generate distorted ideas, distress, over-amplification, illness worry, grief, and so on.

It is important to note here that such strategies work on the clinician's side as well.

One important method of cognitive and cognitive-behavioral therapy resides in its use of "collaborative therapeutic relationship," as demonstrated, for instance, by Wills and Sanders [3]. There, both therapist and patient work together to observe what is going on now and then, to talk about the patient's well-being, to consider and try to find a possible and effective way of solving the difficulties they are facing. A spirit of collaboration leads both of them to active listening, acceptance, and unconditional positive regard, which are all key concepts of the client-centered therapy by Rogers [4].

Although it is important for the therapist to have insights for conceptualization of the patient's difficulties, it is not necessary to be so interpretative and directive toward the patient. Through their collaborative and open talks, the patient's thoughts, feelings, and behaviors are reflected on themselves, in order to find appropriate solutions. Above all, it works on the patient's interpersonal schemata in a humanistic way, thus avoiding the occurrence of the patient's distrust of the doctor.

Finally, I would like to say the following. Let us now place the five problems discussed above on one dimension in that order; you will find the dimension is "the peripheral part of patient's body"—"the human existence as a whole," and that problems (1)–(5) are all related to one another. If we try to extract on without giving any effect on the others for treatment, we fail. We have to treat the patient as a whole entity, and also have to focus on the relationship between him and ourselves. Holistic views seem to be necessary and most important for us is to be a "final doctor" to the patient.

## References

1. Wise TN (1997) The worried patient: clinical management of the patient with hypochondriasis. J. Pract. Psych. Behav. Health July:223–232
2. Beck AT (1976) Cognitive therapy and the emotional disorders. International Universities Press, New York
3. Wills F, Sanders D (1997) Cognitive therapy. Transforming the image. Sage Publications, London
4. Rogers CR (1957) The necessary and sufficient conditions of therapeutic change. J Consult Psychol 21:95–103

# Problems in Pharmacologic Management of Somatoform Disorders

Jack D. Burke Jr.[1], Kimberly C. Burke[1], and Glen Couchman[2]

Key words. Somatoform disorders, Pharmacology, Management, Diagnosis, Treatment

## Introduction

Several problems have made it difficult to determine the effectiveness of pharmacologic management of Somatoform disorders [1]. However, results from recent studies of the Somatoform disorders are hopeful and may provide a basis for conducting trials to assess the role of medications in managing these conditions.

## Current Problems in Studying Somatoform Disorders

### Reliability and Validity vs Prevalence

Somatization disorder, which has been derived from Briquet's syndrome as delineated by Perley, Guze [2, 3] and their colleagues in St. Louis, is the best studied of the Somatoform disorders, and appears to have the best foundation in terms of demonstrated reliability and validity. However, it is less frequent in primary care and general community surveys than had been predicted. For example, the prevalence of ICD-10 Somatization Disorder in a recent WHO International Study of Somatoform Disorders in primary care populations was less than 2% in 7 out of 8 centers.

More common disorders, including Persistent Pain Disorder and Undifferentiated Somatoform Disorder, have been less studied. Their criteria use concepts that may be affected by cultural and other factors related to the characteristics of a health care system [4]. For that reason, they have more uncertain boundaries and require more judgment by the clinician who assigns the diagnosis. Variability across cultures, and differences between clinical and research diagnoses of these disorders, combine to

[1] Department of Psychiatry and Behavioral Science, and [2]Department of Family Medicine, Texas A&M University College of Medicine and 2401 Scott and White Clinic/Hospital, South 31st Street, Temple, TX 7650 8, USA

make it difficult to know how well findings from any particular, culture-specific study can be generalized to other populations.

## Variations in Diagnostic Criteria

Even for the best-studied Somatoform disorder, Somatization, inconsistencies have led to variability in research and clinical practice in the past two decades. All three editions of the Diagnostic and Statistical Manual of Mental Disorders since 1980 have criteria for Somatization disorder that differ from the original Briquet's syndrome criteria, from ICD-10 criteria, and from each other. The changes have been introduced because the original Briquet's criteria proved too complex to use in clinical practice and in many research studies.

For other disorders, such as Undifferentiated Somatoform Disorder, in both DSM-IV and ICD-10 the criteria are necessarily non-specific in terms of the number and pattern of symptoms required. In some research studies, use of the Somatic Symptom Index introduced by Escobar and colleagues [5] in the NIMH Epidemiologic Catchment Area study has been useful, but it is also a rating of number of lifetime symptoms, and appears even less specific than the criteria sets for specific Somatoform disorders.

## Differential Diagnosis

A fundamental problem in this group of disorders is to rule out general medical conditions that may produce these presentations. In some conditions, like Persistent Pain disorder, the difficulty may be in determining when the patient's distress is greater than would be accounted for by the underlying medical problem. The level of certainty of these diagnoses in clinical settings may be low.

Another problem in assessing treatment options is to determine whether the diagnostic category is too heterogeneous to permit broad conclusions about treatment effectiveness. Within the category of Persistent Pain disorder, patients with conditions like headache, backache, joint pain, and abdominal pain may not respond to the same degree to the same medications.

## Comorbidity

Patients with a Somatoform disorder appear likely to have other psychiatric disorders as well [6–8]. Some evidence suggests that patients with both Major Depression and Somatization may be less likely to benefit from anti-depressants than patients with Major Depression alone [9]. This finding is consistent with the recent report that patients with coexisting depressive disorders appear to have the greatest functional impairment of patients with somatoform disorders [10].

## Adverse Effects of Drugs

Unpleasant side effects of medications may limit the patient's willingness to continue with therapy. However, some evidence indicates that selective serotonin reuptake inhibitors are well tolerated in depressed patients with pre-existing gastrointestinal complaints [11].

## Outcome Measures

The persistent nature of Somatoform disorders raises questions about the duration of any clinical trials to demonstrate effectiveness of pharmacologic agents. Trials of 6 weeks' duration, which have been common in studying many psychiatric disorders, may not be adequate for this group of conditions [12, 13].

The intermittent presentation of symptoms over time has led to proposals to study other outcome variables, such as impaired functioning or pattern of using health services, rather than symptom formation or severity.

## Implications of Medication Use

Some clinicians have expressed concern that prescribing medications for Somatoform disorders may reinforce the patient's tendency to somatize, by suggesting that a somatic intervention is appropriate [14, 15]. This view is consistent with the suggestion that the most appropriate pharmacologic agent for some patients with a Somatoform disorder may be a placebo [16]. The high rate of response to placebo has been demonstrated recently in an on-going study of hypochondriasis [17].

# Promising Pharmacologic Agents

## Tricyclic Antidepressants

Tricyclic antidepressants are widely used for pain relief, especially in neuropathic pain, migraine headache prophylaxis, and in patients with coexisting depression and somatizing or hypochondriacal symptoms [1, 18–21].

## SSRI Antidepressants

SSRI antidepressants are commonly used in treatment of Body Dysmorphic disorder (a discrete disorder in DSM-IV, and one form of Hypochondriasis in ICD-I 0) [22]. Results from a 12-week trial suggest that high-dose fluoxetine may also be useful in hypochondriacal patients without depressive disorders, a group usually considered treatment refractory [23]. A subsequent report from this same group noted that this patient population demonstrated a high placebo response, so the apparent benefit of the medication may have been due to non-specific factors [13].

Results from case reports and trials with small samples have generally suggested SSRI antidepressants are useful in managing neuropathic pain [24], headaches [25–27], rheumatic pain [28], and non-specific conditions like fibromyalgia [29]. However, they have been found less effective than tricyclic antidepressants in some studies [30, 31], and no more effective than placebo in some recent double-blind studies [32, 33].

## Other Antidepressants

Animal studies have found evidence that both nefazodone [34] and venlafaxine [35] provide pain relief, and clinical reports have indicated that these new antidepressants are being used in management of chronic pain [18].

Mianserin has been shown effective in reducing abdominal pain in patients with "functional gastrointestinal disorder," compared to placebo [36]. But it appears to be less effective or ineffective in other chronic pain conditions [27, 31, 37].

## Anticonvulsants

Divalproex has been found to be effective in migraine prophylaxis [38]. Gabapentin has been shown in animal models to reduce the effects of neuropathic pain [39, 40]. A series of clinical reports has also suggested that it is effective in relieving neuropathic pain [41–44], but caution has been raised that prospective, double-blind, placebo-controlled studies are needed to establish both efficacy and safety [45]. A report of anxiety and restlessness after 1 week of gabapentin therapy for pain relief in two patients with brain injury also raises caution about the need to monitor adverse effects in patients using the medication for neuropathic pain [46].

## L-Sulpiride

This atypical anti-psychotic agent has been shown to enhance acupuncture analgesia in animal models [47], although an earlier study had been inconclusive [48]. A randomized, double-blind cross-over study comparing sulpiride and paroxetine for chronic tension headache showed slight effects for both agents, but suggested that sulpiride might be more useful than paroxetine [49].

A double-blind study of levo-sulpiride in patients with somatoform disorders showed benefit after 6 weeks [13]. A variety of studies in patients with gastrointestinal discomfort and dyspepsia have shown that L-sulpiride improves these conditions [50–53]. In hospitalized schizophrenic patients, the same effects on somatic concerns have been demonstrated, as sulpiride was more effective than bromperidol in relieving hypochondriacal and neurotic complaints [54].

# Recommendations

Epidemiologic studies have shown that the Somatoform disorders can be found in different cultures, even if their relative distributions vary across cultures and health care systems. Promising findings for many different psychoactive medications provide hope that pharmacologic management may prove useful for many of the patients with these conditions. However, methodologic problems need to be resolved before definitive studies can be conducted. At this point, several points may be helpful for investigators designing studies: (a) studies need to include placebo controls, in view of the likely benefit from non-specific factors; (b) clinical trials need to have sufficient duration to demonstrate sustained benefits for conditions that have a fluctuating course with intermittent symptoms; (c) investigations in the near future will continue to need to define target symptoms among homogeneous groups, since the diagnostic criteria for specific Somatoform disorders cannot yet be specified with certainty; finally, (d) outcome measures will need to include both measures of the patient's distress as well as measures of functional impairment and use of health services.

# References

1. Escobar JL (1996) Overview of somatization: diagnosis, epidemiology, and management. Psychopharm Bull 32:589–596
2. Perley MJ, Guze SB (1962) Hysteria—the stability and usefulness of clinical criteria: a quantitative study based on a follow-up period of six to eight years in 39 patients. N Engl J Med 266:421–426
3. Guze SB (1975) The validity and significance of the clinical diagnosis of hysteria (Briquet's syndrome). Am J Psychiatry 132:138–141
4. Barsky AJ, Borus JF (1995) Somatization and medicalization in the era of managed care. JAMA 274:1931–1934
5. Escobar JI, Burnam A, Karno M, Forsythe A, Golding JM (1987) Somatization in the community. Arch Gen Psychiatry 44:713–718
6. Smith GR (1992) The epidemiology and treatment of depression when it coexists with somatoform disorders, somatization, or pain. Gen Hosp Psychiatry 14:265–272
7. Noyes R, Kathol RG, Fisher MM et al (1994) Psychiatric comorbidity among patients with hypochondriasis. Gen Hosp Psychiatry 16:78–87
8. Kuch K, Cox BJ, Woszczyna CB et al (1991) Chronic pain in panic disorder. J Behav Ther Exp Psychiatry 22:255–259
9. Hoencamp E et al (1994) Predictors of (non)response in depressed outpatients treated with a three-phase sequential medication strategy. J. Affect Disord 31:235–246
10. Hiller W, Rief W, Fichter MM (1997) How disabled are patients with somatoform disorders? Gen Hosp Psychiatry 19:432–438
11. Linden RD, Wilcox CS, Heiser JF et al (1994) Are selective serotonin reuptake inhibitors well tolerated in somatizing depressives? Psychopharmacol Bull 30:151–156
12. Demopulos C, Fava M, McLean NE et al (1996) Psychosom Med 58:314–320
13. Altamura AC, Mauri MC, Regazzatti G et al (1991) L-sulpiride in the treatment of somatoform disturbances: a double-blind study with racemic sulpiride. Minerva Psichiatr 32:25–29
14. Elks ML (1994) On the genesis of somatization disorder: the role of the medical profession. Med Hypotheses 43:151–154
15. Kouyanou K, Pither CE, Wessely S (1997) Iatrogenic factors and chronic pain. Psychosom Med 59:597–604
16. Grandjean P et al (1997) Placebo response in environmental disease: chelation therapy of patients with symptoms attributed to amalgam fillings. J Occup Environ Med 39: 707–714
17. Fallon BA, Schneier FR, Marshall R et al (1996) The pharmacotherapy of hypochondriasis. Psychopharm Bull 32:607–611
18. Galer BS (1995) Neuropathic pain of peripheral origin: advances in pharmacologic treatment. Neurology 45(Suppl 9):S17–S25
19. Vrethem M, Boivie J, Holingren H et al (1997) A comparison of amitriptyline and maprotiline in the treatment of painful polyneuropathy in diabetics and nondiabetics. Clin J Pain 13:313–323
20. Godfrey RG (1996) A guide to the understanding and use of tricyclic antidepressants in the overall management of fibromyalgia and other chronic pain syndromes. Arch Intern Med 156:1047–1052
21. Ziegler DK, Hurwitz A, Preskorn S et al (1993) Propranolol and amitriptyline in prophylaxis of migraine. Pharmacokinetic and therapeutic effects. Arch Neurol 50:825–830
22. Phillips KA, Kim JM, Hudson JI (1995) Body image disturbance in body dysmorphic disorder and eating disorders. Obsessions or delusions? Psychiatr Clin North Am 18:317–334
23. Fallon BA, Liebowitz MR, Salman E et al (1993) Fluoxetine for hypochondriacal patients without major depression. J Clin Psychopharmacol 13:438–441

24. Sindrup SH, Grodum E, Gram LF et al (1991) Concentration-response relationship in paroxetine treatment of diabetic neuropathy symptoms: a patient-blinded dose-escalation study. Ther Drug Monit 13:408–414
25. Foster CA, Bafaloukos J (1994) Paroxetine in the treatment of chronic daily headache. Headache 34:587–589
26. Saper JR, Silberstein SD. Lake AE et al (1994) Double-blind trial of fluoxetine: chronic daily headache and migraine. Headache 34:497–502
27. Adly C, Straumanis J, Chesson A (1992) Fluoxetine prophylaxis of migraine. Headache 32:101–104
28. Rani PU, Naidu MU, Prasad VB et al (1996) An evaluation of antidepressants in rheumatic pain conditions. Anesth Analg 83:371–375
29. Goldenberg D, Mayskiy M, Mossey C et al (1996) A randomized, double-blind crossover trial of fluoxetine and amitriptyline in the treatment of fibromyalgia. Arthritis Rheum 39:1852–1859
30. Max MB (1994) Treatment of post-herpetic neuralgia: antidepressants. Ann Neurol 35(Suppl):S50–S53
31. McQuay HJ, Trainer M, Nye BA et al (1996) A systematic review of antidepressants in neuropathic pain. Pain 68:217–227
32. Wolfe F, Cathey MA, Hawley DJ (1994) A double-blind placebo controlled trial of fluoxetine in fibromyalgia. Scand J Rheumatol 23:255–259
33. Max MB, Lynch SA, Muir J et al (1992) Effects of desimpramine, amitriptyline, and fluoxetine on pain in diabetic neuropathy. N Engl J Med 326:1250–1256
34. Pick CG, Paul D, Eison MS et al (1992) Potentiation of opioid analgesia by the antidepressant nefazodone. Eur J Pharmacol 211:375–381
35. Lang E, Hord AH, Denson D (1996) Venlafaxine hydrochloride (Effexor) relieves thermal hyperalgesia in rats with an experimental mononeuropathy. Pain 68:151–155
36. Tanum L, Malt UF (1996) A new pharmacologic treatment of functional gastrointestinal disorder: a double-blind placebo-controlled study with mianserin. Scand J Gastroenterol 31:318–325
37. Onghena P, DeCuyper H, Van Houdenhove B et al (1993) Mianserin and chronic pain: a double-blind placebo-controlled process and outcome study. Acta Psychiatr Scand 88:198–204
38. Rothrock JF (1997) Clinical studies of valproate for migraine prophylaxis. Cephalalgia 17:81–83
39. Gillin S, Sorkin LS (1998) Gabapentin reverses the allodynia produced by the administration of anti-GD2 ganglioside, an immunotherapeutic drug. Anesth Analg 86:111–116
40. Hunter JC, Gogas KR, Hedley LR et al (1997) the effect of novel anti-epileptic drugs in rat experimental models of acute and chronic pain. Eur J Pharmacol 324:153–160
41. Rosner H, Rubin L, Kestenbaum A (1996) Gabapentin adjunctive therapy in neuropathic pain states. Clin J Pain 12:56–58
42. Sist TC, Filadora VA, Miner M et al (1997) Experience with gabapentin for neuropathic pain in the head and neck: report of ten cases. Reg Anesth 22:473–478
43. Houtchens MK, Richert JR, Sami A, Rose JW (1997) Open label gabapentin treatment for pain in multiple sclerosis. Mult Scler 3:250–253
44. Rosenbert JM, Harrell C, Ristic H, Werner RA, de Rosaryo AM (1997) The effect of gabapentin on neuropathic pain. Clin J Pain 13:251–255
45. Wetzel CH, Connelly JF (1997) Use of gabapentin in pain management. Ann Pharmacother 31:1082–1083
46. Childers MK, Holland D (1997) Psychomotor agitation following gabapentin use in brain injury. Brain Inj 11:537–540
47. Wang HH, Xu SF (1993) Effect of D1 and D2 dopamine receptor antagonists on acupuncture analgesia. Shen Li Hsueh Pao 45:61–68

48. Xu SF, Cao XD, Mo WY, Xu ZB, Pan YY (1989) Effect of combination of drugs with acupuncture on analgesic efficacy. Acupunct Electrother Res 14:103–113
49. Langemark M, Olesen J (1994) Sulpiride and paroxetine in the treatment of chronic tension-type headache. An explanatory double-blind trial. Headache 34:20–24
50. Guslandi M (1990) Antiemetic properties of levo-sulpiride. Minerva Med 81:855–860
51. Mansi C, Savarino V, Vigneri S et al (1995) Gastrokinetic effects of levosulpiride in dyspeptic patients with diabetic gastroparesis. Am J Gastroenterol 90:1989–1993
52. Arienti V, Corazza GR, Sorge M et al (1994) The effects of levosulpiride on gastric and gall-bladder emptying in functional dyspepsia. Aliment Pharmacol Ther 8:631–638
53. Corazza GR, Biagi F, Albano O et al (1996) Levosulpiride in functional dyspepsia: a multicentric, double-blind, controlled trial. Ital J Gastroenterol 28:317–323
54. Yamagami S, Hirayama E, Mui K, Okuno M, Kioka T, Soma T et al (1993) A single-blind comparison of bromperidol and sulpiride in hospitalized schizophrenics. Acta Psychiatr Belg 93:236–244

# Approach to the Treatment of Somatoform Disorders in General Practice

Glen Couchman

*Summary.* In the United States, the current treatment approaches to somatoform disorders are largely unsuccessful because of the physician's difficulty in correctly and efficiently making the diagnosis, as well as by the barriers created by traditional United States medical school training in the biophysiological approach to illness with a clearcut mind/body separation. Future success in the treatment of this disorder is dependent upon improving physicians' ability to diagnose the condition, as well as training physicians on the best approach to meet these patients' psychosocial needs.

*Key words.* Somatoform disorders, Treatment, General practice, Diagnostic criteria

The approach to the treatment of somatoform disorders in general practice can be summed up as generally unsatisfactory. I say that based on both the physician's perspective as well as the patient's perception. From a general practice physician's point of view making the diagnosis of a somatoform disorder is sometimes very difficult. It is a diagnosis that is not used very frequently by primary care physicians for a variety of reasons. But, when they do make the diagnosis, it is usually based on pattern recognition rather than the application of specific diagnostic criteria. The concept of somatization disorder as a diagnosis becomes apparent to general practice physicians when they realize that a patient has demonstrated, over time, a presentation with multiple vague complaints and no truly established etiology. These patients are particularly unsatisfying for general practice physicians as time constraints are a major factor in their daily schedule. These patients, in particular, require more than the usual 10–15 minutes that is typically allotted for routine general practice office visits. Physicians typically resort to focusing their attention on symptom relief with specific drug therapy, as this is their standard approach to most conditions. Further evidence that the patients are viewed in a negative light is the fact that they are frequently labeled as "difficult patients," "whiners," or "doctor shoppers."

Similarly, from the patient's perspective, in general practice their overall experience with the health care system is unsatisfactory. The current environment in the United

Department of Family Medicine, Texas A&M University College of Medicine and Scott and White Clinic and Hospital, 2401 South 31st Street, Temple, TX 76508, USA

States includes a great deal of mass media attention to public health issues including cancer prevention, reduction of cardiovascular risk factors, smoking cessation, and weight loss programs. This media attention aggravates somatic patients' already heightened awareness of bodily concerns. It tends to increase visits to doctors' offices in an attempt to seek explanations for their symptoms. General practice physicians then attempt to rule out disease processes as explanations for these symptoms and typically reassure and dismiss the patients with very little attention to the patient's underlying psychosocial needs. This recurring cycle of concerns, physician encounters, and dismissals tends to eventually undermine the patients' confidence in the medical system in general.

We know that somatoform disorder patients are very common in the general practitioner's office. It has been estimated that one-third of appointments in primary care result in no specific pathology being identified. As mentioned, physicians usually stumble onto this diagnosis by pattern recognition after exhaustive workups and multiple failed therapeutic trials which were directed solely at symptom elimination. It is not uncommon that these patients will ultimately end up in a general practitioner's office with rather fashionable and sometimes exotic diagnoses like environmental hypersensitivity after visiting the allergist; chronic fatigue syndrome after their visit to the internist; fibromyalgia following the rheumatology consultation; irritable bowel syndrome from the gastroenterologist; mixed vascular tension headaches and benign positional vertigo diagnosed by the neurologist; and finally, temporomandibular joint syndrome as per by the dentist. Unfortunately, directing specific treatment at any of these entities does little to help the patient develop insight into their underlying excessive concern over somatic symptoms.

Barry Blackwell reflected that the best approach for physicians is to follow the *Serenity Prayer* when dealing with these patients. This prayer basically asks for the courage to change the things that can be changed, to have the serenity to accept those that cannot be changed, and the wisdom to know the difference. Clearly, the treatment of these patients is very difficult. The successful approach to these patients requires that the physician establish a caring relationship with the patient. He must express interest and empathy in their symptoms and gain the patient's confidence. This can be accomplished by reviewing the patient's previous workup and conducting a thorough but not excessive physical examination shortly after the patient presents. This helps to build trust and conveys interest, as well as validating the patient's concerns. Once this relationship is established, then the physician can begin to explore psychosocial stressors. It is imperative that comorbid conditions like depression, substance abuse, and anxiety disorders be identified and appropriately treated. It is appropriate and probably essential that the physician acknowledge that specific physical causes cannot be found to explain the patient's ailments, as long as the patient has been reassured that this does not mean there is no help available.

Eventually, the patient should be encouraged to analyze how his/her symptoms are affecting their life. They should be encouraged to look for psychosocial links to their symptoms. It is appropriate to offer benign treatments to these patients that are directed at symptom relief. Commonly, low doses of nonsteroidal antiinflammatories are helpful, as well as low doses of antidepressants and/or recommendations for vitamins and antioxidants. It is important that the physician does not underestimate the placebo effect of any of these recommendations. The patient should be encouraged initially to have frequently scheduled visits. This prevents the patient from having to develop new symptoms to justify an appointment. It is hoped that these frequent visits will allow the patient to rebuild a sense of control over his/her symptoms and rebuild their confidence. Lastly, psychology or psychiatry consultation is sometimes helpful for these patients, but it is imperative that the primary care physician continues to be involved in the patient's care. It is important to avoid the message to the patient of a mind/body split in symptom origination.

Let me briefly review the experience we have had with patients from a general practice in Waco, Texas. 1073 patients from a Family Practice office were screened with the World Health Organization screener for somatoform disorders. 120 of these patients were then sampled and tested with the Composite International Diagnostic Interview (CIDI) and the WHO Somatoform Disorder Schedule (SDS). These patients were then followed over a 2-year period of time and their medical records were reviewed. The overall prevalence rate for any somatoform disorder was 26.9%, with the most common being persistent somatoform disorder at 14.2%. Approximately 6% of the patients met criteria for undifferentiated somatoform disorder. None of these patients had a diagnosis of somatoform disorder recorded in the medical record. Over 50% of patients diagnosed with a somatoform disorder on the SDS had a clinical diagnosis of depression recorded in their medical records. Truly, the focus of their care was on their depression. Serotonin reuptake inhibitor medications were being used in the majority of these patients. Alcohol was not identified as a medical/social problem by our study physicians, and yet 9% of the population met criteria for alcohol abuse. None of the patients identified as having a somatoform disorder by formal testing developed any medical illness to explain their somatic complaints during the follow-up period (mean 18.6 months).

# Approaches to the Treatment of Somatoform Disorders in Liaison Psychiatry

Takashi Hosaka[1], Takeshi Sato[2], and Kenji Yamamoto[1]

*Summary.* Somatoform disorders commonly are supposed to be seen in the clinical field of consultation–liaison (C-L) psychiatry; however, a few patients are referred to psychiatry. From the perspective of C-L psychiatry, the authors propose three therapeutic models for somatoform disorders, i.e., (1) physician-oriented with psychiatric advice, (2) psychiatrist-oriented, and (3) cooperative physician/psychiatrist-oriented. The third model especially is recommended because the patient can undergo physical examinations until the relationship between somatic complaints and psychosocial factors is recognized through the third model. Moreover, the psychiatrist can build an alliance with a patient, while the patient completes a "testing phase" to determine whether the psychiatrist can be relied on or not. As such, the third model is useful and can be the aim at least at the initial phase. Each model has strengths and limitations as well. The most important thing in treating such patients in any model is to see the patient as a whole person who is suffering from distress.

*Key words.* Consultation–liaison psychiatry, Somatoform disorder, Somatization, Psychiatric referral, Doctor shopping

## Introduction

Consultation–liaison (C-L) psychiatry was first introduced in Japan in 1977, and it has become one of the major clinical fields in the country since the Japanese Society of General Hospital Psychiatry (JSGHP) was founded in 1988 [1]. However, according to a survey by Kuroki et al., only half of the general hospitals in Japan are furnished with psychiatric departments [2].

Although it is known that patients with somatoform disorders are likely to visit nonpsychiatric departments, it is still controversial where and how to treat them. Somatoform disorders commonly are supposed to be seen in the clinical field of C-L

---

[1] Department of Psychiatry and Behavioral Science, Tokai University School of Medicine, Bohseidai, Isehara, Kanagawa 259-1193, Japan
[2] Department of Psychiatry, Saga Medical School, Nabeshima, Saga, Saga 849-8501, Japan

psychiatry, because there may be many patients with unexplained physical symptoms, and these patients may be referred to C-L psychiatrists for "no organic lesions explaining their physical complaints." Also, it is important to discuss how to treat the patients with somatoform disorders from the viewpoint of medical economics, and also to prevent adverse consequences derived from unnecessary examinations and treatments. As such, the therapeutic approach for somatization patients is one of the major topics in the clinical field of C-L psychiatry.

In this chapter, therefore, the prevalence of somatoform disorders and the psychiatric referral of patients with such disorders were investigated, and the therapeutic approaches are discussed from the viewpoints of C-L psychiatry.

# Methods

## Study 1: Psychiatric Prevalence in Primary Care

Using the Japanese version of the General Health Questionnaire (GHQ) and the Japanese modified Diagnostic Interview Schedule (DIS-JM), patients visiting a general medicine outpatient clinic at Saga Medical School Hospital were assessed according to the DSM-III-R during a 12-month period [3].

## Study 2: Psychiatric Prevalence Among "Doctor-Shopping" Cases

To describe the clinical characteristics of patients with doctor-shopping behavior (doctor-shopping patients) among Japanese patients in primary care, patients from the general medicine outpatient clinic of Saga Medical School Hospital were asked to complete an original questionnaire and a GHQ-30 during a 12 month-period [4]. A random sample of patients was interviewed according to the DSM-JM. In this study, doctor-shopping patients were defined as those who had visited two or more medical facilities prior to visiting the general medicine clinic at this hospital with the same complaints.

## Study 3: Classification of Comorbid Psychiatric Disorders

When physically ill inpatients developed psychiatric symptoms as well, the physicians in charge consult a psychiatrist, especially when the symptoms are moderate or severe. The psychiatric consultant, if necessary, sees the patients on a regular basis and prescribes some tranquilizers during their stay at the hospital. This study investigated the classification of psychiatric disorders of such comorbid cases from 1992 through 1996 at Tokai University Hospital.

## Study 4: Psychiatric Referral in Primary Care

Patients from the general medicine outpatient clinic of Saga Medical School Hospital who were not referred to psychiatrists, although they had psychological problems and needed psychiatric consultation, were evaluated by psychiatrists during a three-month period [5].

## Results

### Study 1: Psychiatric Prevalence in Primary Care

Figure 1 shows the lifetime psychiatric prevalence among the patients who visited the general medicine clinic at a medical school hospital. Excluding tobacco dependence, the psychiatric prevalence was 30.6%. The most frequent diagnosis was alcoholism, which was followed by psychosexual dysfunction, major depressive episode, phobia, and others. Somatization disorders were observed among 2.4% of the 170 outpatients.

### Study 2: Psychiatric Prevalence Among "Doctor-Shopping" Cases

The psychiatric lifetime prevalence among the 'doctor shopping' cases is demonstrated in Figure 2. This revealed the prevalence among the "doctor-shopping" cases was 52.5%, which was significantly higher than the non-"doctor-shopping" cases. Concerning the kinds of the psychiatric disorders, somatization disorders are encountered significantly more frequently among the "doctor-shopping" cases, of which the rate is 7.5%.

### Study 3: Classification of Comorbid Psychiatric Disorders

During these 5 years, there were 1570 cases treated concomitantly by psychiatrists during their stay at hospitals. The frequency of somatoform disorders was 40 (2.5%) among them, which is shown in Figure 3.

### Study 4: Psychiatric Referral in Primary Care

During a 3-month period in a primary care setting, 59 (1.0% of total ambulatory patients) needed psychiatric consultation, but actually only 29 patients were referred

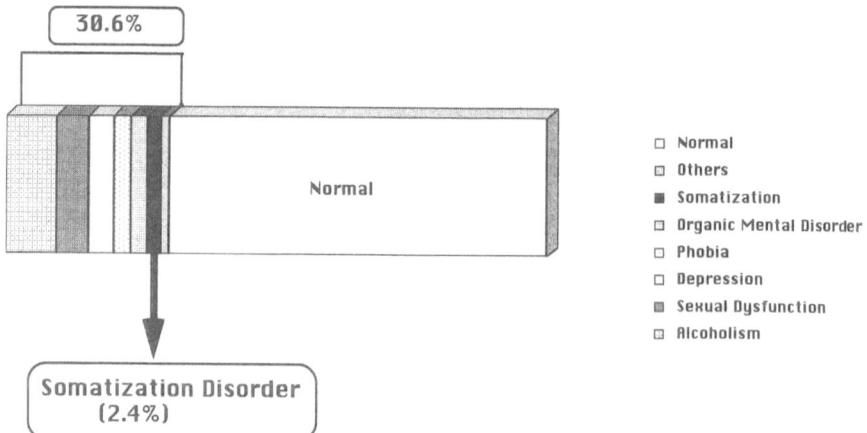

FIG. 1. Psychiatric prevalence in primary care

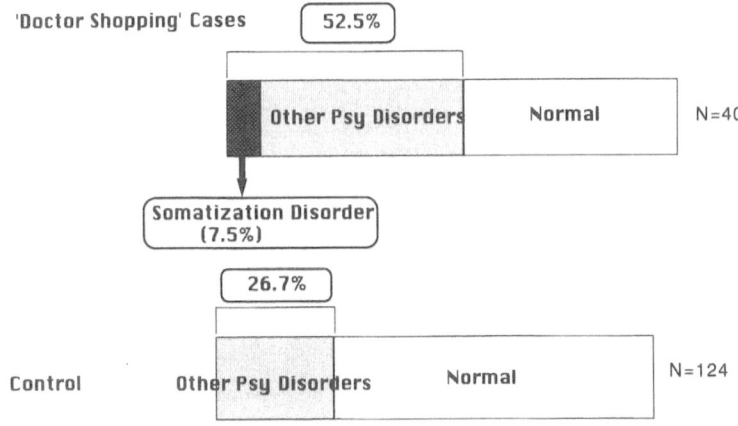

FIG. 2.  Psychiatric prevalence among "doctor-shopping" cases

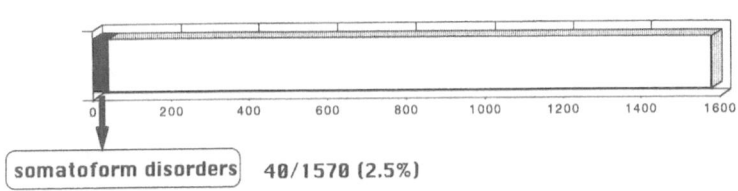

FIG. 3.  Comorbid psychiatric disorders among physically ill inpatients

to psychiatry. Among 30 who were not referred, nine patients (30.0%) were supposed to have somatoform disorders (Figure 4).

## Discussion

Some articles revealed the prevalence of somatoform disorders among patients visiting nonpsychiatric clinics. Gureje et al. reported that on the basis of scores on the General Health Questionnaire and interviews using the Composite International Diagnostic Interview, only 1.1% of primary care clinic patients fulfilled the DSM-III-R criteria for somatization disorder, but 4.7% and 10.8% met the criteria for somatoform pain disorder and undifferentiated somatoform disorder, respectively [6]. Labott et al. reviewed 1908 pulmonary consultation reports for evidence of somatization, which revealed its frequency was 2% [7]. These prevalences are similar to our data.

Concerning the resistance to psychiatric referral, Steinberg et al. conducted a review of medical records to identify the patients with prominent psychiatric problems relating to their hospitalization. It was found that physician resistance to consultation was

**59/5841 (1.0%) needed psychiatric referral**

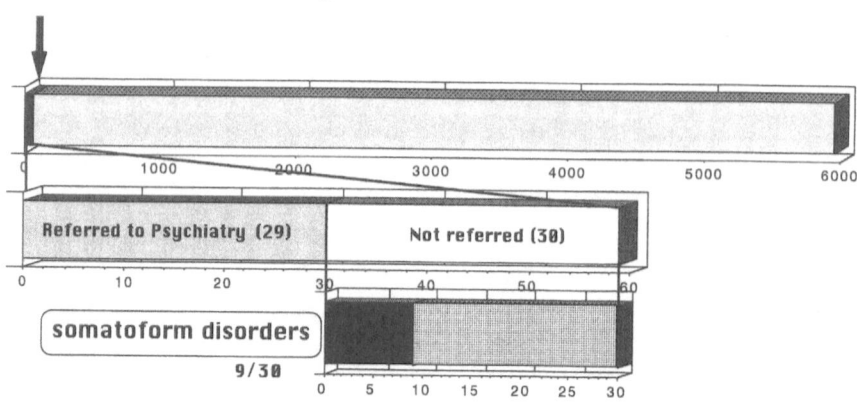

FIG. 4. Psychiatric referral in primary care. Fifty-nine patients needed psychiatric consultation, but actually only 29 patients were referred. Among 30 who were not referred, 9 patients were supposed to have somatoform disorders

involved in more than 50% of the cases not referred, usually because the physicians believed that there were no psychiatric problems or that psychiatry could not help, and less often because the physician thought that the patient might become upset or the patient-doctor relationship would be destroyed [8].

The therapeutic approaches to such patients should be considered from the viewpoint of medical economics. The per capita expenditure for health care of patients with multiple physical symptoms but no apparent physical disease (somatization disorder) is up to nine times the average per capita amount. According to Smith et al., after the psychiatric consultation, the quarterly health care charges in the treatment group declined by 53%. They concluded that psychiatric consultation in the care of patients with somatization disorders reduced subsequent health care expenditures without inducing changes in health status or patient satisfaction with their health care [9].

All of these data suggest that the patients with somatoform disorders are less likely to be referred to C-L psychiatry. As a matter of fact, psychiatric referral does not always produce good outcomes.

From the perspective of C-L psychiatry, the therapeutic models for somatoform disorders are proposed which are classified into the following: (1) physician-oriented with psychiatric advice, (2) psychiatrist-oriented, and (3) cooperative physician/ psychiatrist-oriented, as shown in Figure 5. Each model has strengths and limitations as well.

In the first model, the C-L psychiatrists can advise the physician in charge as a consultant. As mentioned, the patients with somatoform disorders do not accept the relationship between their somatic symptoms and psychological states. They believe that they are physically ill, but not mentally ill. Therefore, they do not like to be referred to a psychiatrist. They often complain of physical symptoms and require repeated examinations to rule out, or to find out their physical disease. If their requests are

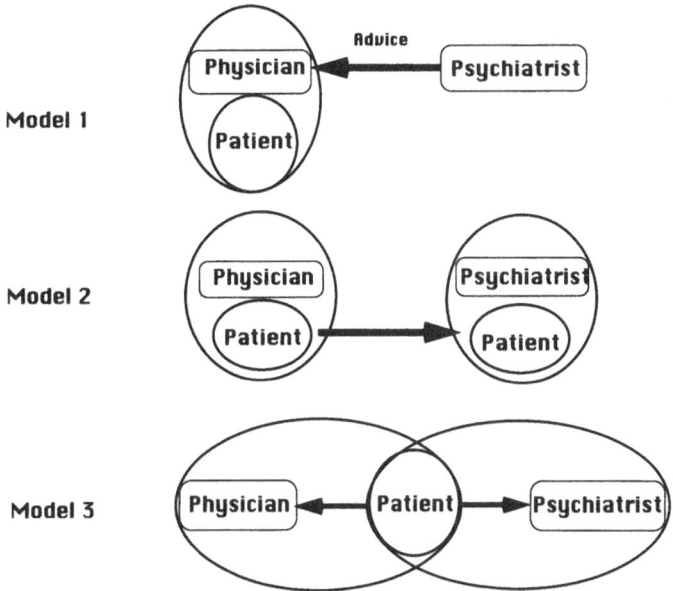

FIG. 5. Therapeutic models for treating somatoform disorders. *1*, physician-oriented with psychiatric advice; *2*, psychiatrist-oriented; *3*, cooperative physician/psychiatrist-oriented

rejected by the doctor, they visit another doctor, which leads to "doctor shopping." The first model is effective for most of the patients with somatoform disorders, because they want to keep regular contact with nonpsychiatric physicians. In this model, C-L psychiatrists can initially advise primary physicians of general management strategies, which will be followed by more specific strategies.

This model can be used for research purposes. We have joined a psychosocial conference at a rehabilitation setting, where the doctors, nurses, PTs, OTs, speech therapists, MSWs, and psychiatrists discuss difficult patients who have psychosocial problems. For example, we have experienced multidisciplinary treatment for several patients with conversion disorders. Some of these patients were successfully treated by rehabilitation staff without referring them to psychiatry. This model can be applied to pain clinics, gynecology, cardiology, etc.

In the second model, transition of the treatment setting is difficult and requires technical skills. It is the role of primary doctors to explain to the patients that their physical symptoms are related to psychosocial factors and that they would be better treated by a psychiatrist. But they should avoid statements making the patients feel rejected and abandoned. After referral, the C-L psychiatrist, in order to establish an alliance with a patient, should sometimes perform a further physical examination. Furthermore, the C-L psychiatrists should accept the patient's ambivalence about seeing a psychiatrist by saying, for example, "You are here, but I know you want to be treated by a nonpsychiatric doctor."

In the third model, the patient is treated by both a nonpsychiatric physician and a psychiatrist. In this model, it is relatively easier for a primary physician to consult a psychiatrist, because the patient would experience less abandonment from a primary physician. "Abandonment" is a key word in the treatment of patients with somatoform disorders.

In order to investigate resistance to psychiatric referrals, the inpatients who had been referred to me were reviewed by their primary physicians. Out of 50 cases, only 4 patients still had negative impressions of the psychiatric referral. Two patients were alcoholic, 1 was severely psychotic, and 1 had an antisocial personality disorder [10]. Among the 46 patients who responded favorably to psychiatric referral, ten patients had somatoform disorders. This study was done at a general hospital without a psychiatric department. During that study, the author worked as a part-time psychiatric consultant. That hospital had no psychiatric outpatient clinic, psychiatric beds, nor full-time psychiatrists. In such a structure, patients with somatoform disorders would not feel abandoned by the primary physician even when referred to psychiatry. Actually, they can persist in being a patient for the primary physician. In treating these patients, it is very important not to make them feel abandoned.

Through this model, the patient can undergo further physical examinations until recognizing the relationship between somatic complaints and psychosocial factors. Also, through this model, the psychiatrist can build an alliance with a patient, while the patient completes a "testing phase" to determine whether the psychiatrist can be relied on or not. As such, the third model is useful and can be aimed at least at the initial phase.

As therapeutic approaches to patients with somatoform disorders, the authors proposed three clinical models from the viewpoints of C-L psychiatry. Each model has strengths and limitations as well. The most important thing in treating such patients in any model is to see such a patient as a whole person who is suffering from distress.

## References

1. Hosaka T, Iwasaki Y (1997) Consultation-liaison psychiatry in Japan. In: Rundell JR, Wise MG (eds) Textbook of consultation-liaison psychiatry. American Psychiatric Press, Washington DC, pp 244–246
2. Kuroki N, Fukui Y, Shiraishi T et al (1996) Economic issues for general hospital psychiatry (In Japanese with English abstract). Jpn J Gen Hosp Psychiatry 8:1–11
3. Sato T, Takeichi M (1993) Lifetime prevalence of specific psychiatric disorders in a general medicine clinic. Gen Hosp Psychiatry 15:224–233
4. Sato T, Takeichi M, Shirahama M et al (1995) Doctor-shopping patients and users of alternative medicine among Japanese primary care patients. Gen Hosp Psychiatry 17:115–125
5. Takeichi M, Sato T, Kimura Y (1991) Studies on general medicine clinic psychiatry—II. Evaluations of cases with mental disorders not referred to psychiatrist (in Japanese). Jpn J Psychiatr Treat 6:985–991
6. Gureje O, Obikoya B (1992) Somatization in primary care: pattern and correlates in a clinic in Nigeria. Acta Psychiatr Scand 86:223–227
7. Labott SM, Preisman RC, Popovich J, Iannuzzi (1995) Health care utilization of somatizing patients in a pulmonary subspecialty. Psychosomatics 36:122–128
8. Steinberg H, Torem M, Saravay SM (1980) An analysis of physician resistance to psychiatric consultations. Arch Gen Psychiatry 37:1007–1012

9. Smith GR, Monson RA, Ray DC (1986) Psychiatric consultation in somatization disorder. A randomized controlled study. N Engl J Med 314:1407–1413
10. Hosaka T (1989) Physicians' attitudes toward psychiatric consultation. Jpn J Psychosom Med 29:351–358

# Approaches to the Treatment of Somatoform Disorders in Internal Medicine

Shinobu Nomura, Tomifusa Kuboki, and Gaku Yamanaka

*Summary.* This chapter discusses the prevalence of somatoform disorders and their treatment approaches in internal medical settings. The subjects of this study were 424 new outpatients in 1997 on our department. In the diagnosis distribution by Axis I of DSM-IV, eating disorders were the largest in number (19.4%), followed by somatoform disorders (18.2%). The number of somatoform disorder patients was 77 (male 28, female 49). In somatoform disorders, somatoform disorder not otherwise specified (NOS) was seen most often (32.5%), followed by pain disorder (22.1%), conversion disorder (19.5%), hypochondriasis (14.3%), and undifferentiated somatoform disorder (11.7%). The treatment for somatoform disorders included mainly supportive psychotherapy and pharmacological treatment. Other therapies included autogenic training and behavior therapy. The pharmacological treatments for somatoform disorders were mainly antianxiety drugs, partial antidepressants, and sleep inducers. In the management of somatoform disorders, both physiological and psychological approaches should be considered. Medication such as antianxiety drugs may be effective in alleviating patients' symptoms. In addition, a psychotherapeutic approach might be necessary to resolve their complaints.

*Key words.* Psychosomatic medicine, Database, DSM-IV, Psychotherapy, Stress management

## Introduction

Our department, Psychosomatic Medicine, is based on internal medicine and also aims to practice psychological treatment approaches. In Japan, seven universities have departments of psychosomatic medicine.

In our department, we treat about 1300 psychosomatic and psychogenic patients per year. Patients with physical symptoms usually visit a general physician rather than a psychiatrist at first. When no physiologic cause for the symptom can be found or the

Department of Psychosomatic Medicine, School of Medicine, University of Tokyo, 3-28-6 Mejirodai, Bunkyo-ku, Tokyo 112-8688, Japan physician recognizes the discrepancy between patient's complaints and objective findings, psychosomatic or psychiatric consultation are requested. But these patients are so many that diagnostic and therapeutic approaches on general clinics for somatoform disorders should be considered more seriously.

In such a context, we have recorded and accumulated a database on diagnosis and treatment of outpatients since 1990 [1, 2]. In order to standardize the assessment of diagnosis, we adopted the classification of the Diagnostic and Statistical Manual of Mental Disorders (DSM-III-R [3] and IV [4]), and discussed the differential diagnosis in cooperation with our staff.

The purpose of this chapter is to discuss the prevalence of somatoform disorders and their treatment approaches in internal medical settings.

# Materials and Methods

## Subjects

The subjects of this study were 424 new outpatients in 1997 on the Department of Psychosomatic Medicine, University of Tokyo. There were 150 male patients (mean age 36.0 ± 13.8 years old), and 274 female patients (mean age 35.0 ± 17.1 years old). All subjects were referred from other departments of our hospital and other hospitals or clinics.

## Methods

At the first intake interview, physicians diagnosed outpatients according to DSM-IV, and recorded the diagnosis with the initial treatment plans in the database. To minimize assessment error, we discussed diagnoses and treatment plans in cooperation with our staff, every week. By the statistical study based on this database, we discussed the prevalence and treatment approaches of the somatoform disorders in our clinic.

# Results

The diagnosis distribution by Axis I of DSM-IV is shown in Figure 1. Eating disorders were the largest in number (19.4%), followed by somatoform disorders (18.2%), anxiety disorders (15.6%), mood disorders (13.0%), psychological factors affecting medical conditions (11.3%), and others.

Anxiety disorders included panic disorder, agoraphobia, social phobia, generalized anxiety disorder, and others. Mood disorders included major depression, dysthymic disorder, and depressive disorder not otherwise specified (NOS). Psychological factors affecting medical conditions included the psychosomatic diseases in a narrow sense such as essential hypertension, irritable bowel syndrome, hyperventilation syndrome, spasmodic torticollis, and others.

The number of somatoform disorder patients was 77 (male patients 28, mean age 36.8 ± 14.9 years old, and female patients 49, mean age 48.5 ± 17.6 years old). As shown in Figure 2, somatoform disorder NOS was seen mostly (32.5%), followed by pain disorder (22.1%), conversion disorder (19.5%), hypochondriasis (14.3%), and undiffer-

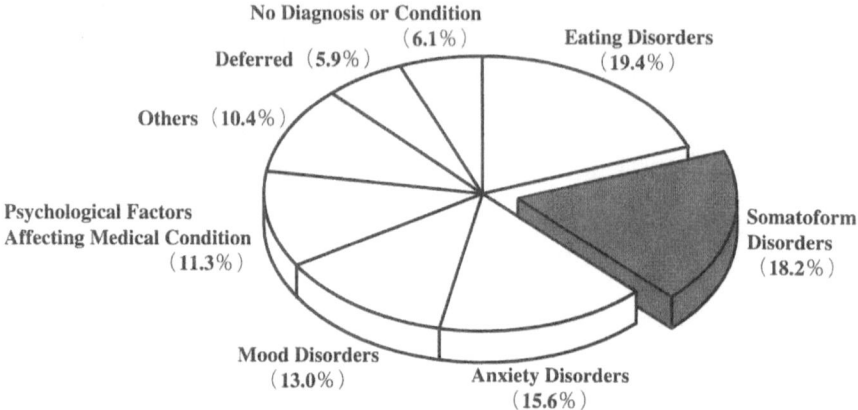

FIG. 1. Distribution of diagnoses by Axis I of DSM-IV

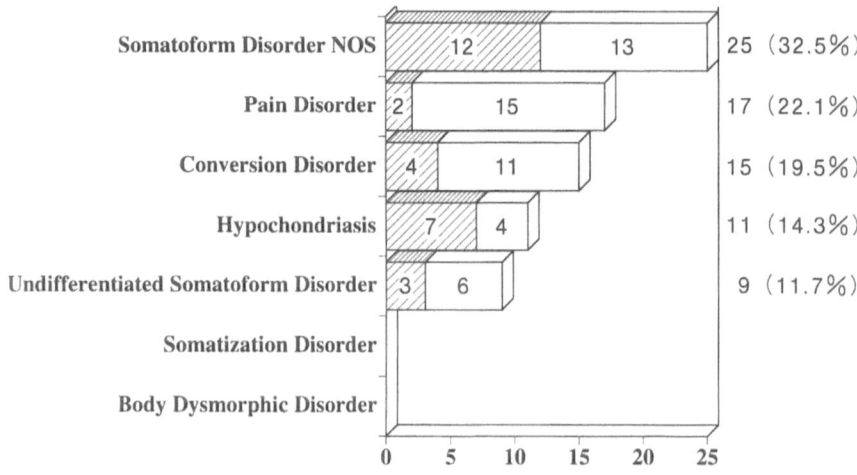

FIG. 2. Distribution of somatoform disorders. Values indicate the number of patients (*shaded*, male; *open*, female) with percentages in parentheses

entiated somatoform disorder (11.7%). Somatization disorder and body dysmorphic disorder were not seen.

Regarding the personality disorder diagnoses by Axis II, there were few personality disorders in somatoform disorders, which included only three histrionic and one NOS personality disorders. Three histrionic personality disorders were consistent with conversion disorder in Axis I.

Table 1 shows the severity of psychosocial stressors scale by Axis IV of DSM-III-R in somatoform disorders, anxiety disorders, and mood disorders, respectively. In somatoform disorders, "Moderate" was largest in number, followed by "mild". But, in

TABLE 1. Severity of psychosocial stressors scale of somatoform, anxiety, and mood disorders (%)

| Code term | Somatoform | Anxiety | Mood |
|---|---|---|---|
| 1 None | 10.5 | 6.8 | 0 |
| 2 Mild | 26.3 | 43.2 | 34.3 |
| 3 Moderate | 42.1 | 20.5 | 29.5 |
| 4 Severe | 8.8 | 9.1 | 11.4 |
| 5 Extreme | 5.3 | 9.1 | 8.6 |
| 6 Catastrophic | 0 | 2.3 | 2.9 |
| 0 No information | 7.1 | 9.1 | 5.7 |

This scale is based on Axis IV of DSM-III-R. All data are given as
percentages.

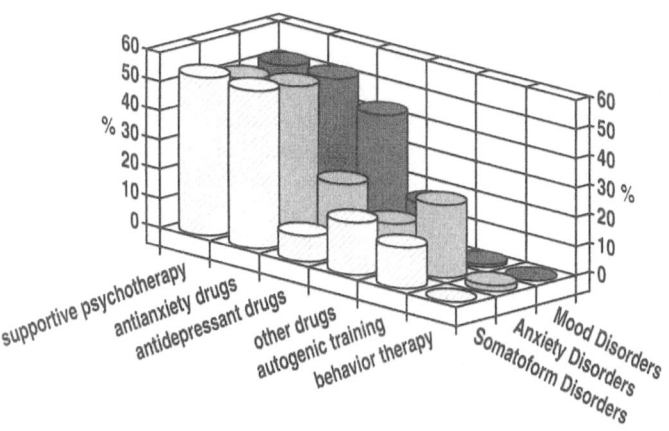

FIG. 3. Treatment approaches for somatoform, anxiety, and mood disorders

both anxiety and mood disorders, "mild" was largest in number. And there were few
strong stressors such as "severe," "extreme," and "catastrophic," in all three groups.

Figure 3 shows the treatment approaches for somatoform, anxiety, and mood disorders. Main treatment plans included supportive psychotherapy and pharmacological treatment in all three groups. Other therapies included autogenic training and
behavior therapy. As a matter of course, there were more antidepressant prescriptions
for mood disorders, and more autogenic training for anxiety disorders. The pharmacological treatments for somatoform disorders were mainly antianxiety drugs, partial antidepressants, and sleep inducers. Behavior therapy was rarely undertaken for
somatoform disorders in our clinic.

## Discussion

Among the total subjects of this study, those in their twenties and teens were more
prevalent than other age groups in female patients. This result was thought to be due
to many eating disorder patients, which were more prevalent in young women. The

reason why eating disorders were most in number is that our department is one of the speciality hospitals for these disorders.

The distribution of diagnoses on our clinic was similar to our previous data of several years [2]. And the prevalence of somatoform disorders was consistent with other reports [5]. In the results of this study, it was characteristic that female patients were larger in number than male, especially regarding pain disorder and conversion disorder. The reason why somatizattion disorder was not seen may be that it was difficult to meet its criteria.

The correlation between severity of psychosocial stressor and somatic symptoms was not as strong as some investigators pointed out [6]. We consider also that recognition or perception of stressors may be more sensitive in patients with somatoform disorders than in healthy people, and that various factors may influence some stress reactions. But, in order to understand the psychopathology of patients, it is important to clarify the relationships between psychosocial stressors and stress reactions. In DSM-IV, severity of psychosocial stressors scale was changed into psychosocial and environmental problems. But we think that the former is more useful than the latter, and use Axis IV of DSM-III-R even now.

As a summary, we would like to mention the treatment approaches for somatoform disorder in internal medical settings from our clinical experiences.

## Supportive Psychotherapy

At the initial interview, it is important that a physician should listen to patients' complaints with empathy and differentiate a functional disorder from an organic disease. At the same time, it is also necessary to ask after psychosocial factors such as stressors and coping style, family relations, and occupational distress. This process contributes to make a good doctor-patient relationship, that is to say, a collaboration with patients. This is the first and important step to an adequate treatment.

By supportive psychotherapy we mean no specific psychotherapy but a general psychological approach, which includes listening to patients' complaints, and to accept them, and to support their effort to be well. The goal of this approach may be to be aware of the relationships between his/her discomfort and psychosocial distress, and his/her symptoms' role in social life.

## Physical Examination

A patient with physical symptoms usually visits a general physician at first and may seek some organic disease which explains the symptoms. Therefore, the doctor may do some medical examinations necessary and explain the results to his patients. So, it should be discussed whether a physical examination and findings could fully explain the patient's complaints. To understand that a patient's complaints are not due to any organic disease, physical examinations play an important role.

For the "doctor-shopping" patients, in order not to do excessive examinations, it is important to make contact with the referring doctor.

## Pharmacological Treatment

Pharmacological treatment is useful for resolution of a patient's discomfort, even if it may be symptomatic. Medication for somatoform disorders includes mostly antianxiety drugs, as indicated by the result of our database. Antidepressants for depression and sleep inducers for insomnia can be used in part. Although antidepressants may reduce the threshold of pain, we are not willing to prescribe it because of their side effects.

## Stress Management and Relaxation Technique

According to Lipowski [7], somatization refers to a process of expressing emotional or psychological distress through somatic symptoms. Therefore, stress management may be one of the main strategies for somatization, which includes modification of cognitive appraisal and coping style, and alleviation of excessive stress reactions by relaxation techniques. As a relaxation technique, we use autogenic training more frequently than progressive muscle relaxation or biofeedback.

# Conclusion

In the management of somatoform disorders, both physiological and psychological approaches should be considered. Medication such as antianxiety drugs may be effective in alleviating patients' symptoms. In addition, a psychotherapeutic approach might be necessary to resolve their complaints. Among many psychotherapies, supportive psychotherapy and relaxation tecniques are often used in our clinic. We believe that cognitive behavior therapy should be tried more frequently for these disorders.

Because the prognosis of somatoform disorders was not discussed in this study, we cannot declare that any treatment approach is superior to any other therapy. Therefore, in the future, a controlled prospective study should be carried out.

## References

1. Nomura S, Ide M, Kumano H et al (1991) Study of the data base in psychosomatic department, preliminary report (in Japanese). Jpn J Psychother 3:85–93
2. Nakao M, Nomura S, Yamanaka G et al (1998) Assessment of patients by DSM-III-R and DSM-IV in a Japanese psychosomatic clinic. Psychother Psychosom 67:43–49
3. American Psychiatric Association (1987) Diagnostic and Statistical Manual of Mental Disorders, 3rd edn—revised. American Psychiatric Press, Washington
4. American Psychiatric Association (1994) Diagnostic and Statistical Manual of Mental Disorders, 4th edn. American Psychiatric Press, Washington
5. Issac M, Janca A, Burke KC et al (1995) Medically unexplained somatic symptoms in different cultures: a preliminary report from phase I of World Health Organization International Study of Somatoform Disorders. Psychother Psychosom 64:88–93
6. Skodol AE (1991) Axis IV: a reliable and valid measure of psychosocial stress? Comprehens Psychiatry 32:503–515
7. Lipowski ZJ (1988) Somatization: the concept and its clinical application. Am J Psychiatry 145:1358–1368

# The Use of Japanese Herbal Medicine in the Treatment of Somatoform Disorders

Hiroko Mizushima[1] and Shigenobu Kanba[2]

*Summary.* It has been observed that Japanese herbal medicine (Kampo medicine), with its philosophy that every disease is psychosomatic in origin and that herbs affect both the psyche and the soma, sometimes has a dramatic effect on somatoform disorders, although there has been no systematic study examining the effects of Kampo on somatoform disorders. We conducted a preliminary study in the Keio Kampo Clinic, which revealed that 65% of the patients had unexplained physical symptoms. This study suggests that Kampo plays an important role in the treatment of somatoform disorders in Japan. In Kampo medicine, every patient is prescribed a Kampo formula according to his/her *Sho. Sho* is equivalent to a syndrome, but it comprises psychic and somatic symptoms and signs obtained by a set of traditional physical examinations that take the patient's constitution into account. Thus, somatoform patients are treated in the same way as nonsomatoform patients, which may give them more satisfaction.

*Key words.* Herbal medicine, Kampo, Somatoform disorders, Unexplained physical symptoms, Traditional medicine

## Introduction

Although there has been no systematic study examining the effects of Japanese herbal medicine (Kampo medicine) on somatoform disorders, it has been observed that Kampo sometimes has a dramatic effect on somatoform disorders. In this article, we will give an outline of Kampo medicine, and then explain the possible benefits in applying Kampo to somatoform patients. Lastly, we will introduce briefly our preliminary and ongoing studies.

[1] Department of Neuropsychiatry, Keio University School of Medicine, 35 Shinanomachi, Shinjuku-ku, Tokyo 160-8582, Japan

[2] Department of Neuropsychiatry, Yamanashi Medical University, Yamanashi 409-38, Japan

# History and Current Status of Kampo

Kampo, Japanese herbal medicine, used to be the official medicine in Japan. It was originally developed in ancient China and came to Japan via Korea in the sixth century. Kampo developed dramatically in Japan from the sixteenth to the eighteenth centuries, when several original Japanese prescriptions were invented. In 1875, the Japanese government chose Western medicine as that which should be practiced by doctors and taught in medical schools. This led to a decline in the practice of Kampo; however, a few physicians continued the study and practice of the traditional medicine. In recent decades, Kampo medicine has become recognized for its efficacy and safety. Patients as well as physicians have reconsidered the value of its holistic and humane values. As a result of the gradual acceptance of the role of Kampo medicine, the Ministry of Health and Welfare of Japan now covers about 150 Kampo prescriptions under the National Health Insurance Plan. In a 1993 survey of 2000 physicians by the Japan Medical Association, 77% reported using Kampo, compared with only 28% in 1979.

In Kampo prescriptions, several plants are mixed, and sometimes animal and mineral constituents are included in order to get the maximum effect and to keep adverse effects at a minimum. There are approximately 200 kinds of medicinal herbs, animals, and minerals that are commonly used in Kampo prescriptions, and they are used in numerous combinations. More than 200 formulas are used routinely in Japan.

Traditionally, the patients themselves boil the preparations to extract medicinal compounds. This procedure is believed to be the most effective, and there are a number of people who are still boiling their preparations daily. However, for the convenience of the users, about 150 different formulas are now available as powdered extracts, and are used just like other chemical compounds.

The improvement induced by Kampo is usually mild and slow, but it can be dramatic and rapid. Adverse effects are rare. Those that do occur are mostly allergic reactions to natural substances.

The ten most common diseases for which Kampo formulas are prescribed are: chronic hepatitis, common cold, constipation, menopausal syndrome, essential hypertension, autonomic imbalance, allergic rhinitis, osteoarthritis, atrophic gastritis, chronic sinusitis, and bronchial asthma. In chronic hepatitis, common cold, menopausal syndrome, autonomic imbalance, osteoarthritis, and chronic sinusitis, Kampo often shows a better effect than modern Western medicine. For essential hypertension, allergic rhinitis, and bronchial asthma, Kampo shows long-acting preventive effects without significant adverse effects. For bronchial asthma, allergic rhinitis, and atopic dermatitis, Kampo formulas are included in the treatment guidelines of the Japanese Society of Allergology. Other than these diseases, Kampo is commonly used for irritable bowel syndrome, chronic pain syndrome, and other disorders which are considered to be included under somatoform disorders.

# Fundamental Philosophy and Therapeutic Theory of Kampo

The fundamental philosophy of Kampo treatment is the enhancement of the body's natural healing power. Kampo medicine traditionally teaches that health can be maintained by a correct lifestyle, food intake, and natural medicines. Herbs are believed to

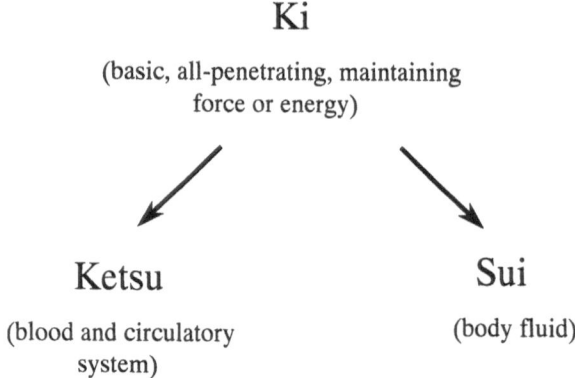

FIG. 1. The Ki-Ketsu-Sui theory

affect both the psyche and the soma. The treatment not only aims at improving or maintaining physical health but also takes into account the patient's psychic and mental balance. In Kampo medicine, every disease is psychosomatic in origin. Furthermore, the human being is regarded as a microcosm reflecting the macrocosm.

Kampo theory is completely independent of that of modern Western medicine. One of the most unique theories is the Ki-Ketsu-Sui theory (Fig. 1).

In Kampo medicine, human body functions are believed to be controlled by three components, Ki, Ketsu, and Sui. Unhealthy conditions are explained by impairment of one or a combination of the three components. The first component, Ki, is basic, all-penetrating, vital energy that is the source of all other forms of energy. Ki is equivalent to Chi in Chinese, Prana in Aryuveda, and Vis Vitalis in the traditional European medical system. Disturbances of Ki are classified as Ki-deficiency, Ki-depression, or Ki-regurgitation. Depression is considered to be due to Ki-deficiency or Ki-depression, and the panic disorder is considered to be a regurgitation of Ki. The second component, Ketsu, is equivalent to the blood and circulatory system. Disturbances of Ketsu are classified as either a deficiency or stagnation. Ketsu-deficiency is seen in anemia, and Ketsu-stagnation is seen in menopausal syndrome, dysmenorrhea, premenstrual syndrome, Raynaud's phenomenon, and similar ailments. The third component, Sui, is equivalent to the body fluids. Disturbances of Sui are disorders of body fluid metabolism, which are seen in such diseases as osteoarthritis, allergic rhinitis, and dizziness.

Since Kampo medicine regards human beings as a unit, these three components are thought to interact with each other. Especially, Ki is considered to be the most essential and thought to be the source of nourishment and stimulation for the other two components.

## *Sho:* Diagnosis in Kampo

The specific prescription is traditionally selected by judging the *Sho* of a patient. *Sho* is equivalent to a syndrome, but it comprises both psychic and somatic symptoms and signs obtained by a set of traditional physical examinations that focus on the constitution, general physical condition, pulse, abdominal signs, and the appearance of the tongue. Every patient has a specific *Sho*, and is prescribed a corresponding invariant Kampo formula.

## Possible Benefits in Applying Kampo to Somatoform Patients

There appear to be mainly two benefits in applying Kampo to somatoform patients. The first point is that somatoform patients are treated in the same way as nonsomatoform patients, which may give them more satisfaction. Somatoform patients tend to believe that their symptoms are really somatic and not psychic, so they are usually unwilling to seek psychiatric care. This leads to confusion in medical care settings and to poor treatment outcome for somatoform patients, as is generally known.

Figure 2 shows the difference in the process of deciding the treatment for the two kinds of medicine. In modern Western medicine, the treatment is decided in two steps. The first step is determining the diagnosis from the results of examinations, and the second step is determining the treatment from the diagnosis. On the other hand, in Kampo medicine, the treatment is decided in only one step, since the diagnosis, *Sho*, is itself an indication of the appropriate Kampo formula.

When we apply these systems to somatoform patients, the difference is clear (Fig. 3). In modern medicine, we find no or not enough objective findings during examinations, and the diagnosis is made as somatoform disorder, and then we have to explore treatments. Most of the patients who are recommended to take psychiatric care refuse treatment and move to other hospitals to seek additional examinations. In Kampo medicine, everyone has certain objective findings during the traditional examination, and the diagnosis is made as a specific *Sho*, which indicates a Kampo formula at the same time. Thus, somatoform patients are treated in the same way as nonsomatoform patients.

The second beneficial point is that a Kampo formula targets multiple symptoms defined by one's *Sho*. Such multiple actions of Kampo can be attributed partly to the complicated pharmacology of natural substances, and partly to the combination of

modern medicine    ( two steps)

examination $\longrightarrow$ diagnosis $\longrightarrow$ treatment

Kampo medicine    (one step)

examination $\longrightarrow$ diagnosis $=$ treatment

FIG. 2. Decision-making process in deciding treatment

## modern medicine

examination   ⟶  diagnosis ⟶ treatment

no objective findings    somatoform

disorder      ?

## Kampo medicine

examination ⟶ diagnosis ＝ treatment

certain objective     certain     prescription

findings       *Sho*     of Kampo

FIG. 3.  Treatment of somatoform patients by modern and Kampo medicine

multiple substances. Considering that the nature of somatoform symptoms is not clearly known yet, Kampo, which improves both somatic and psychic symptoms, may be a desirable remedy.

## Preliminary Study

We conducted a preliminary study [1] to investigate the effects of Kampo on somatoform disorders. In this preliminary study, the percentage of patients with medically unexplained physical symptoms among Kampo patients and their psychological well-being were examined.

The subjects were 100 patients who sought Kampo treatment for the first time at Keio University Hospital. A Japanese checklist derived from the Somatoform Disorders Schedule version 1.1 was used to check the symptoms. To assess their psychological well-being, the Subjective Well-being Inventory (SUBI) [2] was performed. The subjects' clinical records were examined afterwards to rule out symptoms which could be medically explained.

SUBI is an inventory used to evaluate psychological well-being and ill-being independently. Psychological well-being is scored on the SUBI positive scale, and psychological ill-being is scored on the SUBI negative scale. SUBI has been shown to be useful in screening for psychiatric disorders in the general population in Japan [3].

Patients with medically explained physical symptoms and patients with unexplained physical symptoms were 26% and 65% of the total, respectively. The remaining 9% were either patients without any physical symptoms who sought infertility treatment or patients who visited the clinic for their psychiatric symptoms such as anxiety and depression. As for SUBI scores, patients with unexplained physical symptoms scored significantly lower on both subscales of SUBI, which indicates that patients with unexplained physical symptoms are in a worse mental condition. Among

TABLE 1. Major reasons for seeking Kampo treatment

| | Patients with explained symptoms (%) | Patients with unexplained symptoms (%) |
|---|---|---|
| Modern medicine is not safe enough | 73.1 | 53.8 |
| Kampo would be effective | 65.4 | 53.8 |
| Effects of modern medicine are not satisfactory enough | 30.8 | 27.7 |

the patients with unexplained physical symptoms, there was a tendency for a negative correlation between the number of unexplained symptoms and SUBI subscale scores. Considering the fact that SUBI is a useful instrument in screening for psychiatric disorders, most of the patients with unexplained physical symptoms may be psychiatrically disordered, which suggests that they should be diagnosed as having somatoform disorders. It could then be said that Kampo is already playing an important role in the treatment of somatoform disorders in Japan.

Table 1 shows the patients' major reasons for seeking Kampo treatment. The efficacy and safety of Kampo were the major reasons, and this tendency was similar in both groups of patients.

## Ongoing Study

Here we introduce briefly our ongoing study. This study has three purposes. (1) Subtyping patients with unexplained physical symptoms into somatoform patients and nonsomatoform patients. What is meant by this statement is that classifying patients as having unexplained physical symptoms does not automatically mean that they have somatoform disorders. In some cases, it is possible that the symptoms cannot be explained by modern diagnostic technology but can be explained with the concepts of Kampo, since we sometimes uncover objective findings sufficient to explain the severity of the symptoms when we perform the traditional Kampo examinations. (2) Evaluating the effects of Kampo on the physical symptoms in the two subgroups. (3) Evaluating the effects of Kampo on mental condition in the two subgroups.

The subjects of this study are patients who seek Kampo treatment for their unexplained physical symptoms. NEO-PI [4] is used to evaluate the patients' personality, the Hospital Anxiety and Depression Scale (HADS) [5] is used to evaluate the patients' anxiety and depression, GAF [6] is used to evaluate the global function of the patients, and psychiatrists make a diagnosis based on interviews.

Although the number of patients is not enough yet because this study has just started, we can already see certain tendencies. Approximately one-third of the patients have anxiety and depression, both within normal limits. Thus, it is suggested that patients with unexplained physical symptoms could be separated into some subgroups including the nonsomatoform group, as we have hypothesized in planning this study. We are now increasing the number of patients, and are following HADS scores and severity of symptoms during the course of Kampo treatment, which may lead to a better understanding of the pathology of somatoform disorders and to more effective uses of Kampo.

## References

1. Mizushima H, Ono Y, Kanba S, Yamada K, Yorozu T, Yamada H, Fukuzawa M, Ishii K, Ota H, Murata T, Asai M (1997) Somatoform disorders among patients who visit Kampo Clinic (in Japanese). Jpn J Oriental Med 48:23–29
2. Sell H, Nagpal R (1992) Assessment of subjective well-being. In: WHO regional office for South Asia (ed) World Health Organization regional health paper, SEARO, No. 24. New Delhi
3. Ono Y, Yoshimura K, Yamauchi K, Momose T, Mizushima H, Asai M (1996) Psychological well-being and ill-being: WHO Subjective Well-being Inventory (SUBI) (in Japanese). Jpn J Stress Sci 10:273–278
4. Costa PT Jr, McCrae RR (1992) Revised NEO Personality Inventory (NEO PI-R) and NEO Five-Factor Inventory (NEO-FFI) professional manual. Psychological Assessment Resources, Odessa, FL
5. Zigmond A, Snaith R (1983) The hospital anxiety and depression scale. Acta Psychiatr Scand 67:361–370
6. American Psychiatric Association (1994) Diagnostic and statistical manual of mental disorders, fourth edition; DSM-IV. American Psychiatric Association, Washington

# Therapeutic Effects of Acupuncture Combined with Psychotherapy for Patients with Somatoform Disorders

Dongfen Hou[1] and Shizong Song[2]

*Summary.* The objective of the study reported in this chapter was to observe the therapeutic effect of acupuncture for the treatment of somatoform disorders. One hundred and twenty outpatients and inpatients with somatoform disorders were randomly assigned to an acupuncture plus psychotherapy group and a psychotherapy group. Cognitive psychotherapy was used in both treatment groups. Treatments lasted for 8 weeks. Hamilton Rating Scale for Depression (HRSD), the Hamilton Rating Scale for Anxiety (HRSA), and the Four-Grade Clinical Assessment were used to assess the clinical effectiveness. The percentage of patients responding to acupuncture plus psychotherapy was significantly higher than that of patients treated with psychotherapy ($P < 0.01$). The HRSD and HRSA total scores decreased much more in patients treated with acupuncture plus psychotherapy than in patients treated with psychotherapy alone ($P < 0.05$, $P < 0.01$, respectively). Acupuncture plus psychotherapy had better therapeutic effects for patients with somatoform disorders than psychotherapy alone.

*Key words.* Acupuncture, Psychotherapy, Somatoform scales, Treatment

## Introduction

Somatoform disorders constitute a very important mental health problem in general hospitals. In our clinical practice of traditional Chinese medicine, many patients with somatoform disorders come to our outpatient clinic or even to be hospitalized. However, no established therapy has been available for them. In China, acupuncture is widely used and accepted by patients. We also found that patients with somatoform disorders reading accepted acupuncture. Our present study was to investigate the therapeutic effects of acupuncture combined with psychotherapy for patients with somatoform disorders.

---

[1] Department of Acupuncture and Moxibustion, Second Affiliated Hospital of Tianjin Traditional Chinese Medicine College, Tianjin 300150, P. R. China
[2] Department of Neurology, The General Hospital of Tianjin Medical University, Tianjin 300052, P. R. China

# Patients and Methods

## Subjects

All patients met the diagnostic criteria for ICD-10 somatoform disorders [1]. Patients were either inpatients the in Department of Acupuncture or outpatients in the outpatient clinic.

## Clinical Assessments

The Hamilton Rating Scale for Depression (HRSD) [2] and the Hamilton Rating Scale for Anxiety (HRSA) [3] were used to assess clinical effectiveness. Four-Grade Clinical Assessment (completely cured; markedly improved; improved; unchanged or worse) was also used for the assessment of clinical improvement. Patients who were completely cured and markedly improved were regarded as treatment responsive. Patients who were improved, unchanged, or worse were considered unresponsive.

## Research Procedure

Patients with somatoform disorders were wash-out for 1 week. During that period, various tests including routine blood tests, ECG, EEG, liver, and renal functions were done. Patients were randomly divided into two treatment groups: one receiving psychotherapy alone, the other with acupuncture as well as psychotherapy. Treatments were given for 8 weeks. All the patients received the same cognitive psychotherapy. Treatments were given twice a week. Acupuncture was given to patients five times a week. Acupoints of Shang Xing, Bai Hui, Shen Men (both sides), and Nei Guan (both sides) were selected according to the theory of traditional Chinese medicine. The twirling reinforce method was employed. Each time the needle was manipulated for 1 min, then the needle was left in place for 20 min.

## Statistical Analysis

$\chi$-Square and $t$-tests were used for data analysis.

# Results

## General Material

One hundred twenty patients with somatoform disorders were recruited, with 60 patients in each treatment group. The age, sex, and the course of illness were not different between two groups (Table 1).

## Therapeutic Effect of Acupuncture

Patients' improvement after acupuncture treatment according to the Four-Grade Clinical Assessment was found as following: in acupuncture combining psychotherapy group: 44 (73.3%) patients responded to acupuncture plus psychotherapy, while

TABLE 1. General data of 120 patients with somatoform disorders

| | Sex | | Age (years) (mean ± SD) | Course (years) (mean ± SD) |
| --- | --- | --- | --- | --- |
| | Male | Female | | |
| Acupuncture + psychotherapy | 36 | 24 | 25.6 ± 11.5 | 4.2 ± 7.0 |
| Psychotherapy | 34 | 26 | 24.6 ± 11.8 | 4.1 ± 6.6 |

TABLE 2. Total score changes of Hamilton Rating Scale for Depression after treatment

| | $n$ | Baseline (mean ± SD) | After treatment (mean ± SD) |
| --- | --- | --- | --- |
| Acupuncture + psychotherapy | 60 | 22.5 ± 6.2 | 13.9 ± 7.6 |
| Psychotherapy | 60 | 23.4 ± 6.6 | 17.3 ± 8.5* |

* $P < 0.05$, Student $t$-test, comparing between groups.

TABLE 3. Total score changes of Hamilton Rating Scale for Anxiety after treatment

| | $n$ | Baseline (mean ± SD) | After treatment (mean ± SD) |
| --- | --- | --- | --- |
| Acupuncture + psychotherapy | 60 | 21.4 ± 6.2 | 14.3 ± 3.2 |
| Psychotherapy | 60 | 20.8 ± 6.3 | 16.9 ± 3.4** |

** $P < 0.01$, Student $t$-test, comparing groups.

28 (46.6%) patients responded to psychotherapy alone. There was a significant difference between the two groups ($P < 0.01$).

Both the Hamilton Rating Scale for Depression and Hamilton Rating scale for anxiety scores showed that acupuncture plus psychotherapy was significantly better then psychotherapy alone ($P < 0.05$, $P < 0.01$, respectively) (see Tables 2 and 3).

## Discussion

In China, patients with somatoform disorders often receive medical treatments in department of internal medicine, neurology, or gynecology of general hospitals. The somatoform patients occupy about 18.2% of total outpatients in general hospitals (F. Meng et al., unpublished data). There is no established therapy or treatment for somatoform disorders. In our clinical practice, we found that the disorders were difficult to cure. Some patients spent large funds for medication and suffered a lot from the disorders. The disorders were a great burden for the individual patients, society, and the family. Many countries have paid attention to the treatment and rehabilitation of somatoform disorder.

Our results showed that acupuncture plus psychotherapy had a better therapeutic effect for patients than psychotherapy alone. During our research, we found patients with somatoform disorders were ready to accept acupuncture treatment.

The present research was done in a general hospital of traditional Chinese medicine. In traditional Chinese medicine, there is a theory of "Unity of Physique and Vitality," which meants that the disorders can be treated from regulating the whole body function of the patients. By the use of acupuncture to regulate the heart and tranquilize vitality, we were able to offer effective treatment for patients with somatoform disorders.

## References

1. World Health Organization (1992) The ICD-10 Classification of mental and behavioral disorders: clinical descriptions and diagnostic guidelines. World Health Organization, Geneva, pp 132–173
2. Hamilton M (1967) Development of a psychiatric rating scale for primary depression. Br Soc Clin Psychol 6:278–296
3. Hamilton M (1959) The assessment of anxiety by rating scale. Br J Med Psychol 32:50–55

# The Economic Burden of Somatoform Disorders

Keita Yamauchi and Naoki Ikegami

*Summary.* While there have been few economic studies on somatoform disorders, many economic analyses have been done concerning depression, which is also a common mental illness seen in primary care settings. A large proportion of the total costs of depression are accounted for by the indirect costs, especially the morbidity costs. The background behind this distribution is as follows. First, depression results in the reduction in productivity due to absenteeism from work and decreased work performance. Second, most individuals with depression do not seek any treatment. Of those who seek help, most consult primary care physicians because of their somatic symptoms, and those physicians tend to make an inaccurate diagnosis and perform unnecessary medical tests and treatments. Because there are some similarities between depression and somatoform disorders, such as their high prevalence, impairment in productivity, and health care resource use arising from unexplained somatic symptoms, the economic aspects of somatoform disorders may share similar characteristics to that of depression. The viewpoint from health economics would have an important role in clarifying the significance of somatoform disorders, and in developing an appropriate treatment system linking psychiatric care and primary care.

*Key words.* Depression, Somatoform disorders, Practice pattern, Help-seeking behavior, Cost

## Introduction

Health economic analysis is needed for developing an efficient and appropriate health care system under resource constraints. Moreover, health economic studies play an important role in the provision of more rational treatment and intervention. Unfortunately, there have been few economic studies on somatoform disorders. However, many economic analyses have been done concerning depression, which has similarities to somatoform disorders, such as a high prevalence in the community and

Department of Health Policy and Management, Keio University School of Medicine, Shinanomachi 35, Shinjuku-ku, Tokyo, Japan

primary care settings, and utilizing health care resources arising from unexplained somatic symptoms. Therefore, we would like to consider the economic aspects of somatoform disorders by looking at the economic analysis of depression. In this paper, first, we explain the concept of cost. Second, we point out its characteristics in depression. Finally, returning to somatoform disorders, we consider somatoform disorders from the viewpoint of health economics.

## The Concept of Cost-of-Illness

When comparing the burden of a particular disease to society, the prevalence rate in the community, the number of deaths from that disease, and the health care expenditure incurred have usually been used as a measure. However, in recent years, the need to take into account the economic burden, namely cost-of-illness, has come to be recognized. In health economics, the costs of disease are generally divided into two categories, direct costs and indirect costs, which are defined as follows.

Direct costs are the value of the resources used to prevent, detect, and treat a health impairment. In other words, direct costs represent the value of all the goods, services, and other resources that are consumed in the course of a health care intervention. For example, costs of drugs, laboratory tests, supplies, health care personnel, and medical facilities are categorized as direct costs. In addition, nonhealth care resources that are used for providing health care intervention are also categorized as direct costs, for example, the costs of transportation to and from a clinic and the time family members provide at home care setting.

Indirect costs are the value of reduced, or loss of productivity as a consequence of illness. They consist of mortality costs and morbidity costs. Mortality costs are costs associated with loss of productivity due to premature death. If an individual did not die prematurely from disease, he or she would continue to be productive for a number of years. Mortality costs are estimated on the basis of the loss of lifetime earnings. Morbidity costs, which are defined as costs associated with lost or impaired ability to work due to morbidity, consist of two factors. The first is costs associated with the excess absenteeism from work, as well as with loss of employment and early retirement. The second is costs associated with a reduction in productivity while at work.

In addition to direct costs and indirect costs, intangible costs are usually regarded as a third category. Intangible costs are those associated with pain, suffering, discomfort, and reduction in quality of life occurring as a result of illness or treatment. However, due to technical difficulties in measuring the monetary equivalent of intangible costs, most studies measure only the direct and indirect costs.

## Costs of Depression

### Distribution of the Costs of Depression

Greenberg et al. estimated the annual costs of depression in the United States in 1990 (Fig. 1) [1]. The total costs were estimated to be approximately $43.7 billion per year. Of the total costs, $12.4 billion were attributed to direct costs and $31.3 billion were attributed to indirect costs. The indirect costs consisted of $7.5 billion attributed to

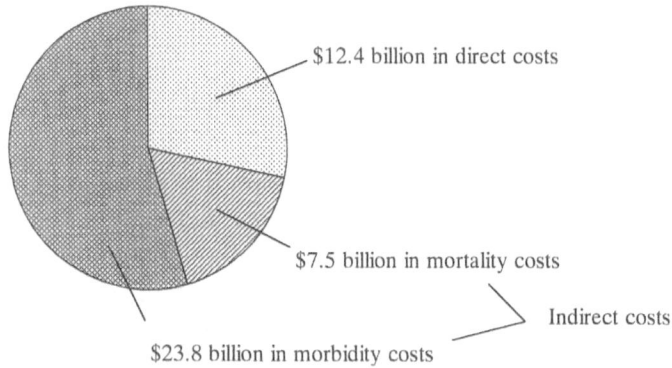

FIG. 1. The annual costs of depression in the United States in 1990 [1]

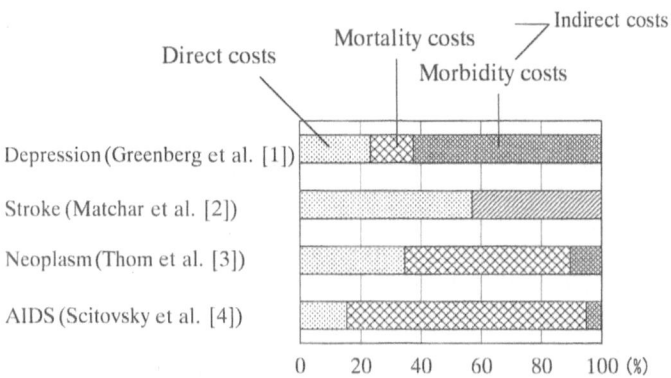

FIG. 2. Distribution of the costs of major diseases in the United States

mortality costs and $23.8 billion attributed to morbidity costs. It is significant that the major proportion of the total costs are accounted for by the indirect costs, especially the morbidity costs. The indirect costs accounted for 72% of the total costs, and 76% of the indirect costs were attributed to morbidity costs.

To clarify the characteristics of the costs of depression, comparing its distribution to other major diseases would be useful. Caution is needed when comparing estimates in different studies because the methods cannot be completely consistent. To minimize this difference, we have compared the estimated annual costs of several diseases within the United States. Figure 2 shows that a large proportion of the total costs of depression can be attributed to indirect costs and that the indirect costs can be mostly attributed to morbidity costs [2–4]. On the other hand, in stroke, more than half of the total costs can be attributed to direct costs, due to its onset later in life. With regard to AIDS, the mortality costs comprise a large proportion of the total costs because of the relatively short survival period from the onset of the disease, as well as the earlier onset in life. This comparison shows that it is important to pay attention to indirect costs when considering the economic burden of depression. If only direct costs are calculated, the costs and the social burden of depression will be underestimated.

## The Characteristics of the Costs of Depression

As an explanation of why morbidity costs comprise a large component of the total costs of depression, the following two factors have been pointed out.

The first is that depression results in the reduction in productivity due to absenteeism from work and decreased work performance [5-8]. For instance, DEPRES (Depression Research in European Society), a survey of depression in the community conducted across six European countries, showed that the number of days of work lost due to illness was more for depressed subjects than for non-depressed subjects [9].

The second is that most individuals with depression do not receive optimal treatment due to inappropriate help-seeking behavior and inappropriate practice patterns [10-12]. Although there is a high prevalence of depression in the community, half of the individuals suffering from depression do not seek any treatment. Of those who do seek help, most consult primary care physicians because of their somatic symptoms [9, 13]. However, primary care physicians fail to detect depression in up to half of the patients. They also fail to provide appropriate treatment [14]. For instance, DEPRES showed that 57% of subjects with depression sought treatment, and 89% of those seeking treatment consulted a primary care physician. Concerning treatment, of the total number of subjects with depression, 31% took medication, of whom only 25% received antidepressant therapy.

Several studies have tried to explain why depression is under-diagnosed by primary care physicians. Most patients with depression have somatic symptoms, upon which they tend to selectively focus and complain [15, 16]. At the same time, because physicians have generally received training oriented towards the biological or somatic aspects of disease, they also tend to focus on the somatic symptoms [17]. As a result, primary care physicians tend to perform costly and unnecessary medical tests and to overtreat physical symptoms. These inappropriate help-seeking behavior and practice patterns result not only in an increase in the direct costs associated with overexamination and overtreatment for somatic complaints, but also in the indirect costs due to the prolongation of distress.

The fact that most patients receive inappropriate treatment should be emphasized. Since depression is highly treatable, it is possible to reduce the overall costs by improving help-seeking behavior and practice patterns. Although the direct costs may not be reduced because costs of inappropriate treatment are replaced by costs of appropriate treatment, huge indirect costs could be potentially reduced by early detection and optimal treatment.

# Economic Burden of Somatoform Disorders

As noted at the beginning, there are few studies on the cost of somatoform disorders. However, somatoform disorders may share similar characteristics to that of depression. First, somatoform disorders are among the most prevalent of mental illnesses in the community. Second, most people with somatoform disorders consult primary care physicians, who tend to diagnose incorrectly, undertake unnecessary examinations, and overtreat physical symptoms [18]. Third, somatoform disorders may lead to impaired social and occupational functioning, which results in reduced productivity [19, 20]. Concerning prevalence rates of somatoform disorders as defined by ICD-10 or DSM-IV in the community and primary care settings, few surveys have been made except for somatization disorder, one of the subcategories of somatoform disorders [21, 22]. But according to Janca et al., it is estimated that about 5% of the general population and 30%–40% of people who seek medical care have medically unexplained somatic symptoms [23].

The above suggest that the economic aspects of somatoform disorders may share similar characteristics to that of depression. That is, indirect costs, especially morbidity costs, may account for a large proportion of the overall costs. In addition, inappropriate treatment may contribute to a greater utilization of health care resources and an increase in indirect costs due to the prolongation of distress.

Unfortunately, further economic analysis of somatoform disorders is not possible because there are not enough concrete data. A basic survey for the economic analysis should be made with detailed estimates of the costs of somatoform disorders, focusing on the reduction in productivity, patterns of help-seeking behavior, and practice patterns. If the prevalence of somatoform disorders in the community and primary care settings and its economic burden can be identified, public health experts and primary care physicians would be compelled to recognize its significance and take appropriate steps. The resulting more appropriate help-seeking behavior, diagnosis, and treatment would make a major contribution to developing an ideal system that links psychiatric care and primary care.

## References

1. Greenberg PE, Stiglin LE, Finkelstein SN et al (1993) The economic burden of depression in 1990. J Clin Psychiatry 54:405–418
2. Matchar DP, Duncan PT (1994) Cost of stroke. Stroke Clin Updates 5:9–12
3. Thom TJ (1996) Economic costs of neoplasms, arteriosclerosis, and diabetes in the United States. in vivo 10:255–260
4. Scitovsky AA, Rice DP (1987) Estimates of the direct and indirect costs of acquired immunodeficiency syndrome in the United States, 1985, 1986, and 1991. Public Health Rep 102:5–17
5. Wells KB, Stewart A, Hays RD et al (1989) The functioning and well-being of depressed patients: results from the medical outcome study. JAMA 262:914–919
6. Broadhead WE, Blazer DG, George LK et al (1990) Depression, disability days, and days lost from work in a prospective epidemiologic survey. JAMA 264:2524–2528
7. Conti DJ, Burton WN (1994) The economic impact of depression in a workplace. JOM 36:983–988
8. Ormel J, VonKorff M, Utun TB et al (1994) Common mental disorders and disability across cultures: results from the WHO collaborative study on psychological problems in general health care. JAMA 272:1741–1748
9. Lepine JP, Gastpar M, Mendlewicz J et al (1997) Depression in the community: the first pan-European study DEPRES (Depression Research in European Society). Int Clin Psychopharmacol 12:19–29

10. Regier DA, Hirschfeld RM, Goodwin FK et al (1988) The NIMH depression awareness, recognition and treatment program: structure, aims and scientific basis. Am J Psychiatry 145:1351–1357
11. Hirschfeld JP, Gastoar M, Mendlewicz J et al (1997) The National Depressive and Manic-Depressive Association consensus statement on the undertreatment of depression. JAMA 277:333–340
12. Katz SJ, Kessler RC, Lin E et al (1998) Medication management of depression in the United States and Ontario. J Gen Intern Med 13:77–85
13. Regier DA, Narrow WE, Rae DS et al (1993) The de facto US mental and addictive disorders service system: epidemiologic catchment area prospective 1-year prevalence rates of disorders and services. Arch Gen Psychiatry 50:85–94
14. Katon W, von Korff M, Lin E et al (1992) Adequacy and duration of antidepressant treatment in primary care. Med Care 30:67–76
15. Simon G, Gater R, Kisely S et al (1996) Somatic symptoms of distress: an international primary care study. Psychosom Med 58:481–488
16. Katon W, Kleinman A, Rosen G (1982) Depression and somatization: a review part I. Am J Med 72:127–135
17. Court C (1995) Report urges better psychological care. BMJ 310:1027
18. Quill TE (1985) Somatization disorder: One of medicine's blind spots. JAMA 254:3075–3079
19. Escobar JI, Golding JM, Hough RL et al (1987) Somatization in the community: relationship to disability and use of services. Am J Public Health 77:837–840
20. Spitzer RL, Kroenke K, Linzer M et al (1995) Health-related quality of life in primary care patients with mental disorders: Results from the PRIME-MD 1000 study. JAMA 274:1511–1517
21. Escobar JI, Burnam A, Karno M et al (1987) Somatization in the community. Arch Gen Psychiatry 44:713–718
22. Gureje O, Simon GE, Ustun TB et al (1997) Somatization in cross cultural perspective: a World Health Organization Study in primary care. Am J Psychiatry 154:989–995
23. Janca A, Isaac M, Costa e Silva JA (1995) World Health Organization international study of somatoform disorders: background and rationale. Eur J Psychiatry 9:100–110

# Economic Aspects of Somatoform Disorders in Japan

Kimio Yoshimura[1], Kenji Nakamura[2], Fumiko Maeda[3],
Naoko Saito[1], Hiromi Sakazume[4], Rumi Ishii[5], Nobuo Araki[6],
and Yutaka Ono[3]

*Summary.* This preliminary descriptive study examined somatoform disorders from the viewpoint of health economics in Japan. It was based on research carried out in Japan as a part of the WHO International Study of Somatoform Disorders. Subjects were 372 consecutive new patients aged 18 to 60 years, who visited a medical doctor at a general hospital from October 1994 to July 1995. They were screened by the Screener for Somatoform Disorders (SSD), a brief self-administered questionnaire. Patients suspected of having a somatoform disorder by the SSD were then interviewed by trained psychologists using the Somatoform Disorder Schedule (SDS). Eighty-one patients were screened. Seventy-two patients (19%) had one or more medically unexplained somatic symptoms by the SDS. Fifty-six patients (78%) consulted a general practitioner for their somatoform symptoms in the last year before the interview. Fifty-three patients (74%) were provided with some kind of treatment, mainly medication, for their somatoform symptoms in the last year although only about half of them felt it effective. Thirty-eight (53%) patients consulted a general practitioner three times or more during the previous year. Twenty-eight patients (39%) with somatoform symptoms could not carry out their usual daily activities fully. Most of the patients (93%) with unexplained physical symptoms consulted a doctor for their somatoform symptoms and/or could not carry out their daily activities fully. When considering total cost as the sum of direct and indirect costs, practically everyone with somatoform symptoms suffers from the economic burden. It is important not only medically but also economically to diagnose and treat patients with somatoform symptoms in primary care settings.

*Key words.* Somatoform disorders, Economic burden, Cost, Somatoform Disorder Schedule (SDS)

[1] Cancer Information and Epidemiology Division, National Cancer Center Research Institute, 5-1-1 Tsukiji Chuo-ku, Tokyo 104-0045, Japan
[2] Ministry of Health and Welfare, Japan
[3] Department of Neuropsychiatry, Keio University School of Medicine
[4] Graduate School of Business Administration, Keio University
[5] Welfare Center of Meguro, Japan
[6] Nippon Kokan Hospital

# Introduction

Somatoform disorder is explained as "the presence of physical symptoms that suggest a general medical condition and are not fully explained by a general medical condition."[1] Individuals with unexplained physical symptoms, if not properly treated, overuse health care services [2–7]. In somatoform disorder, "the symptoms cause clinically significant distress or impairment in social, occupational, or other areas of functioning" [1]. From the economic point of view, such overuse and impairments are strongly associated with the cost of somatoform disorders. A number of studies have previously focused on the cost of somatoform disorders [8, 9].

The aim of this study was to investigate somatoform disorders from the viewpoint of health economics in Japan. It was based on research carried out in Japan as a part of the WHO International Study of Somatoform Disorders. We focused on the utilization of health care services and the decline of daily activities among those who have somatoform symptoms. The former is considered as direct cost, and the latter as indirect cost.

# Subjects and Methods

Subjects were 372 consecutive new patients aged 18 to 60 years, who visited a medical doctor at Nippon Kokan Hospital from October 1994 to July 1995. Nippon Kokan Hospital is located in the urban district of Kawasaki city in Kanagawa prefecture, Japan.

Subjects were screened by the Screener for Somatoform Disorders (SSD) [10]. The SSD is a brief self-administered questionnaire developed by the WHO for screening somatoform disorders. Patients suspected of having somatoform disorders by the SSD were then interviewed by trained psychologists using the Somatoform Disorders Schedule (SDS) [11]. The SDS, also developed by the WHO, is a structured interview schedule used to diagnose somatoform disorders, anxiety disorders, depressive disorders, and alcohol dependence. In addition, patients' activities during the last month before the interview and their health care utilization during the last year were taken into consideration. The utilization of health care obtained by the interview was investigated as an index of direct cost. This includes whether or not they consult a general practitioner, frequency of consultation, content of treatment, and subjective therapeutic response. The reduction of daily activities reflects indirect cost. Chi-squared tests or Fisher's exact tests were used where appropriate to test statistical significance.

# Results

Eighty-one patients were suspected of having somatoform symptoms by the SSD. These patients were then interviewed by psychologists using the SDS. Seventy-two patients (19%) had one or more medically unexplained somatic symptoms. One patient was diagnosed as anxiety disorder, six as depressive disorders, and five as alcohol dependent. Eight patients (11%) with somatoform symptoms had a comorbidity of other mental disorders (1 with anxiety disorder, 4 with depressive disorders, and 3 with alcohol dependence).

TABLE 1. Frequency of consulting general practitioners in the last year among patients with somatoform symptoms ($n = 72$)

| | | |
|---|---|---|
| None | 16 | 22% |
| Subtotal (once or more) | 56 | 78% |
| Once | 9 | 13% |
| Twice | 9 | 13% |
| Three times or more | 38 | 53% |
| Total | 72 | 100% |

TABLE 2. Number of patients who received specific types of treatment for somatoform disorders

| | | |
|---|---|---|
| Medication | 53/72 | 74% |
| Surgery | 4/72 | 6% |
| Psychotherapy or counseling | 0/72 | |
| Acupuncture | 1/72 | 1% |
| Other alternative treatment | 4/72 | 6% |
| Ritual cure | 0/72 | |
| Traditional healing | 0/72 | |
| Other treatment | 0/72 | |
| No treatment | 19/72 | 26% |

Table 1 shows the frequency of consulting a general practitioner in the last year among patients with somatoform symptoms. Fifty-six patients (78%) consulted a general practitioner in the last year for their somatoform symptoms. The number of patients who saw a general practitioner once and twice were 9 (13%) each. Thirty-eight (53%) patients consulted a general practitioner more than twice in the last year. All 8 patients with a comorbidity of anxiety disorder, depressive disorder, or alcohol dependence consulted general practitioners, and these patients did not consult a psychiatrist at all.

The treatment received by the patients with one or more somatoform symptoms is shown in Table 2. Fifty-three patients (74%) were provided with medication, 4 had surgery, 1 had acupuncture, and 4 had other alternative treatments. Only 19 patients (26%) received no treatment at all.

Twenty-six patients answered that their symptoms improved after some kind of treatment, whereas 27 patients answered that their symptoms had worsened or had no change. The effect of treatment for each kind of treatment is shown in Table 3. Approximately half of those who received medication answered that the treatment was effective. All of those who received surgery answered that it was effective. However, statistical significance was not evident ($P = 0.12$) for all these results. There was no significant difference in the frequency of consultation between the improvement group and the worsening or no-change group among patients who consulted a general practitioner.

TABLE 3. Effectiveness of different treatments

|  | Improvement | Worsened/no change |
|---|---|---|
| Medication | 25 | 22 |
| Surgery | 4 | 0 |
| Acupuncture | 0 | 1 |
| Other alternative treatment | 4 | 0 |

TABLE 4. Number of patients whose activity decreased during the last month because of their somatoform symptoms

| | |
|---|---|
| Unable to carry out fully their usual daily activities | 28/72 (39%) |
| Had to stay in bed most of the day for 1 or more days | 17/72 (24%) |

Table 4 shows the number of patients whose activity declined during the last month because of their somatoform symptoms. Twenty-eight patients (39%) were unable to carry out their usual daily activities fully during the last month because of their somatoform symptoms. Seventeen patients (24%) answered that they had to stay in bed most of the day for 1 or more days during the last month because of their somatoform symptoms.

Of the 72 patients with somatoform symptoms, only 5 patients (7%) did not consult a general practitioner for their somatoform symptoms and were able to carry out their usual daily activities fully. That is to say, 93% of patients with unexplained physical symptoms consulted a general practitioner about their somatoform symptoms and/or could not carry out their daily activities fully.

## Discussion

This preliminary descriptive study indicates the following: (1) three-quarters of the patients with medically unexplained somatic symptoms consulted a general practitioner before they visited Nippon Kokan Hospital; (2) three quarters of the patients with somatoform symptoms were provided with some kind of treatment, mainly medication, for their somatoform symptoms in the last year although only about half of them felt it effective; (3) about half of the patients with somatoform symptoms consulted a general practitioner three times or more during the last year; (4) about one third of the patients with somatoform symptoms could not carry out their usual daily activities fully; (5) most of the patients (93%) with unexplained physical symptoms consulted a doctor for their somatoform symptoms and/or could not carry out their daily activities fully.

In this study, 19% of subjects had one or more somatic complaints for which no organic etiology could be found. Previous studies observed that 20% to 84% of patients in general medical settings present medically unexplained physical symptoms [12, 13]. The prevalence of patients with somatoform symptoms varies greatly among studies, partly due to the difference in study design. Still, it can be seen that there is a considerable number of patients with somatoform symptoms.

Consulting a general practitioner twice may be useful if the patient demands a second opinion. However, three or more repetitive consultations for the same complaint seem to constitute an overuse of health services. It is a burden for the patients not only in terms of time, but also in terms of money.

One half of those who received treatment did not find it effective. Most received medication as treatment, and treatment other than with medication was rare. It may be useful to investigate further what kinds of drugs were actually used. Craig et al. reported that the physical symptoms of somatizers were less likely to improve than those of patients with pure physical illness or those whose physical and psychiatric symptoms had only a chance association, and that one third of the somatizers continued to experience their physical symptoms at the point of 2-year follow-up [14]. Speckens et al. showed that 76% of patients with unexplained physical symptoms in a general medical outpatient clinic reported that they had recovered or improved [15]. Low therapeutic response may imply inappropriate treatment and hence will produce an overuse of health resources. As can be seen from this study, the high proportion of patients seeing a general practitioner, the low recovery rate, and the high frequency of seeing the doctor infer that the patients with somatoform disorders consume a great number of health resources, ultimately leading to high direct cost.

One third of the patients with somatoform symptoms could not carry out their usual daily activities fully in this study. This confirms findings of previous studies, i.e., that restricted daily activities lead to substantial social and occupational disability and impaired functioning [5, 6, 16]. This is regarded as indirect cost.

When considering total cost as the sum of direct and indirect costs, practically everyone with somatoform symptoms suffers from the economic burden. It is important not only medically but also economically to diagnose and treat patients with physical symptoms that are not fully explained by a general medical condition in primary care settings.

Smith et al. have verified the validity of psychiatric consultation for the management of these patients in a clinical trial [9]. The intervention improved physical functioning and reduced medical charges in patients with somatoform symptoms. Effective management for somatoform disorder patients includes regular visits, careful physical examination, and avoidance of hospitalization [7].

In Japan, general practitioners are far from familiar with the concept of somatoform disorders as well as other psychiatric disorders. In this study, all eight patients with a comorbidity of anxiety disorder, depressive disorder, or alcohol dependence consulted general practitioners, without consulting a psychiatrist at all. This result suggests that mental disorders of these patients were not recognized as mental disorders by general practitioners. General practitioners need to be aware of the concept of somatoform disorders in order to manage patients with somatoform disorders properly. This may be the preliminary step needed to avoid wasting medical resources associated with somatoform disorders.

We have been examining the economic burden of somatoform disorders on the basis of a hospital-based study. Although a population-based study is necessary in order to obtain more knowledge about somatoform disorders among the general population, there are a number of problems to overcome beforehand (e.g., the difficulty in ruling out organic disorders) [17].

Three years have passed since we conducted this research. We are now conducting a follow-up study. From this follow-up study, the course and outcome of these patients with somatoform disorders will be identified.

## References

1. American Psychiatric Association (1994) Diagnostic and statistical manual of mental disorders, fourth edn. American Psychiatric Association, Washington, pp 445–469
2. Bass C, Benjamin S (1993) The management of chronic somatisation. Br J Psychiatry 162:72–80
3. Sato T, Takeichi M, Shirahama M, Fukui T, Gude JK (1995) Doctor-shopping patients and users of alternative medicine among Japanese primary care patients. Gen Hosp Psychiatry 17:115–125
4. Smith GR Jr, Monson RA, Ray DC (1986) Patients with multiple unexplained symptoms. Their characteristics, functional health, and health care utilization. Arch Intern Med 146:69–72
5. Escobar JI, Golding JM, Hough RL, Karno M, Burnam MA, Wells KB (1987) Somatization in the community: relationship to disability and use of services. Am J Public Health 77:837–840
6. Simon GE, VonKorff M (1991) Somatization and psychiatric disorder in the NIMH epidemiologic catchment area study. Am J Psychiatry 148:1494–1500
7. Zhang M, Booth BM, Smith GR Jr (1998) Services utilization before and after the prospective payment system by patients with somatization disorder. J Behav Health Serv Res 25:76–82
8. Shaw J, Creed F (1991) The cost of somatization. J Psychosom Res 35:307–312
9. Smith GR Jr, Rost K, Kashner TM (1995) A trial of the effect of a standardized psychiatric consultation on health outcomes and costs in somatizing patients. Arch Gen Psychiat 52:238–243
10. Isaac M, Tacchini G, Janca A (1994) Screener for Somatoform Disorders (SSD) version 2.0. World Health Organization, Geneva
11. Tacchini G, Janca A, Isaac M (1994) Somatoform Disorders Schedule (SDS) version 2.0. World Health Organization, Geneva
12. Van Hemert AM, Hengeveld MW, Bolk JH, Rooijmans HG, Vandenbroucke JP (1993) Psychiatric disorders in relation to medical illness among patients of a general medical out-patient clinic. Psychol Med 23:167–173
13. Kellner R (1985) Functional somatic symptoms and hypochondriasis. A survey of empirical studies. Arch Gen Psychiatry 42:821–833
14. Craig TK, Boardman AP, Mills K, Daly-Jones O, Drake H (1993) The south-London somatisation study. I. Longitudinal course and the influence of early life experiences. Br J Psychiatry 163:579–588
15. Speckens AE, Van Hemert AM, Bolk JH, Rooijmans HG, Hengeveld MW (1996) Unexplained physical symptoms: outcome, utilization of medical care and associated factors. Psychol Med 26:745–752
16. Zoccolillo M, Cloninger CR (1986) Somatization disorder: psychologic symptoms, social disability, and diagnosis. Comp Psychiatry 27:65–73
17. Faravelli C, Salvatori S, Galassi F, Aiazzi L, Drei C, Cabras P (1997) Epidemiology of somatoform disorders: a community survey in Florence. Soc Psychiatry Psychiatr Epidemiol 32:24–29

# Part 4
# Summary and Outlook

# Rhetorics of the Body: Medically Unexplained Symptoms in Sociocultural Perspective

Laurence J. Kirmayer

*Summary.* Medically unexplained symptoms place patients in a distinctive social predicament. Their conditions are ambiguous and so their expectations for treatment and recovery are uncertain. Their symptoms may be attributed by clinicians to psychological traits or conflicts, and the reality and legitimacy of their suffering and disability may be challenged. To maintain medical attention and support, and legitimate their distress, patients must be skilled in rhetoric. Rhetorical practices shape the presentation of somatic symptoms in primary care, specialty medicine, and psychiatry. Beyond this clinical context, somatic symptoms may have rhetorical value as: (1) an index of disease or disorder; (2) an indication of psychopathology; (3) a symbolic expression of intrapsychic or interpersonal conflict; (4) a culturally coded "idiom of distress"; (5) a metaphor for experience; (6) a strategy for expressing social discontent; and (7) a mechanism through which people attempt to reposition themselves in their local worlds. The clinical treatment of somatoform disorders, as well as the responses of the disability and compensation systems, can be analyzed in terms of their influence on these different levels of meaning. Analysis of the rhetorical power of institutional practices to transform the meaning of somatic distress can guide the development of new clinical and social strategies to help individuals with medically unexplained somatic distress.

*Key words.* Somatization, Discourse, Causal attribution, Culture, Treatment

## Rhetorics of the Body

Around the world and across diverse cultural groups, somatic symptoms are the most common individual expression of social problems and emotional distress [1]. Despite this ubiquity, as a result of the mind-body dualism inherent in the Western cultural

---

Division of Social and Transcultural Psychiatry, McGill University, and Culture and Mental Health Research Unit, Institute of Community and Family Psychiatry, Sir Mortimer B. Davis—Jewish General Hospital, 4333 Côte Ste-Catherine Road, Montréal, Québec H3T 1E4, Canada
Preparation of this chapter was supported by a grant from the Fonds de la recherche en santé du Québec.

concept of the person and in biomedical practice itself, bodily expressions of emotional distress, in the absence of medical disease, have been considered to be a special category of psychopathology, the somatoform disorders, and are attributed to specific psychological mechanisms of "somatization" [2]. This partition of somatoform disorders from anxiety, depressive, and dissociative disorders does not reflect the natural covariation of symptoms in syndromes which often cut across these categories (a fact misleadingly labeled "comorbidity"). However, the existence of a distinct category of somatoform disorders suits the institutional role of psychiatry and other mental health practitioners in general hospital and primary care settings. In these medical contexts, psychiatrists are called upon to diagnose and treat patients whose problems fall between the cracks of a nosological system increasingly organized by laboratory markers of physiological disturbance. The term "somatization" turns the ambiguity and uncertainty of medically unexplained symptoms into the presumptive clarity of a distinct form of psychopathology. Any serious analysis of the problem should probably begin by reversing this rhetorical move and turning "somatization" back into its "raw observable": medically unexplained symptoms.

Of course, medically unexplained symptoms are not a natural category but a culturally and historically contingent reflection of the current state of medical practice. As medical knowledge advances, and as diagnostic fashions change, some symptoms or problems are satisfactorily explained while other previously accepted explanations may fall into disrepute, with fresh uncertainty raised about the significance of common symptoms. The recent history of fibromyalgia syndrome presents a case in point. This common syndrome of muscular aches and pains was once termed "fibrositis" and symptoms were implicitly attributed to an inflammatory process [3]. No consistent musculoskeletal pathology has ever been documented, however, so the syndrome has been redefined as a form of pain disorder. Multiple anatomical sites sensitive to pressure ("tenderpoints") have been taken as pathognomonic but these are found in other conditions. The status of fibromyalgia as a valid medical explanation for aches and pains today is less contested than 20 years ago, despite the absence of any great advance in our understanding of pathophysiology or treatment. The current situation varies for other common unexplained symptoms: for example, abdominal pain often is confidently attributed to irritable bowel syndrome which itself is taken to be a consequence of a disturbance in gut motility (though there may not be confirmatory changes in bowel habit or other measurable disorder); in contrast, persistent fatigue may be labeled "chronic fatigue syndrome" but this remains a hotly contested diagnostic entity. Many other functional somatic symptoms and syndromes have plausible physiological explanations but these are not consistently accepted as valid medical diagnoses [4].

An integrated model of somatization considers the role of individual physiological and psychological factors in generating and amplifying bodily sensations and misattributing ordinary sensations to somatic disease, resulting in activity avoidance and disability [5]. Whatever the underlying basis or ultimate explanation of their symptoms, though, patients with medically unexplained symptoms face a distinct social predicament. The response of clinicians, family, friends, and employers as well as the compensation and disability systems is influenced by the lack of a clearcut medical explanation. Social responses may contribute to patients' recovery or exacerbate their distress and disability. The dilemmas posed by unexplained distress demand close analysis since they may yield insights into pathogenesis and chronicity as well as effective intervention.

This chapter will focus on interpersonal and social aspects of symptom experience and illness behavior in the somatoform disorders. A social perspective examines the influence of ideologies and institutions on "body practices" and discourse [6, 7]. Body practices include the many ways that we handle the body throughout individual development and across many different situations, in families, the workplace, recreation, and in clinical settings. Different ways of handling the body shape illness experience during infancy and childhood, and influence adult illness behavior [8–10].

The focus in this chapter, however, will be primarily on discourse, which includes everyday conversation, interactions with clinicians, and accounts provided in lay and professional literature. In all of these situations, people are called upon to narrate and explain their bodily experience. They do this by taking up some of the many narrative strands available from their own past experience, mass media, and medical encounters. They then give accounts aimed to alleviate their own distress and to explain or justify their predicament to others. The basic notion of discursive psychology relevant to rethinking the somatoform disorders is that narratives of bodily experience and illness not only reflect their specific social and cultural background, they contribute directly to our subsequent bodily experience [11–13].

Discourse that aims to influence others falls into the domain of rhetoric [14]. While patients with clearcut medical conditions are readily granted the sick role, patients with medically unexplained symptoms often must convince others of the reality, seriousness, and urgency of their symptoms and suffering. To obtain validation of their illness at home and at work, and to maintain medical interest in their vexing problems, they must be skilled rhetoricians. This rhetorical enterprise then becomes a major feature of the illness behavior and experience of sufferers. Family interaction, clinical diagnostic practices, treatment interventions, workman's compensation, and disability systems, can all be examined in terms of their rhetorical goals and strategies. This level of analysis can help to identify social issues or problems where interventions may prevent, or improve the outcome of, common somatic syndromes.

## The Predicament of Medically Unexplained Distress

Somatic symptoms that have no obvious basis in injury or disease are variously labeled as medically unexplained, "not yet diagnosed," "functional" (in contrast to "organic"), or " psychosomatic." Clinicians commonly attribute unexplained symptoms to psychological factors or social stress. There are significant stressful events and psychological conflicts in most people's everyday life so this sort of attribution is easy to make. Unfortunately, the causal role of any given psychosocial factors is usually impossible to confirm in an individual case owing to the epistemological limitations of the clinical situation [15]. A wealth of experimental work suggests that psychological factors can influence the full range of physiological processes that give rise to distress. Despite this conceptual and empirical union of the psyche and soma, the implicit dualism of biomedicine makes a significant ontological distinction between "real" disease (with demonstrable physical pathology) and "imaginary" illness, which arises exclusively from patients' cognitive processes [16]. Thus, while the term "psychosomatic" includes the possibility of a psychophysiological basis for symptoms, in practice it often amounts to a dismissal of illness as "all in the head." This dualism persists not because of any rigidity of biomedicine itself but because it is woven into broader cultural concepts of the person that are slow to change.

Medically unexplained symptoms therefore present a kind of double jeopardy for patients: their problems are ill-understood and, often, poorly treated. As a result, patients experience a high degree of uncertainty or ambiguity about the meaning of their symptoms, the correct course of action to take, and the likely outcome. This ambiguity results in a continuing search for definite diagnosis and effective treatment. It may lead to frequent changes in care providers or the pursuit of multiple sources of care at once. The resultant confusion and contradiction further heightens ambiguity and uncertainty, which are in themselves sources of anxiety.

At the same time, unexplained symptoms may be readily attributed to psychological factors with pejorative implications. While such common psychophysiological disturbances as hyperventilation or sleep disorders can explain many somatic symptoms, many mental health practitioners prefer more purely psychological or interpersonal explanations. Psychological explanations generally convey connotations of problems being at once less serious, less deserving of the conventional sick role, more due to the patients' own bad actions or character flaws and therefore, more directly damaging of their social identity. As a result of this potential stigma, patients are naturally eager to avoid psychiatric labeling and seek a medical or other external, environmental explanation for their distress.

At the same time, psychological attributions serve a basic clinical goal: to provide a diagnostic label or explanation for every patient's problem. The dividend for clinicians is that because psychological and psychiatric diagnoses tend to imply that patients are responsible for their own problems, the clinician is relieved of some of the frustration or anxiety he or she is likely to feel due to continuing diagnostic uncertainty and the limitations of current biomedical treatments.

The ambiguity and ambivalence of the clinical response to medically unexplained symptoms creates a crisis of legitimation for patients and clinicians [17]. The search for legitimation drives the help-seeking of these patients, who tend to consult many care providers, and contributes to their frequent evaluation of these encounters as frustrating and disappointing.

This is illustrated by results from a study we conducted of patients with three common functional somatic syndromes (FSS) (fibromyalgia (FMS), irritable bowel (IBS), and chronic fatigue (CFS)) compared to patients with clear-cut medical diagnoses (non-FSS) with some similar symptoms (rheumatoid arthritis (RA), inflammatory bowel disease (IBD), and multiple sclerosis (MS)) [18]. Forty consecutive patients with each of the diagnoses were recruited from the practices of medical specialists. As shown in Table 1, patients with FSS sought more sources of help than did the non-FSS patients. This difference was mainly due to the chronic fatigue group. CFS patients had tried significantly more different types of treatment than all other groups. However, CFS patients found treatments less helpful than did RA, IBS, IBD, and MS patients. FMS patients and IBS patients tended to find treatments less helpful than did their corresponding non-FSS comparison groups, RA and IBD. All of the FSS groups found their sources of help less understanding of their condition than did the non-FSS patients. Interestingly, the mean number of helpful sources

TABLE 1. Lifetime health care utilization of functional somatic syndrome (FSS) and non-FSS groups

| FSS (n = 127) Mean (SD) | non-FSS (n = 138) Mean (SD) | Significance test |
|---|---|---|
| Total number of sources of health care ever used[a] | | |
| 9.8 (3.1) | 8.2 (2.7) | $t = 4.49$; df $= 263$, $P < 0.001$ |
| Total number of sources used for current diagnosis | | |
| 8.0 (4.3) | 6.7 (3.2) | $t = 2.74$; df $= 230.12$, $P < 0.01$ |
| Proportion of sources found to be helpful[b] | | |
| 0.51 (0.25) | 0.68 (0.28) | $t = 4.93$; df $= 263$, $P < 0.001$ |
| Degree to which sources understand condition[c] | | |
| 2.01 (0.80) | 2.61 (1.05) | $t = 5.18$, df $= 254.81$, $P < 0.001$ |
| Total number of treatments tried[d] | | |
| 6.3 (3.5) | 5.6 (2.5) | $t = 2.08$; df $= 226.81$, $P < 0.05$ |
| Proportion of treatments found helpful[e] | | |
| 0.65 (0.27) | 0.81 (0.21) | $t = 5.49$; df $= 237.1$, $P < 0.05$ |

[a] Lifetime utilization counting distinct practitioners or settings (e.g., self care, family friends, hospital emergency room, rheumatologist, gastroenterologist, general practitioners, physiotherapist, chiropractor, acupuncturist, etc.).
[b] Rated helpful (1) or not (0) on single dichotomous item and averaged over total number of sources ever used.
[c] "How you feel people there [at each type of provider] understood your problems" rated on 4-point Likert scale from "not at all" (1), "somewhat" (2), "well" (3), "very well" (4).
[d] Use of distinct types of treatment including: analgesics, antibiotics, steroids, antiinflammatory medication, dietary advice, exercise, relaxation training, etc.
[e] Rated helpful (1) or not (0) on single dichotomous item and averaged over total number of treatments used.

in the two groups is similar. This suggests that the excess health care utilization of FSS patients is commensurate with their perception that much of the care they receive is not helpful.

In other results (not shown), FSS patients were more likely than non-FSS patients to have received and to be making current use of psychological or psychiatric care. Those FSS patients receiving psychological care tended to find it less useful than did their non-FSS counterparts. As well, they rated the mental health practitioner they were seeing as much less understanding of their problem than did the non-FSS patients. Patients with CFS reported higher levels of family burden and stigma associated with their condition than did any other group. Patients with FSS were more likely than non-FSS patients to report that care providers had made them feel that their problems were somehow not real, were due to emotional factors, and that they were somehow to blame for their illness.

Legitimation is a problem not only in the clinical setting but in the workplace and for the insurance system that seeks some reliable way to determine who is deserving of compensation for their illness and who can be justifiably denied. As Beaulieu [17] has shown in a study of these same chronic fatigue patients, their families, physicians, and insurance providers, all of the implicated groups are involved in similar dilemmas of setting boundaries on ill-defined conditions that they fear will make limitless demands on limited resources. This raises the stakes in a situation of conflicting interests and unequal power. The vociferous claims of patient advocacy groups and the rigid rejection of psychological explanations for distress are both causes and consequences of this highly charged social context.

Clearly, patients with medically unexplained symptoms face specific obstacles to effective coping with their distress [19]. The persistent ambiguity of the meaning of medically unexplained symptoms prevents settling on a fixed interpretation and course of action that would allow less thought and attention to symptoms. Instead, ambiguity promotes continued cognitive effort to figure out the meaning of symptoms and assess just how alarmed one should be—and whether one is overlooking some potential diagnostic or treatment approach. At the same time, the relative lack of lay medical information organized by symptom rather than diagnosis limits information-seeking unless patients can fit their symptoms into a well-known disease or disorder. The tendency to receive psychological attributions for symptoms lurks constantly in the background as a way to "explain away" symptoms at the cost of the patient's self-esteem, often without any direct translation into more effective coping strategies. Finally, the absence of other sufferers with validated illness against whose experience one can gauge one's own success in coping, leaves doubt about whether one is exaggerating or minimizing distress. Patients then must provide their own measure of the appropriateness of distress and disability, which can only be vouchsafed by articulate expressions of their suffering. The only way they can shift attention away from efforts to demonstrate the gravity of their illness is to have it fully acknowledged and legitimated.

## The Social Amplification of Somatic Distress

Beyond the psychological impact of having an ill-defined condition, powerful social factors may shape illness experience and behavior. It is difficult to subject these large-scale factors to experimental manipulation or even to conduct epidemiological studies that isolate the significant social factors, since this requires systematic comparison of different health and social systems which inevitably differ in many more ways than the specific factors of immediate interest. However, case studies give evidence of the dramatic influence of social factors on the course of medically unexplained distress.

From 1983 to 1987, Australia witnessed an epidemic of upper limb regional pain among workers in occupations requiring repetitive movements of wrist and forearm (e.g., computer keyboard operators) [20]. The first workman's compensation claims for repetitive strain injury (RSI) were made in 1983 and the number increased dramatically from 1984 to 1985, leveled off in 1986, and then declined equally rapidly to preepidemic levels by 1988.

Typical symptoms included disabling hand, arm, shoulder, and neck pain along with numbness, paresthesias, and headache. Initial symptoms were diffuse with only a minority of patients having well-defined syndromes (e.g., carpal tunnel, tenosynovitis, epicondylitis) and there were rarely any clinical signs. The regional pain syndromes were often accompanied by anxiety, depression, and "preoccupation with the significance of the symptoms." Significantly, RSI did not appear in other industrialized countries using the same technologies (in the United States, concern about the ill effects of video display terminals was more prominent). This points to the role of some local, presumably social, factors giving rise to the condition or, at least, to widespread awareness of it.

Medical opinion turned the everyday problem in living of "muscle strain" into a discrete pathological entity with recognized potential for serious disablement. This reframing included a specific set of attributions to repetitive movements in work settings, which were endorsed by medical specialists as well as by the National Occupational Health and Safety Commission.

As the epidemic progressed it became apparent that the majority of sufferers had no definite evidence of injury or other pathology. Several observers began to liken RSI to a form of mass psychogenic illness akin to conversion disorder or epidemic forms of health anxiety. Cases tended to occur in clusters and were more common among women. However, the problem tended to be chronic and disabling rather than presenting as acute anxiety, and most of the symptoms could not be accounted for by hyperventilation. Among those still convinced of a physical basis but concerned about unwarranted levels of disability, suggestions were made for relabeling the problem as a chronic pain syndrome or "localized" fibromyalgia complicated by conflict over returning to work.

Musculoskeletal pain is common in the general population, and occupational activities may well cause or aggravate such pain with gross evidence of injury. The existence of a diagnostic category provides a schema to organize bodily sensations, search for additional symptoms consistent with the pain, and maintain attention on symptoms to monitor their waxing and waning. Medical legitimation of symptoms as part of a syndrome may set up a series of contingencies including clinical care, release from work, and workman's compensation that, inadvertently, reinforce attention to the symptoms, sick role behavior, and disability. "Once involved in litigation the claimant was placed in the untherapeutic situation of having to demonstrate illness or disability for the 2 to 3 years that settlement took" ([20], p. 647).

The social amplification of RSI went beyond this familiar dilemma of the disability system. The occupational health movement in Australia used the issue of RSI to press for improvements in work conditions [21]. Economic forces also probably played a significant role in the origins of the epidemic. RSI emerged at a time of increasing unemployment, which some labor unions linked directly to the introduction of computer technology. Mass media also depicted RSI as a widely prevalent and seriously disabling disorder. Occupational health workers, union leaders, and mass media thus all contributed to making the notion of RSI salient and credible [21].

RSI became an emblem of other social problems in Australia: work dissatisfaction, the socioeconomic plight of migrants, concerns about the impact of automation in the workplace, as well as idiosyncratic issues of individuals. RSI functioned rhetorically as "a polysemic metaphor not only for what ailed the Australian workforce but for what ails Australian society" ([22], p. 185). Ironically, "the social movement characteristics of RSI . . . (were) used as a basis for attacking its legitimacy" ([21], p. 229). The tacit assumption seemed to be that a real problem would be recognized without the need for advocacy. Once a problem becomes the focus of lobbying, its validity is suspect. Arguments for the causal role of social factors, while pointing to problems in the workplace and the larger economic system, also implied that RSI was not really a medical problem. In a further irony, social constructivist perspectives helped to dismantle the case for RSI being a "real" biomedical disorder by undermining the significance of efforts of RSI proponents to wield scientific methods to prove its existence [21]. Ultimately, the challenge to the status quo posed through RSI was neutralized by psychological attributions: RSI was transformed from an indication of poor conditions in the workplace to a sign of individual vulnerability or even culpability.

A second example of the social shaping of medically unexplained distress is found in the area of allergy and toxicology, in the form of multiple chemical sensitivity, total allergy syndrome, twentieth century disease, or environmental illness [23, 24]. People with these conditions describe a wide range of symptoms involving headache, fatigue, weakness, paresthesias, impaired concentration, skin rashes, breathing difficulties, and the gamut of neurological, mood, and behavioral symptoms. They attribute their symptoms to the immunologic or toxic effects of environmental substances and characteristically report multiple sensitivities; in the majority of cases, however, no consistent relationship to antigens or toxins can be established. Sufferers often must make drastic changes in lifestyle and activity to avoid exposure to materials that trigger symptoms.

Environmental illness (EI) has become a prevalent concern in Halifax, Nova Scotia (C. Fletcher, personal communication, 1998). After a major outbreak of work-related EI at a local hospital, the provincial government funded a specialized clinic, the Nova Scotia Environmental Health Center, which currently has a waiting list of some 1500 people. Lobbying of self-help and advocacy groups (e.g., the Community Advisory Resources for the Environmentally Sensitive) has led to the creation of "scent-free areas" in public places, where people are asked to avoid the use of aftershave, cologne, or perfumes, because these may have negative health effects.

Although EI has been described in most industrialized settings, its apparent high prevalence in Nova Scotia is attributed by many sufferers to prevailing weather patterns along the Atlantic seaboard which carry airborne chemicals from the large industrial centers of the eastern United States. Once an economic and transportation center of Canada, Halifax has suffered decline in this century. The current sense of economic, political, and geographic marginality fits with the image of the teeming megalopolises of the eastern seaboard carelessly dumping effluents into the air. A collective sense of identity as a vulnerable and forgotten people interacts with specific notions about the unhealthy effects of urbanization to amplify concerns about effects of pollution, chemicals, and other modern effluvia. Just as in the early stages of the RSI epidemic, the clinical and governmental responses to the problem may increase the legitimacy, salience, and prevalence of the condition.

Both RSI and EI can be understood, in part, as problems of symptom attribution. From the point of view of biomedicine, in most cases the explanations of symptoms in terms of environmental factors appear to be misattributions. However, the symptoms fit prevailing illness models, and the sense of bodily vulnerability is supported by wider social concerns. Of course, not every individual exposed to these ideas gets RSI, EI, or some other functional somatic syndrome. Identifying individuals at risk involves consideration of pre-existing psychopathology and social stressors. It also requires consideration of how illness representations spread throughout a population—a sort of "epidemiology of representations" that examines the circulation and contagion of ideas and anxieties [25]. Whether a particular illness representation becomes popular and gets taken up by many people depends on many different social factors, including: (1) the aptness of representations in terms of coexisting cultural representations and practices; (2) which agents promote the representation (not only individuals with power and authority but lay groups, corporations and institutions); (3) how the representation is deployed, i.e., used technically and rhetorically in day-to-day and clinical encounters; (4) how it is transformed through use. This takes us beyond an epidemiological perspective to a social-ecological one in which we recognize that there are a range of powerful interests at work able to deploy and advance specific interpretations and to counter, invalidate, and sabotage others.

## Implications for Treatment

The ways we talk about the body and explain its afflictions are drawn from a fund of cultural knowledge that includes different systems of medicine, and lay knowledge about common ills, as well as religious and moral ideas. These explanations, in turn, have widespread social effects. Adopting a social perspective on the amplification of bodily distress adds an important dimension to our assessment and treatment of patients with medically unexplained symptoms.

The most basic implication of a social perspective has to do with how we conceive of somatic symptoms. Bodily experience is embedded in a sociocultural matrix of cognitive representations and social practices [26]. As a result, the experience of symptoms responds to social contingencies. So, too, does the reporting of symptoms: any account of bodily distress must be understood as a narrative constructed in a specific social context for a particular purpose. The need for this social perspective is evident from the outcome of efforts to measure the lifetime prevalence of medically unexplained symptoms in epidemiological studies. For example, the WHO Cross-National Study of Mental Disorders in Primary Care [27] found low test-retest reliability with the somatization disorder section of the Composite International Diagnostic Interview (CIDI) on 1-year follow-up (Gureje, personal communication, 1998). This low reliability can be viewed either as a methodological limitation of existing interview instruments or as a substantive finding about memory and symptom experience. The somatization disorder section of the CIDI asks about the lifetime prevalence of medically unexplained somatic symptoms. Surprisingly, some respondents who met criteria for somatization disorder initially could not remember having had many somatic symptoms on a later second interview. A higher correlation was found between the current level of symptoms reported on the initial interview and subsequent symptom level. Thus, current symptoms predict later symptoms, but memory of symptoms does not predict later memory of symptoms. Clearly, as has been found in many other domains, memory is malleable and influenced by current context. Quite likely it is helpful to forget one ever had certain symptoms when feeling better, in order to get on with one's life. Alternatively, people may neglect to mention symptoms from the past to an interviewer when they are trying to have their current problems taken seriously. Particularly in clinical settings, respondents may feel that acknowledging a long litany of complaints form the past will lead to dismissal of their current problems as simply "more of the same." On either interpretation, however, the low test-retest reliability of the CIDI is revealing something important about how people adapt to medically unexplained symptoms, and this deserves further study with appropriate social psychological methods that approach self-reports as cognitive and social constructions rather than as unbiased summaries of past experience.

The relevance of the social and cultural shaping of the bodily experience for our understanding of somatoform disorders goes beyond problems of measurement to the pathogenesis of somatoform disorders. Both hypochondriacal worry and the disability that accompanies many functional somatic syndromes like chronic fatigue are thought to be due to activity restriction secondary to perceptions of the body as vulnerable and activity as harmful [28]. However, the meaning of bodily vulnerability itself must be seen in cultural context. F. Noda (personal communication, 1998) has pointed out that many Japanese experience the normal body as vulnerable to illness. This notion of vulnerability does not have the same connotations as vulnerability in North America. In North American health psychology, vulnerability is equivalent to weakness, and weakness is unequivocally bad. The healthy body should be intact, solid, impermeable, and strong. As a result, any deviation from this state of health is anxiety-provoking. Noda suggests that in Japan the body is conceived of as fragile, weak, and prone to ills. While this view may encourage low-level health concerns and interest in health precautions, it may actually diminish anxiety when acute illness brings about loss of bodily control and strength. This might explain why, despite relatively high levels of introspectiveness or self-consciousness, there is not more overt hypochondriasis or pathological somatization in Japan. Other studies suggest that culturally mediated patterns of illness behavior may contribute to chronicity and disability. For example, Greek immigrants in Sweden have been observed to severely restrict their activity when they suffer low back pain because they fear that pain indicates ongoing injury so that, if they persist in their work or daily routines, permanent damage may ensue [29].

Beyond these social mechanisms of symptom amplification and disablement, a sociocultural perspective has much to offer the clinician who treats patients with medically unexplained symptoms. Social factors are important at the initial phase of treatment because they must be acknowledged to build trust and a working alliance with patients who may have been rejected by many care providers and blamed for their condition. In the mid-phase of treatment, social factors may help to explain why reattribution training and cognitive-behavioral approaches are insufficient to bring improvement in some patients. In the final phase of treatment, careful consideration of the social context may identify factors that can undermine therapeutic gains and contribute to relapse.

The first task in the treatment of patients with medically unexplained symptoms involves helping them past the "either/or" dilemma posed by the fundamental dualism of biomedicine. Patients will fail to return to see practitioners who treat their somatic problems as entirely psychological. However, most patients do not entirely reject psychological aspects to their distress. Indeed, to do so marks a patient as overly defensive compared to patients with medically explained conditions and may lead to greater skepticism and rejection by clinicians. The patient who is a skillful rhetorician will acknowledge some degree of psychological distress while insisting that there is some residual physical problem that requires attention.

Treatment, too, is a rhetorical enterprise. Depending on the clinician's orientation and the patient's style of self-presentation, somatic symptoms may be interpreted variously as: (1) an index of physical disease or disorder (e.g., fibromyalgia or chronic fatigue); (2) an indication of psychopathology (affective, anxiety, or somatoform disorder); (3) a symbolic expression of intrapsychic or interpersonal conflict (the classic example is the psychodynamic interpretation of conversion symptoms); (4) a culturally-coded "idiom of distress" (e.g., *dhat* syndrome in India, in which ethnophysiological theory leads to concerns about semen loss as the cause of a myriad of symptoms); (5) a metaphor for bodily, personal or social events; (6) a strategy for expressing social discontent; and (7) a mechanism through which people attempt to reposition themselves in their local worlds [30]. Every clinical encounter involves explicit or implicit diagnostic actions by the clinician that may reinforce or shift the interpretation of somatic symptoms across these parallel categories. The acceptability of a diagnosis, as well as its therapeutic efficacy, depends on the social significance of this shift in meaning.

The clinician must begin by joining with the patient to acknowledge the somatic nature and reality of the symptoms. After this basic acknowledgment, it is possible to gradually introduce psychological and social strategies to improve coping with somatic symptoms and reduce disability and distress. Once patients see that something effective is being done to alleviate their somatic distress, they are often ready and willing themselves to introduce other psychological and social issues for psychotherapeutic attention.

Awareness of the social dimensions of the patient's predicament would counsel clinicians to develop the therapeutic alliance and relieve distress through several basic steps: (1) acknowledge the bodily nature and extent of the patient's suffering through careful exploration of its particulars; (2) legitimate the illness as something not caused by the patient's willful action; (3) provide a coherent explanation of the symptoms in terms the patient can understand and can, in turn, explain to others without loss of face; (4) arrange to be consistently available over the long term, rather than dismissing the patient once a diagnosis is made; (5) train the patient in cognitive-behavioral strategies for symptom re-attribution, coping with distress, and reduction of disability [31]; (6) when this individually oriented treatment is not sufficient, identify interactional factors that may account for treatment resistance and chronicity and intervene in the family or larger social circle [32, 33].

A social perspective has obvious implications for the prevention of medically unexplained syndromes, which may occur in epidemic form. Drawing on the Australian experience with RSI, Hall and Morrow argue that "the major lesson for the specialist medical profession is to be wary of creating diagnostic labels in the absence of reliable evidence" [20]. At the same time, patients often feel great relief when they have a label for a problem and may persist in searching for one if the clinician simply says they are "unexplained." A balance between providing reassuring explanations and accepting uncertainty must be found both through clinical relationships that provide a container for working through the consequences of persistent distress, and through public health education that acknowledges both the strengths and limitations of conventional and alternative forms of medicine.

The most far-reaching implication of a sociocultural perspective is that our own diagnostic categories can be viewed as cultural constructions [34]. In this light, we ought to temper our enthusiasm for refining the nosology of somatoform disorders with the realization that the diagnostic category itself may create part of the problem it seeks to resolve. By hiving off a group of patients as having somatic illness of psychiatric origin, we put them in a potentially stigmatizing position that may threaten the doctor-patient alliance and impede subsequent treatment. It is worth considering that some other systems of medicine do not make a strong ontological distinction between physical and mental disorders [35]. Introducing the concept of somatoform disorders in this setting may reproduce a form of dualism that aggravates the problem. Of course, the dualism of biomedicine is tied to larger cultural ideologies of the person [16]. Further study is needed to understand how this medical dualism works in cultures where the prevailing concept of the person has different historical origins and does not fit so closely with the tacit assumptions of biomedicine.

## Conclusion: The Future of Somatoform Disorders

The symposium "Rethinking Somatoform Disorders" at Keio University, on which this book is based, brought together diverse perspectives and approaches to the problem of somatization. The title of the symposium was borrowed from Arthur Kleinman's *Rethinking Psychiatry* [36]—a seminal text in cultural psychiatry that urges that we take a step back from everyday clinical practice to examine the cultural origins and implications of psychiatric theories and practice. By putting issues of nosology, psychopathology, and treatment in cultural context, we can begin to identify our tacit assumptions and generate fresh ideas. In that spirit, the Keio meeting raised many questions about the construct of somatization.

Discussion at the meeting pointed out the pragmatic and epistemological difficulties with somatoform diagnoses. There was concern among participants that the category of somatoform disorders had the potential to limit or misdirect both research and clinical practice. A more agnostic term for part of the domain of study would be "medically unexplained symptoms." This reorientation, suggests the following directions for future research.

1. *The development of psychophysiological models of functional somatic disturbances.* The most prevalent forms of somatization do not fit the full-blown syndromes described in DSM-IV. Instead they represent the common functional somatic symptoms and syndromes noted by every medical specialty [5, 31]. It is likely that many of the somatic symptoms now viewed as medically unexplained eventually will receive explanations in terms of perturbations of physiology and function that are simply too complex, subtle, or sporadic to be consistently identified with current methods [4]. Having physiological explanations for symptoms will improve treatment and lessen the stigma attached to these disorders.

2. *The relationship of somatic symptoms to the regulation and communication of emotional distress.* Contrary to the implication of the term, somatoform disorders are commonly associated with depression, anxiety, and other forms of emotional distress. There is a need to more closely examine the personal and social circumstances under

which the experience and reporting of somatic symptoms serves as an alternative to the expression of emotional distress. Psychodynamic theorists have argued for an either/or relationship in which adequate emotional symbolization, processing, and expression of conflict prevents somatic disease and distress [37]. Alternatively, suppression, repression, or dissociation of affectively charged events can lead to somatic distress. Epidemiological studies, on the other hand, tend to show strong correlations between emotional and somatic distress [38]. These studies, however, do not constitute a fair test of the psychodynamic hypotheses because they lump together people with different patterns of response and rely entirely on self-reports, which may confound good health with a defensive style or strategic self-presentation [39]. A new generation of experimental studies examining the impact of the disclosure and narrative recounting of emotional conflict and traumatic events has the potential to clarify the connections between emotion suppression and somatic distress [40–42].

3. *The role of cognitive processes in symptom interpretation and coping.* There is much evidence that cognitive processes play a central role in the translation from bodily sensations to disabling somatic symptoms [2, 5]. Among these processes, symptom and illness attributions appear to be pivotal [43]. Attributions have both cognitive and social effects [26]. Future work can examine the interplay of personal and social spheres in the generation, stabilization, and consequences of specific patterns of symptom attribution. This leads to considerations of the tradeoff involved in different diagnostic fashions or cultural systems of interpretation [1].

Taken seriously, this cognitive social psychological approach has implications for psychiatric nosology. In place of a discrete group of somatoform disorders, greater attention could be given to the somatic component of all forms of psychiatric distress, with the inclusion of a category of problems related to illness behavior or coping with symptoms that would cut across all forms of disorder, as Pilowsky has suggested [44]. This more inclusive approach would avoid the mind-body split implicit in our current notion of somatization. It would still allow for the recognition of certain special processes, like dissociation, which may give rise to somatic symptoms in the absence of structural anatomical pathology [45].

4. *The impact of social and cultural factors including the health care system.* As reported elsewhere in this volume, there is now good evidence from cross-national studies, particularly those of the WHO on primary care and on somatoform disorders, that somatization in its various forms is ubiquitous and not exclusively associated some specific type of culture or health care system [27]. These same studies, though, have uncovered regional variations in symptomatology, diagnostic practice, and treatment that demand further study and explanation [1].

Perhaps it should come as no great surprise that the WHO cross-national study on somatoform disorders, which looked at health care through the lens of local biomedical and psychiatric practitioners, found somatoform disorders to be prevalent and to pose similar problems of social stigma and legitimation across cultures. Patients everywhere find biomedical and psychiatric approaches to medically unexplained symptoms to be stigmatizing and often ineffective.

There is an unfortunate legacy of the construct of somatization disorder that tends to view somatic distress as intrinsic to the person rather than as having an intelligible course and response to life events and psychosocial factors. This last requires close attention to the lived experience of patients through ethnographic research. We need to understand the process of negotiation and the social consequences, outside the consulting room, of specific interpretations and responses to somatic distress.

A focus on individual patients opens onto the broader comparative study of health care systems. What is still largely unexamined is how somatic distress is influenced by social and cultural variations in the availability of alternative and traditional systems of medicine, religious healing, family networks, and the economic institutions of work, insurance, and disability systems. We need to better understand the role of help-seeking and the response of the health care system in the outcome of transient somatic distress and the processes that lead to chronicity.

5. *Effective treatments.* A diagnosis of somatoform disorder often conveys a sense of therapeutic nihilism. However, recent work suggests that many patients with medically unexplained symptoms and syndromes can be substantially helped by treatments that reduce symptomatology, help-seeking, and disability, and improve quality of life [31]. We need further clinical trials of a range of interventions, especially cognitive-behavioral approaches which have shown great promise. Family therapy and social network interventions have not received the systematic evaluation they deserve [32, 33]. The agenda of contemporary psychiatry is heavily influenced by the potential for pharmacotherapy, both because of the promise of simple, widely applicable treatments and the potential profit for pharmaceutical corporations. If there is no drug to treat a problem, it is hard to interest pharmaceutical companies in funding research or education on the issue. In the current climate of limited public funds for health care research, this fact exerts a strong influence on the direction of psychiatric research and practice. Given that psychological and social factors play a significant role in the course of somatic distress, it is important to maintain a vigorous research program on psychosocial treatments.

Future research will likely better establish the physical basis of many "unexplained" symptoms. At the same time, evidence will continue to accrue that symptom perception and experience are not simple reflections of bodily processes but the outcome of complex psychological evaluative processes, interpersonal interaction, and discursive practices. With this broad perspective, it will be possible to think through the impact of diagnostic practices and treatment programs.

Ultimately, advancing our understanding of somatoform disorders requires rethinking our cultural assumptions about more fundamental issues including the mind-body problem and its relationship to other cultural value systems, particularly the concept of the person, and corresponding patterns of attribution of causality, responsibility, and blame. Within biomedicine, psychosomatic theory has provided the dominant paradigm for the study of somatization. Other medical systems more often espouse some version of *sociosomatics*—not just by acknowledging the social causes of disease, but also through understanding and responding to somatic symptoms as meaningful events embedded in a larger social world [46]. If we still wish to reserve a special place for the "theatres of the mind," privileged by psychodynamics and psychosomatic theory, we must recognize that, across cultures, there are different styles of theatre, arrangements of audience and stage, languages of bodily gesture, and narrative conventions that set the drama in motion.

# References

1. Kirmayer LJ, Young A (1998) Culture and somatization: clinical, epidemiological and ethnographic perspectives. Psychosom Med 60:420–430
2. Kirmayer LJ, Robbins JM (1991) Current concepts of somatization: research and clinical perspectives. American Psychiatric Press, Washington
3. Bennett RM (1981) Fibrositis: misnomer for a common rheumatic disorder. West J Med 134:405–413
4. Sharpe M, Bass C (1992) Pathophysiological mechanisms in somatization. Int Rev Psychiatry 4:81–97
5. Kirmayer LJ, Taillefer S (1997) Somatoform disorders. In: Turner S, Hersen M (eds) Adult psychopathology. J Wiley, New York, pp 333–383
6. Strathern A (1996) Body thoughts. University of Michigan Press, Ann Arbor
7. Csordas TJ (1994) Embodiment and experience. Cambridge University Press, Cambridge
8. Benjamin S, Eminson DM (1992) Abnormal illness behaviour: childhood experiences and long-term consequences. Int Rev Psychiatry 4:55–70
9. Walker LS, Garber J, Greene JW (1991) Somatization symptoms in pediatric abdominal pain patients: relation to chronicity of abdominal pain and parent somatization. J Abnorm Child Psychol 19:379–394
10. Whitehead WE, Crowell MD, Heller BR, Robinson JC, Schuster MM, Horn S (1994) Modeling and reinforcement of the sick role during childhood predicts adult illness behavior. Psychosom Med 56:541–550
11. Edwards D (1997) Discourse and cognition. Sage, London
12. Kirmayer LJ (1992) The body's insistence on meaning: metaphor as presentation and representation in illness experience. Med Anthropol Q 6:323–346
13. Yardley L (1997) Material discourses of health and illness. Routledge, London
14. Perelman C (1982) The realm of rhetoric. University of Notre Dame Press, Notre Dame
15. Kirmayer LJ (1994) Improvisation and authority in illness meaning. Cult Med Psychiatr 18:183–214
16. Kirmayer LJ (1988) Mind and body as metaphors: hidden values in biomedicine. In: Lock M, Gordon D (eds) Biomedicine examined. Kluwer, Dordrecht, pp 57–92
17. Beaulieu M (1997) Stigma and legitimation in chronic fatigue syndrome: the role of social location. Department of Sociology, McGill University, Montreal
18. Kirmayer LJ, Robbins JM, Taillefer S (1995) Development of a structured diagnostic interview for functional somatic syndromes: Culture & Mental Health Research Unit, Department of Psychiatry, Sir Mortimer B. Davis–Jewish General Hospital, Montréal
19. Draucker CB (1991) Coping with a difficult-to-diagnose illness: the example of interstitial cystitis. Health Care Women Int 12:191–198
20. Hall W, Morrow L (1988) "Repetition strain injury": an Australian epidemic of upper limb pain. Soc Sci Medicine 27:645–649
21. Bammer G, Martin B (1992) Repetitition strain injury in Australia: medical knowledge, social movement, and de facto partisanship. Soc Problems 39:219–237
22. Reid J, Reynolds L (1990) Requiem for RSI: the explanation and control of an occupational epidemic. Med Anthropol Q 4:162–190
23. Simon GE, Katon WJ, Sparks PJ (1990) Allergic to life: psychological factors in environmental illness. Am J Psychiatry 147:901–908
24. Stewart DE, Raskin J (1985) Psychiatric assessment of patients with 20th-century disease (total allergy syndrome). CMAJ 133:1001–1006
25. Sperber D (1985) Anthropology and psychology: towards an epidemiology of representations. Man 20:73–89
26. Kirmayer LJ, Young A, Robbins JM (1994) Symptom attribution in cultural perspective. Can J Psychiatry 39:584–595

27. Gureje O, Simon GE, Ustun TB, Goldberg DP (1997) Somatization in cross-cultural perspective: a World Health Organization study in primary care. Am J Psychiatry 154:989–995
28. Sharpe M, Chalder T, Palmer I, Wessely S (1997) Chronic fatigue syndrome: a practical guide to assessment and management. Gen Hosp Psychiatry 19:185–199
29. Löfvander M (1997) Illness, disease, sickness: clinical factors, concepts of pain and sick leave patterns among immigrants in primary health care. Department of Clinical Neuroscience and Family Medicine, Division of Family Medicine, Karolinska Institute, Stockholm
30. Kirmayer LJ, Dao THT, Smith A (1998) Somatization and psychologization: understanding cultural idioms of distress. In: Okpaku S (ed) Clinical methods in transcultural psychiatry. American Psychiatric Press, Washington, pp 233–265
31. Mayou R, Bass C, Sharpe M (1995) Treatment of functional somatic symptoms. Oxford University Press, Oxford
32. Griffith JL, Griffith ME (1994) The body speaks: therapeutic dialogues for mind-body problems. Basic Books, New York
33. McDaniel SH, Hepworth J, Doherty WJ (1995) Medical family therapy with somaticizing patients: the co-creation of therapeutic stories. Fam Process 34:349–361
34. Mezzich JE, Kirmayer LJ, Kleinman A, Febrega H Jr, Parron DL, Good BJ, Lin K-M, Manson SM (1998) The place of culture in DSM-IV. J Nerv Ment Dis (in press)
35. Fabrega H (1991) Somatization in cultural and historical perspective. In: Kirmayer LJ, Robbins JM (eds) Current concepts of somatization: research and clinical perspectives. American Psychiatric Press, Washington, pp 181–199
36. Kleinman A (1988) Rethinking psychiatry. Free Press, New York
37. Taylor G, Bagby RM, Parker JAD (1997) Disorders of affect regulation. Cambridge University Press, Cambridge
38. Simon GE, Von Korff M (1991) Somatization and psychiatric disorder in the NIMH Epidemiologic Catchement Area study. Am J Psychiatry 148:1494–1500
39. Shedler J, Mayman M, Manis M (1993) The illusion of mental health. Am Psychol 48:1117–1131
40. Pennebaker JW (1995) Emotion, disclosure, and health. American Psychological Association, Washington, DC
41. Pennebaker JW, Francis ME (1996) Cognitive, emotional and language processes in disclosure. Cognit Emotion 10:601–626
42. Pennebaker JW, Mayne TJ, Francis ME (1997) Linguistic predictors of adaptive bereavement. J Pers Soc Psychol 72:863–871
43. Sensky T (1997) Causal attributions in physical illness. J Psychosom Res 43:565–573
44. Pilowsky I (1997) Abnormal Illness Behaviour. J Wiley West Sussex
45. Lynn SJ, Rhue JW (1994) Dissociation: clinical and theoretical perspectives. Guilford, New York
46. Kleinman A, Becker AE (1998) Sociosomatics: the contribution of anthropology to psychosomatics. Psychosom Med 60:389–393

# Key Word Index